Doing It For Ourselves

A Guide to Aging as a Lesbian or Bisexual Woman

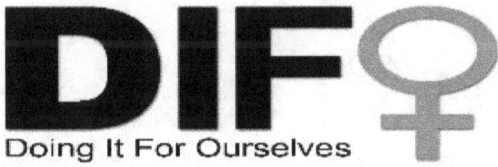

Mickey. Eliason
San Francisco State University

© March, 2015

Table of Contents

Acknowledgments

DIFO was created from federal funding from the Office on Women's Health, Contract Number: HHSP233420095615. Suzanne Haynes was our project officer, and we worked with 4 other funded projects all aimed at improving the health of lesbian/bisexual women. The contract was held at IMPAQ International in Oakland, CA, with staff members Nada Rayyes and Linda Toms Barker playing critical roles in project management and data collection and analysis. Deborah Craig oversaw the logistics of the groups from recruiting to getting women into groups to corresponding about program logistics. Community partners included the San Francisco LGBT Center, The World Institute on Disability, Rainbow Women of Oakmont, and Openhouse, a San Francisco LGBT aging agency.

This book is a collaborative effort that included input from DIFO facilitators, advisory committee members, and participants in focus groups and the program itself. I cannot possibly name everyone who provided input into the content, but here are some of the major contributors: DIFO facilitators have included Joan Hepperly, Simi Litvak, Jana Rickerson, Jan Thomas, and Gloria Soliz. Two incredible women developed the physical activity components of the program: Penny Sablove and Wini Linguvic, and Deborah Craig helped to capture their words and movements into the DIFO physical activity manual and video. We also had a community advisory group that included: Maria Cora, Gloria Soliz, Patty Robertson, Jeanne DeJoseph, Migdalia Reyes, Michele Alcedo, and Sue Dibble. Finally, over 120 women participated in the focus groups and/or early waves of DIFO groups, and all gave us valuable feedback about what works and doesn't work so well. All of these individuals' input led to the materials in this book. Any errors or misinterpretations of the research literature are Mickey's fault.

NOTE: This book is a work in progress, and many chapters are incomplete. I would like this book to be the go-to resource for older lesbian/bisexual women. For that to happen, I need your help in identifying what is missing, what sections don't work for you, who/what I am leaving out, and so on. Please send any comments you have about the book to difobayarea@gmail.com.

About This Book

This book is meant to serve several purposes. It was originally designed as the background information and content for a health education and support group. Doing It For Ourselves (DIFO) was a federally-funded grant project and a research study, and the materials evolved over time with input from participants, facilitators, changes in research findings, and experience. Over and over we heard that there was a need for a health resource book specific to lesbian and bisexual women, because it is such as challenge to find this kind of information on the internet and because other books about LGBT health address general issues that are shared by LGBT people, but may not all be relevant to women. And we heard that aging is another challenge—there is little information that is geared toward the practical aspects of aging as a lesbian or bisexual woman.

This book can be a stand-alone resource. It includes some references to research studies to show that the information is based on the best science that we have available to us, but it also contains practical information based on experiences in DIFO groups, because the best science is still not very good. There are major limitations with the available research, particularly related to who gets studied. Research participants in most studies have more education and are more likely to be white than one would expect from the actual diversity of our communities. The published research does not represent all of the subgroups that make up the lesbian/bisexual women's population in the U.S. We have included the best information that is available to us at this time, but recognize that it is incomplete.

Second, the book contains the workbook for the DIFO program at the end. You can use this information in a formal DIFO group, start a group of your own, or do the exercises on your own. Reading information in a book is only a small set toward improving your health. You will need to take action, and the workbook outlines the action steps needed for change.

The book is organized into 4 parts. Part I provides you with the research on the health problems that have been studied among lesbian and bisexual women. This is the most factual, research-based part of the book. There are many references in this section, although I have tried to hone them down to the ones that are the most relevant or the best research designs. Unlike ten years ago, now there are hundreds of studies that focus on lesbian and bisexual women, although information about older, ethnically diverse, or women with disabilities is still hard to come by. Part II offers ideas for how to understand health problems in lesbian and bisexual women. Too often, mainstream health programs only focus on the individual level, such as what and how much we eat and how much exercise we get. The danger of an individual approach is that we might blame the victim for health problems. Part II shows how complicated health is. The "upstream" social determinants of health include interpersonal relationships, communities, healthcare and other institutions of society that create laws and policies. Part II shows where we might need to campaign for changes or work within our own communities to make them healthier. Part III offers some suggestions for making the individual level changes that might be beneficial. Obviously, these changes are not easy to make, or everyone would eat healthy, move their bodies more, and deal with stress in healthy ways. The upstream factors affect our motivation and ability to engage in healthier practices. Whatever we do, it must be done with self-compassion, recognizing that some influences are beyond our control

Finally, Part IV is the DIFO workbook for those who are enrolled in a group, or want to lead or participate in a group. You can also do the exercises on your own, although one of the main findings of DIFO was that group support was critical in supporting women to make individual changes. If you can, find a buddy or small group to work through the exercises with you. However you use the book materials, I wish you the best in getting and staying as healthy as you can!

PART I:
HEALTH RISKS AND CHALLENGES

Summary: These nine chapters summarize the research on the health status of lesbian and bisexual women and contain information on the risk factors, signs and symptoms, and treatments for common health problems or challenges. The book also addresses the aging process.

Chapter 1: Introduction to Lesbian Health

This book is meant to be a practical guide to healthy living as a lesbian or bisexual woman in our fast-paced, ever changing world. On one hand, societal attitudes about us (and our bisexual male, gay male, and transgender family) have improved substantially in recent years. On the other hand, we still have a long ways to go to overcome homophobia, sexism, racism, ageism, ableism, and other forces of oppression that impact our health and wellbeing. Many of the health problems described here, and the suggestions offered will also apply to others in our communities, such as transgender men and women who live within lesbian communities or others on the LGBTQ spectrum. Sometimes it is best and morally right to be as inclusive as possible, and other times, it is important to spotlight particular segments of the population, as this book does. It is not meant to exclude, just to recognize that the particular situations of our lives can differ and sometimes a culturally-centered approach is needed. Even the focus on "lesbian" and "bisexual" and "women," however, does not mean that we are discussing a homogeneous group. Lesbian and bisexual women are diverse in every possible way and vary by age, race, ethnic group, national origins, religion, language, (dis)ability, political affiliations, educational levels, income, immigration status, and social class. We will explore how the diversity enhances our communities, as well as raises challenges for us as we attempt to create inclusive communities.

The available research on lesbian/bisexual women's health often has not captured the full diversity of our communities for at least three reasons. First, the combined stigmas of racism, ageism, classism, sexism, ableism, and so on, keep many lesbian and bisexual women from participating in research studies. Their voices are often not heard. The more oppressed minority identifications a woman has, the less likely she is to trust researchers (for good reasons). Second, large health surveys that are used to study population health often do not include questions about sexual orientation or gender identity. These studies have been used to identify health disparities in the general population, and when disparities are made public, often there are changes in funding and greater attention is given to reducing the disparities. Lesbian and bisexual women are too often invisible in health research and large health systems record keeping, so we know less about the disparities related to both sexuality and gender. Third, there is really no consensus on the best way to ask questions about sexuality, and many women may use terms other than lesbian, bisexual, or homosexual, the labels often used on research surveys. Women who use other labels might or might not be included in the research.

Research is used in the U.S. to justify changes in funding and policy, so this book will provide some research citations. You can easily read around the research if you are not interested, but references to actual research studies are made in most chapters in case you need to educate your healthcare provider or want to delve deeper into a problem. Parts I and II are heavily referenced but Part III is made up mostly of suggestions that come from the general population research on health behavior change. This is because there is virtually no research on whether lesbian and bisexual women respond to health programs, medications, or treatment/prevention strategies in the same way as other women in the population. In spite of the emphasis in the past 20 years on culturally-specific treatment modalities, these have rarely been studied for lesbian and bisexual women's populations. A recent study of federal funding for LGBT health studies found that the majority of funding went to research on HIV and other sexually transmitted infections among men who have sex, and only a handful of studies were funded to study lesbian or bisexual women (13.5% of the LGBT-focused research) (Coulter, Kenst, Bowen et al., 2014). The federal initiative that funded DIFO was the first government funding to specifically set aside money for lesbian and bisexual women's health.

Before we launch into health problems, this introductory chapter will provide some background information from which to understand how and why lesbian and bisexual women might have greater health challenges than heterosexual women. This section includes a brief historical overview, including the history of lesbian health movements, and a short review of developmental milestones from coming out to developing intimate relationships and families (and sometimes ex-lover networks), communities, and aging. But first, we need to define some terms.

WHO ARE WE AND WHY DO WE HAVE SO MANY LABELS?

This book focuses on individuals who identify as women and as non-heterosexual. But even within those limits, we have enormous diversity in our life experiences and identities. If you read online blog posts, or consume lesbian/bisexual women's fiction, films, and music, you will find a wide variety of terms that some women use to identify themselves or others. Here is a sampling of that language:

Lesbian, bisexual, gay, dyke, dike, womyn-loving womyn, homosexual, sapphite, two-spirit, political lesbian, bull dagger, chapstick lesbian, gay gal, queer, lesbian identified bisexual, transgender, friend of Dorothy, same-gender loving woman, butch, wimmin-loving-wimmin, gay women, gold star lesbian, one of the tribe, femme, vagitarian, lone star lesbian, transmasculine, baby dyke, grrl, fluid, aggressive, granola lesbian, crunchy lesbian, bisexual-identified lesbian, member of the choir, ambisexual, pansexual, family, bi-dykes (or Bykes), lipstick lesbians, dipstick lesbians, hasbians, tortillera, ex-lesbians, barsexuals, lesbian pretenders, phony lesbians, diesel dykes, fake lesbians, marimacha, bi-curious, LUGs (lesbians until graduation), LUTs (lesbians until thirty), sexual minority women, tomboy, tomboi, bottom, women who partner with women, service butch, stud, lezzie, futch, LURD (lesbians until release date), and…what else?

Questions to consider:
--What terms, if any, do you use to describe your own sexuality?
--What terms make you feel uncomfortable or offended? What terms would be inappropriate to use in your own ethnic community? With your family?
--What terms would you use when talking to other community members, but not in public?
--Do words matter? Why? How?
How about gender? What pronouns do you prefer to use? Many of the terms above imply a difference on the gender continuum. Are you familiar with the terms cisgender and transgender?
--Where do you feel you fit best on a gender presentation continuum? Do you identify as butch/femme/or some other gender label?

We will use the shorthand term "lesbian/bisexual" in this program to simplify the writing, but recognize that women in our communities may use a wide diversity of terms.

Definitions of Terms and Concepts

This book is for lesbian and bisexual women, but what does that mean? We have such confusing language and such lack of agreement on terms that sometimes it seems almost impossible to communicate about sexuality and gender. Some definitions are offered here, so that we can use shared definitions of the terms, but we know these definitions will not satisfy everyone. Language is very personal, idiosyncratic, and constantly changing. The terms vary by one's ethnic community, national background, age, geographic region, and so many other factors that it can get very confusing.

Terms related to sexual orientation

One problem is that we still don't really know what sexual orientation is. Is it something genetic or innate that we are born with? Is it something we learn? Or is it some combination of nature and nurture? We don't have any biological measures of it; nor do we really have good self-report measures. We can probably accept from work since at least Alfred Kinsey in the 1940s and 50s, that sexuality is on a continuum, not an either/or situation. Most people are somewhere between exclusively attracted to others of the same sex and exclusively attracted to people of the other sex. In fact, probably more people are closer to the middle than to either extreme. But we also know that sexual orientation is more than just attraction. It also includes behavior. Do we act on our attractions or fantasies? Sometimes yes, sometimes no. Sexual orientation also includes identity, or our core concept of who we are. Identity is probably the most important, and a famous thinker once said, "A lesbian is a woman who says she is a lesbian" (Jill Johnston in Lesbian Nation). Lesbian is used to label women who mostly have relationships with other women and bisexual is used to label women who mostly have relationships with both men and women, but there are also many other terms, for example: dyke, two spirit, queer, same-gender loving, gay women, homosexuals, and euphemisms like "member of the choir," "family," and "that way." When a woman adopts an identity, theoretically she has access to a community of people who use that same label. For lesbian/bisexual women, that community might include other lesbian/bisexual women or LGBTQ people in general or women's communities in general. For shorthand in this book, we will use lesbian/bisexual to refer to women who have regular relationships with or attractions to other women, whether or not they also have relationships with men. There is a growing movement to include asexual as a form of sexual orientation. To be asexual is to have emotional and intimate connections with others, but little or no sexual desire.

Terms related to sex

Notice that we have been using the term woman without commentary thus far. This term is also ambiguous. Some use the term to refer to people with typical female genitalia and internal organs. But feminist theorists of the second wave (1960s-70s) rightly suggested that woman is a social construct. Having a vagina and ovaries does not make a woman; rather, our societal expectations based on gender create the categories of men and women. So in this book, we use woman to refer to a person who calls herself a woman. Some transgender men who still consider themselves lesbians may find parts of this book useful and many transgender women who have relationships with women may also find the book relevant. The gendered body parts matter in only a few ways—for example, with menopause or cervical cancer screening. Most of the time, the problems of lesbian/bisexual women are because of the societal stigma about sexual orientation and gender and not the physical body. Sex, the physical body, is not as important as gender, the social constructions created to distinguish between biological men and women.

Terms related to gender expression

Gender identity refers to how a person identifies along a gender continuum that is based on societal standards for men and women in terms of their appearance and behavior. We can identify as:
- cisgender female (comfortable with the term "woman" that was assigned at birth and still applies),
- transgender (identify as a gender different than was assigned at birth), or
- gender queer (somewhere in between).

On top of that, we can express gender identity in the ways that we present to the world. In lesbian/bisexual communities, a butch/femme continuum is often used, and there are many terms that note where along this continuum any particular woman may fit. Terms related to the more feminine side of the continuum may include lipstick lesbian, femme, high-femme, girly, and so on. Terms that are around the middle include old terms like kiki and androgynous, and also tomboy, boi, and the like. Gender terms for the more masculine side of things include butch, transgender, transmasculine, stud, and bulldagger. The world judges us first on our gender expression because it is visible. Our sexual orientation is hidden, unless we announce it in some way. Women who are butch or androgynous are more likely to be harassed and victimized in public places than are more feminine lesbian and bisexual women. Butch women may also experience more discrimination in healthcare settings (Lehavot and colleagues, 2012).

Terms related to societal stigma

We will keep returning to the central message of this book: **Sexual orientation/identity and gender expression are the not the causes of health problems. Instead how society treats people who are different is the root cause of health disparities**. In this book, we will focus on sexual orientation, gender (or sex), and age as the triad of stigma that all older lesbian/bisexual women share. However, we will also consider how racism, classism, ableism, immigration status, and other forms of oppression affect lesbian/bisexual women. When research shows that there are differences in health purely based on group membership, that is the definition of a health disparity. In regards to the stigma of sexual identity, we will use the term heterosexism the most often. It refers to the privilege that is given to heterosexuality in all the power discourses of society (legal systems, medicine, education, religion, media). Many people use the term homophobia, but it refers to individual level prejudice. It only has power because the institutions of society give it power. Of course, as lesbian or bisexual women, we do face homophobia all the time from people in our lives, but it's more effective in the long run to change the power structures of society than to try to change people one person at a time. In regards to gender expression, we will use the term gender normativity. This is a parallel term to heterosexism, and shows how male/female and masculine/feminine dichotomies are ingrained in society. We are forced to pick one and not acknowledge that gender is a continuum. Gender socialization is one of the most powerful forces in our society today, and starts before we are even born. Feminism focuses on breaking down gender normativity. Many lesbian and bisexual women are feminists because they recognize that sexism, heterosexism, and gender normativity are all connected and they harm all humans.

In the 1970s, women used consciousness-raising groups to educate themselves about the effects of oppression on women's lives. They taught women that what they experienced were not just individual failings or personal short-comings, but shared by many other women. Those early consciousness-raising groups examined the role of sexism on women's daily experiences and led to important books, like Our Bodies, Ourselves (Boston Women's Health Collective, 2005). The DIFO program uses the same idea of consciousness-raising by providing accurate information about health, discussing how external factors affect lesbian and bisexual women's health, and helping each other to find solutions to improve health.

We are all affected by the forces of oppression in society. There are many different forms of oppression, but they operate in similar ways. Oppression is defined as prejudices held by individuals (holding stereotypes that all members of a group have similar, mostly negative characteristics) plus power of societal institutions (the ability to discriminate against, treat badly without penalty, and withhold rights and services).

Figure 1.1. The definition of oppression

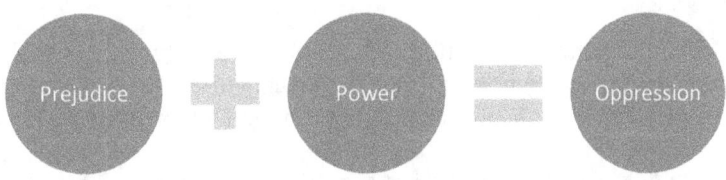

Using this formula, the power of societal laws, policies, and attitudes support and maintain many types of prejudices (definitions from Eliason, Dibble, DeJoseph, & Chinn, 2009):

- *Homophobia* is based on prejudice against people who have same-sex attractions and relationships;
- *Biphobia* is prejudice about people with both same and other-sex attractions;
- *Transphobia* is prejudice about people who differ by gender identities and expressions;
- *Sexism* is prejudice based on one's perceived biological sex;
- *Gender normativity* refers to expectations for how men and women are supposed to look and behave, and is based on the idea that there are only two genders;
- *Racism* is prejudice based mostly on skin color;
- *Classism* stems from prejudice based on income level and social class status;
- *Ableism* is based on negative stereotypes about people who are differently able;
- *Ageism* is based on assumptions about age, and that older people have less worth than younger people;
- *Fatphobia* (also called weight stigma or sizeism) is prejudice based on body size or shape;
- Other prejudices can be based on religion, language, political beliefs, sexual practices (like S&M), and immigration status.

LGB people can be prejudiced about heterosexual people, but since LGB people have no systematic, institutional power, it is merely a negative attitude, not a form of oppression. In a similar fashion, people of color can have negative attitudes about white people, but without power to back it up, it is not racism. Terms like "reverse racism" or "reverse sexism" are just ploys to detract attention from the serious effects of oppression on real people's lives.

Privilege

The flip side of oppression is privilege. Certain factors give us power and privilege in society whether or not we have asked for them. If we belong to the dominant groups (white, male, heterosexual, able-bodied, middle or upper class income), we get unearned privileges (McIntosh, 1990). Complete the table below to see where you might have unacknowledged privilege.

Yes	No	Form of Privilege
		Race or ethnicity (White people have greater privilege)
		Sex (Men have more privilege than women)
		Language (Native English speakers with no accents have the most privilege)
		Gender (People who fit gender stereotypes for appearance have more privilege)
		Age (Younger and middle aged-adults have more privilege than old adults or children)
		Education (College educated have more privilege)
		Income (Middle class or wealthy have more privileges than poor)
		Sexual orientation (Heterosexuals have more privilege than LGB)
		Religion (in the U.S. Christians tend to have more privilege)
		Body Size ("normal" body size (i.e., thin) as defined by beauty and medical standards is privileged)
		Body Functioning ("Normal" body functioning with no visible disabilities is privileged)
		Others:

Recognizing your privilege comes with an obligation to be mindful about how you use that privilege and power for the good of others in our communities, and how it might affect the way you are perceived in groups. Having guilt over one's privileges is not helpful, but examining how we use our privilege is.

Reasons for using "lesbian and bisexual" in this book

There is a lot of overlap among women who currently use the label "lesbian" and those who currently use "bisexual." Some identified as the other at some point in life, and sometimes the behavior of women who use different labels is virtually identical. There is value in being specific and focusing on one or the other at times, because sometimes the lived experiences of women with these labels can be quite different. We discuss both lesbian and bisexual women in this book. We will point out the times when research finds differences, but these are often a matter of degree rather than qualitative differences. The major differences may be philosophical and related to inclusiveness of the so-called "lesbian community." Some lesbian feminist ideologies have rejected bisexual women because of their relationships or attractions to men, or accuse them of bringing "male energy" to women's spaces. Similarly, lesbian feminism has been rejecting of transgender men and women. Many in our communities believe that societal stigma about all of us who have a different gender or sexual identity is a unifying point, and we need to band together to get changes in society. In our social networks, we can choose our friends and with whom we spend our leisure time, but politically, we need each other. Embracing the diversity of our communities in all its forms, can only strengthen us. Communities that are inclusive and reach out to others are healthier than communities that are constantly policing their borders and actively excluding. Being divisive is a waste of our precious energy!

HISTORY OF LESBIAN/BISEXUAL WOMEN'S ORGANIZING

Our history as lesbian and bisexual women tends to be fragmented and hard to find, particularly as it relates to organizing around health. Our movements have tended to be grassroots, involving small women's collectives and mimeographed pamphlets, rallies, and gatherings to share information. It's hard to even pinpoint when lesbian/bisexual women's communities started to form. This chapter focuses on a few moments in history, but there is a need to collect and summarize our history, so that we can celebrate the many accomplishments and learn from pioneering women's experiences.

Many of the famous lesbian and bisexual women in our early history were involved in health movements, including Florence Nightingale (nursing), Jane Addams (social work), and Marty Mann (one of the early advocates in the alcoholism treatment field). Most historians date the contemporary LGBT political movement to the end of World War II. Although the sexologists of the late 1800s had created the categories of lesbian and gay (and to some extent, bisexual and transgender), it was the circumstances after the war that created the possibilities for community organizing. Women had moved to the cities to take over jobs in factories vacated by men who went to war, and some women joined the service for the first time. Men who had attractions to men met each other at war, and when they returned (mostly to port cities like New York, San Francisco, and Boston), they stayed in the city rather than return to the isolation of more remote locations. The strength in numbers allowed LGBT people to start to organize. The first public gay rights group in the U.S. formed in 1950 and was called the Mattachine Society. It was all-male until 1952, when they formed a new group called One, that included women. They also gave money to help support the first lesbian rights organization, the Daughters of Bilitis.

Daughters of Bilitis

Founded in 1955 by Del Martin and Phyllis Lyon in San Francisco, DOB had its origins in the age-old lesbian dilemma: Where can I go to dance? Del and Phyllis first wanted a social outlet for lesbians to dance without fear of police raids and harassment that were so common in the gay bars of the 1950s. They chose the term "Bilitis" from an obscure French poem who named Bilitis as a contemporary of Sappho. They figured no one would know what it meant. In the early days, they were a secretive social group, but they soon matured into a support and education organization. They obtained non-profit status in 1957 and opened chapters in New York City, Los Angeles, Chicago and Rhode Island by 1960. That same year, they hosted the first ever lesbian convention in San Francisco, and moved into a more activist position for the decade of the 1960s. The organization folded in 1972. They are widely known for their newsletter, *The Ladder*, which was published by DOB from 1956 to 1964. It continued for a few years after that when Barbara Grier took over the newsletter as an independent publication. It is hard to imagine today the courage that it took for those early pioneer women to be out and advocate for our rights in the extremely hostile climate of the times, when same-sex desires were illegal, considered mental illness, and viewed as sin. Del Martin died in 2008.

Activism Against the Diagnostic and Statistical Manual (DSM)

One of the defining moments of the new LGBT liberation/political movement was the activism that led to the removal of the diagnosis of homosexuality from the DSM. The Diagnostic and Statistical Manual, the guidebook of mental health disorders used by psychiatrists and other mental health professionals included homosexuality as a diagnostic category from its first edition in 1952, until it was removed as a result of activist work within and outside of psychiatry, in 1973. Part of the success in removing the diagnostic category of homosexuality was because of activists staging a take-over of a session at the American Psychiatric Association conference to force a dialogue among professionals in the field. Since 1973, debates about "reparative therapy" or whether one could be "cured" of a gay, lesbian, or bisexual identity, continued to rage in some quarters. For example, 2010 presidential candidate Michelle Bachman's husband is a psychologist who specialized in reparative therapy. In 2014, California became the first state to legally ban reparative therapy for youth.

The Lavender Menace

Lesbian and bisexual women were also involved in the second wave of the women's movement, and many health issues were central to this organizing, including sexual and reproductive rights, paternalism in healthcare, lack of women participants in clinical trials testing new treatments for health problems, and lack of study of issues specific to women such as menstrual cycle and menopause studies. The ground-breaking, grassroots publication, *Our Bodies, Ourselves* had a paragraph or two about lesbians in its first edition (around 1970).

Many lesbian and bisexual women joined the National Organization of Women (NOW) after it was founded in 1966, but they were pressured to keep silent about their sexuality to avoid tainting the organization that was already considered radical by many people. The president of NOW in 1969, Betty Friedan, referred to lesbians as the "lavender menace" because she thought NOW would be considered a radical man-hating organization if the leadership acknowledged the lesbian/bisexual women in the movement. NOW attempted to distance itself from lesbian causes, and in 1970, lesbian feminist Rita Mae Brown resigned her administrative job at NOW, and along with a small group of women, organized a "zap" for the Second Congress to Unite Women (also in 1970). They prepared a ten-page manifesto called "The Woman-Identified Woman," the document that gave us the famous definition: "A lesbian is the rage of all women condensed to the point of explosion." When the first speaker came to the microphone, they switched off the lights, pulled the plug on the microphone and took over the stage. When the lights came back on, 16 women in Lavender Menace t-shirts and placards invited other lesbian/bisexual women to join them. They engaged the audience in a discussion of how it felt to be excluded, and offered workshops at the rest of the Congress. This may have been a turning-point in the mostly white feminist movement to start being more inclusive, first of lesbian/bisexual women, and then of women of color. A critical event for feminists of color was the publication of Combahee River Collective paper in 1977 that outlined how feminism ignored the major issues of women of color.

In spite of some acknowledgement in feminist organizations, some lesbian and bisexual women felt that the women's movement made them choose between their sexuality and their sex/gender. Some of these women branched out to join LGBT organizations and others became separatists and embraced a uniquely lesbian feminism. Lesbian separatism lead to the formation of lesbian coffee shops, music festivals, bookstores, and many books on ethics and politics by authors such as Mary Daly, Julia Penelope, Sheila Jeffreys, Sarah Lucia Hoaglund, and others. Lesbian feminism is an offshoot of radical feminism, or the belief that supposedly female characteristics such as nurturance, cooperation, and emotional responses are superior to male characteristics such as competition, aggressive, and logic-based responses. Lesbian feminists drew a definitive line in the sand to define themselves as "womyn-born womyn" and excluded bisexual and transgender people from events. One of the ongoing battles that continues today is over the Michigan Women's Musical Festival, which still excludes transgender women. Other debates within lesbian/bisexual women's communities have been over the so-called "sex wars" that challenged whether eroticizing power dynamics as in bondage/domination/sado-masochistic practices, promoted healthy relationships or reproduced abusive/unequal relationships. There was also debate about identity politics (banding together around a particular identity, like lesbian) versus coalition or issues based politics.

Lesbian and bisexual women in fat liberation movements

We were also at the table for the start of the fat positive movement. Judy Freespirit is often considered one of the first to publicly declare a fat positive identity with her essay, The Fat Liberation Manifesto, in 1973 (see a copy of this in Chapter 5). Lesbian/bisexual women were featured in the first anthology on fat as a form of oppression: *Shadows on a Tightrope: Writings by Women on Fat Oppression* (Schoenfielder & Wieser, 1983). Dawn Atkin's edited volume *Looking Queer: Body Image and Identity in Lesbian, Bisexual, Gay, and Transgender Communities* (1998) addressed body image from a uniquely LGBT perspective. Contemporary lesbian and bisexual women are influential in fat studies (Esther Rothblum, editor of *Fat Studies Reader* and the *Fat Studies Journal*, as well as the *Journal of Lesbian Studies*, Linda Bacon, author of *Health At Every Size*, and therapist/writer Deb Burgaard are just a few).

Lesbian/bisexual women in the HIV/AIDS movement

Many lesbian and bisexual women were actively engaged in the efforts to educate the public about HIV/AIDS, and to provide care and support to those affected by HIV. In the early 1980s, the world was changed in dramatic ways by the spread of HIV/AIDS, most rapidly in men who have sex with men. As the epidemic progressed without government intervention, grassroots and activist organizations popped up across the country. AIDS Coalition to Unleash Power (ACT-UP) was one of the few national organizations. Founded in 1987 in New York City, ACT-UP had a women's caucus. Lesbian and bisexual women worked at AIDS organizations, volunteered as helpers, and cared for their gay/bisexual male friends with AIDS. Some think that this experience with advocacy and caregiving for gay men politicized lesbian and bisexual women to start to act up on their own health issues.

Creation of health clinics and education

Some activists focused on lesbian and bisexual women's health, and created clinics or programs specifically for our needs. Some still exist today. For example, in San Francisco, the Lyon Martin Health Clinic opened in 1979 to serve sexual minority women, and currently about 60% of their patient population identify as LB or T. This clinic was named for pioneering lesbian couple Phyllis Lyon and Del Martin. The Mautner Project was founded in 1990, a year after Mary-Helen Mautner died of breast cancer. She had directed her partner Susan Hester, to begin an organization to help other lesbians with life-threatening illnesses. Later, the Mautner project mission broadened to "improving the health of women who partner with women including lesbian, bisexual, and transgender individuals through direct and support services, education, and advocacy." They are currently part of the Whitman-Walker Clinic in Washington, DC, an LGBT-health clinic. There are other LGBT health clinics in the U.S., including Callen-Lorde Clinic in New York, Fenway in Boston, Howard Brown Clinic in Chicago, The Gay and Lesbian Center in Los Angeles, and Alliance Health in San Francisco. The Lesbian Health Research Center was founded in 2000 at the University of California, San Francisco by Suzanne Dibble and Patty Robertson to disseminate research about lesbian health to consumers and healthcare professionals.

Many lesbian/bisexual women have written about their own health issues and provided guidance about how to negotiate the world of healthcare systems and societal attitudes about illness and disability. Here are just a few examples:

- Audre Lorde's *The Cancer Journals* describes how she navigated the health care system during life-threatening illness (actually any of Audre Lorde's books could be used as inspiration for living healthier lives).
- Gloria Anzaldua who died of complications of diabetes, wrote about what life is like on the borders (outside of the mainstream society) in *Borderlands/La Frontera: The New Mestiza*, among other books.
- Dorothy Allison writes and speaks so eloquently about being poor and the consequences on health, and is most known for *Bastard out of Carolina*, a story of survival of child abuse.
- Starhawk writes about the relationships between our gender and sexuality and the earth and the concept of ecofeminism in books such as *The Spiral Dance*.

Lesbian/bisexual women against ageism

We have also been active in all movements to improve the status of individuals as we age. One organization, Old Lesbians Organizing Change, consists mainly of separatist lesbians who are finding ways to continue activism as they age, and make old lesbians visible in the world. Other lesbian and bisexual women work within mainstream aging organizations or LGBT communities to focus on aging issues more broadly. Chris Almvig was one of the founders of SAGE: Services and Advocacy for GLBT Elders in New York City in 1978, an organization that now has affiliates in 17 states. Marcy Adelman, a psychologist in San Francisco, was one of the first to study the needs of LGBT elders, pointing out that even in gay-friendly San Francisco, older LGBT adults felt isolated. She went on to found Openhouse, a nonprofit agency that focuses on housing and other critical issues for LGBT elders.

Mainstream funding for lesbian/bisexual women's health

Unfortunately, federal funding for LGBT health has focused on HIV/AIDS and other sexually transmitted infections to the exclusion of most other topics. A review of all funding from the National Institutes of Health from 1980 to 2009 found that 86% of all funds went to HIV research. In that 25 year span, only 12 studies had developed and tested health programs for lesbian or bisexual women and most of those were aimed at sexual health of younger women (Coulter et al., 2014). A review of research articles on LGBT health shows the same bias. Lesbian/bisexual women are still relatively invisible in the biomedical field. Without support, we learned to do it for ourselves, and continue to do so.

SEXUAL IDENTITIES AND HUMAN DEVELOPMENT

Some research has focused on the milestones of human development, and how they might differ for lesbian and bisexual women compared to heterosexual women, or compared to gay/bisexual men or transgender individuals. Much of this work has focused on two issues: coming out and relationships. What are the stresses and the processes of adopting a minority sexual identity and disclosing it to others? Secondly, how do same-sex relationships differ from other-sex relationships? There has been much less research on other aspects of adult development, such as aging. The issue of developmental tasks of old age will be addressed in the next chapter.

Coming Out

Coming out is the process of exploring and adopting a personal identity, and then making decisions about disclosure. Women can come out at any age and life stage, but as you can imagine, the experience is different if we are age 15 or age 45 or 75. We have different coping mechanisms, different life experiences, and have different priorities, depending on our life stages. When we are youth, family rejection can have more serious physical consequences—getting kicked out of our homes or physically abused—but at any age, family rejection can hurt. Being rejected by children might be just as traumatic as parental rejection.

Whatever age we are, coming out can be a challenging process, because we have to deal with the potential reactions of family, friends, coworkers, bosses, children, members of our churches or spiritual groups, and many others. We have to learn to "manage" our identities—or decide how and when to come out to others, versus keep our sexuality private. Coming out to others is a very personal decision, and we need to honor the choices of other women. It is still not safe to be out in all settings. Keeping a big secret can take its toll on our mental health. It is exhausting and stressful to hide our private lives, and can result in feeling shame and guilt over not being honest. It helps to have a social support network to vent the stress, but if we are not out, that supportive community may not be available.

Intimate Relationships

Another potentially challenging developmental task of the adult is developing intimate relationships and family. Heterosexual women are taught the informal rules of dating and relationship, but as lesbian and bisexual women, there are not clear-cut rules. Until recently, marriage was not an option, so same-sex couples forged their own unique relationships. Some had to negotiate the challenges of having two individuals in relationship who were both socialized in the same gender stereotypes. If women are socialized to be the caregivers, to be self-less, and to use passive-aggressive rather than direct communication, how does that affect the intimate relationship?

Most research finds that female same-sex couples are just as likely to be satisfied with their relationships as other-sex couples, but that they tend to be more egalitarian (more equal in how they make decisions and distribute household tasks). Some of the early literature from therapists suggested that female same-sex couples often suffered from "merger" or "fusion," defined as an "unnatural" degree of closeness. It turns out that female same-sex couples are no more likely than other types of couples to have this pattern (Frost & Eliason, 2013) and many authors objecting to pathologizing emotional closeness. Being too close is generally not the problem; problems arise when each member of a relationship have different desires and expectations about how close they want the relationship to be.

Parenting

Finally, parenting may be another challenge to healthy living. Stresses of raising children in same-sex households can be intense at times in a society that thinks children must be exposed to male role-models in the home. Adult children and grandchildren can present other challenges (and joys!). There is virtually no research on how or whether lesbian and bisexual women grandparent differently than heterosexual women.

Lesbian and bisexual women of color are more likely to have children (and therefore, grandchildren) and could teach us a lot about these issues.

THEORETICAL FRAMEWORKS

Why do we need theories? Well, health is a complicated matter, and we need some systematic way to organize this complex mess and to create ways to improve health. Theories are just handy tools to organize lots of information in a manner that makes sense and helps us to identify what topics or issues should be addressed in health education programs.

At this point, no one theory or model has been used extensively to explain lesbian and bisexual women's health. In the 1970s, lesbian feminism was highly influential (and still is in some subsets of lesbians). Many lesbian and bisexual women identify as feminist and are mostly women-centered in their philosophies. Others adopted queer theory or broader LGBT models, like minority stress. Others use theories or models from other fields and apply them to our circumstances. Theories vary in the lens that they use to view the world. The most simplistic way to understand the difference between various theories is to examine their central focus or lens:

- Feminism: gender or focusing the lens on women's experiences.
- Socialism: class or focusing on the effects of social class status.
- Critical race theory: the lens is on how race or ethnicities are constructed and experienced.
- Queer theory: focus on sexuality and gender combined.
- Minority stress theory: studies how internal and external discrimination from oppressed minority identities (could be race, ethnicity, language, sexuality) impacts health.
- Disability studies: considers how certain body functions get defined as "normal" or "disabled."
- Intersectionality: tries to use multiple lens simultaneously to see how oppressed minority identities interact with each other to produce effects on health.

Upstream Social Determinants of Health
In public health, we talk about "upstream" social determinants of health. This comes from a story about a drowning person in a river. Rescuers help the drowning victim out of the river, but then see another victim, and another. The rescuers on the bank organize and try to save as many as possible, but there are too many to save them all. At one point, one of the rescuers starts heading upriver. The others ask, "Where are you going? We need all the bodies we can get to help these drowning victims." The errant one says, "I'm going upriver to see if I can discover why so many people are falling into the river." She discovers a hole in the bridge a mile upstream that if patched, prevents the problem. In the case of some cancer clusters, the upstream effect might be a chemical pollution of the water source for a town. In our case, the hole in the bridge is a symbol for all the problems in society and communities that create stigma and put lesbian and bisexual women at risk. If it were not for upstream social determinants of health, such as sexism, heterosexism, gender normativity, racism, ableism, and ageism (just a few examples), lesbian and bisexual women would be more like heterosexual women in their health status. These upstream influences, not our sexuality or gender, are the root causes of health disparities. There are so many upstream influences that we need a theoretical container to organize them. That is where the ecological model comes in.

Ecological Model
This book is based on the ecological framework that considers any individual as part of expanding circles of influence from the family and close community to larger community systems and organizations, and broader societal policies and politics (Krieger, 2002, 2012). The ecological model is broad enough to hold components of all the other theories. At each level of the model, minority stress (internalized oppression, experiences of invalidation, harassment, discrimination, and/or violence based on sexual identity or sex/gender) impacts the lives of sexual minority women. At each level, you can apply a feminist lens or a queer theory lens or a critical race lens to understand how women with different identities might experience the world.

Any program that is likely to be successful in preventing or treating chronic health conditions must draw from all levels of the model, considering the sources of minority stress at each level as well as how stigmatized identities may intersect with one another, complicating any simplistic notion of individual risk factors or resiliency. Furthermore, each level of influence may require a different set of strategies to address the health risk. Individual risk factors may require behavior change strategies, interpersonal and community level issues may need changes in community norms or alterations in physical environments, and all change is facilitated by modifications of public policies that reduce stigma. Community, in this model, includes both the physical neighborhoods in which we live or work, the mainstream social institutions in our neighborhood like churches, schools, and the healthcare agencies and institutions, and it also includes LGBT or women's communities. The figure below shows the five levels of the ecological model that are explored in this book.

Figure 1.2. The Ecological Model

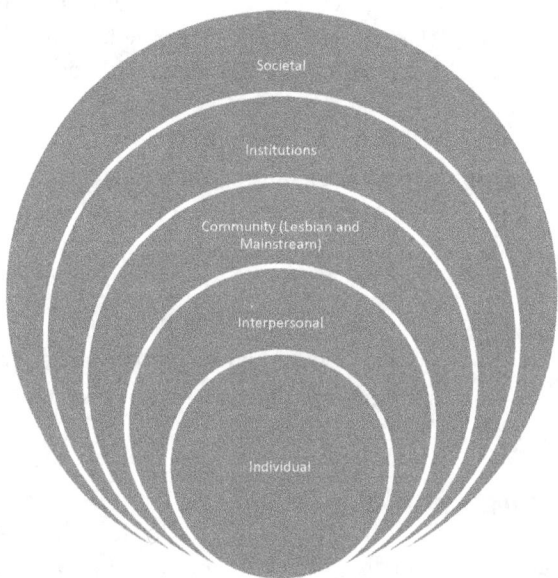

The ecological model is a perfect container for the incorporating many theoretical perspectives because it highlights the intersections of individual, community, and society. But we can also look at intersections within a specific level, like the individual. Part II of this book will break down the risk and protective factors for our health using this model.

In conclusion, this chapter has introduced the history of lesbian/bisexual women's health research and practice, discussed the diverse terminology used to describe ourselves and others, and suggested some theoretical frameworks for viewing how health problems develop, and how we can address them.

REFERENCES

Boston Women's Health Collective (2005). *Our bodies, ourselves.* Boston, MA.

Bowleg, L. (2012). The problem with the phrase women and minorities: Intersectionality an important theoretical framework for public health. *American Journal of Public Health, 102*(7), 1267-1273.

Coulter, R.W.S., Kenst, K.S., Bowen, D.J., et al. (2013). Research funded by the NIH on the health of lesbian, gay, bisexual, and transgender populations. *American Journal of Public Health,* e1-e8 doi:10.2105/AJPH.2013.301501.

Eliason, M.J., Dibble, S., De Joseph, J., & Chinn, P. (2009). *LGBTQ Cultures: What healthcare professionals need to know about sexual and gender diversity.* Philadelphia: Lippincott

Frost, D. & Eliason, M.J. (2014). Challenging fusion in female same-sex relationships: An Inclusion of Other in Self (IOS) approach. *Psychology of Women Quarterly, 38*(1), 65-74.

Krieger, N. (2002). A glossary for social epidemiology. *Epidemiological Bulletin, 23*(1).

Krieger, N. (2012). Methods for the scientific study of discrimination and health: An ecosocial approach. *American Journal of Public Health, 102*(5), 936-945.

Lehavot, K., Molina, Y., & Simoni, J.M. (2012). Childhood trauma, adult sexual assault, and adult gender expression among lesbian and bisexual women. *Sex Roles, 67*, 272-284.

McIntosh, M. (1988). White Privilege. Unpacking the invisible knapsack. Wellesley College.

Chapter 2:
Aging as a Lesbian/Bisexual Woman

We are at a crossroads in history. Many of the "greatest/silent" generation who grew up during the depression and early years of WWII are gone now. They were exposed to the most hostile climate where homosexuality was both criminalized and pathologized by psychiatry. That generation often did not come out, so did not experience a lot of overt discrimination, but suffered the negative consequences of a secret life in the closet. Women who are over 65 now turned into adults just before Stonewall, and directly experienced the civil rights, feminist, and early gay rights movements. Finally, women 65 and younger now are mostly post-Stonewall era. They are the most likely to have lived much of their lives out and proud. Of course, that is a generalization and there are young closeted women and old activist dykes! But what is undeniable is that the generations of lesbian/bisexual women now reaching their elder years are much more likely to have lived open and out lives and will continue to demand to be recognized as they age. We are changing the face of aging just by being out and proud.

Prior to the 1970s, homosexuality was illegal in most states and listed as a mental disorder in the Diagnostic and Statistical Manual of Mental Disorders (DSM). LGBT individuals might have been subject to arrest and incarceration (in jails, prisons, and mental institutions), electric shock treatments, having their names published in newspapers after raids at gay bars, and suffering dishonorable discharge from the military. Times have changed with the Supreme Court striking down laws that make same-sex conduct illegal, the military reversing its policy on LGB people in the military, and same-sex marriage becoming legal in several states. But older adults may still be suffering the effects of the earlier repression and may be suspicious and fearful of revealing their sexuality or gender identity in health care settings (Cronin & King, 2010). Those who have been out, may feel a need to return to the closet if they require home care from strangers or need to be in assisted living or nursing homes.

In many ways, lesbian and bisexual women face many of the same challenges of aging that heterosexual women do. The physical body inevitably changes and sometimes mental health and cognitive abilities start to decline. Many face the challenges of caring for partners as they age. We all face the fears of needing assisted living or nursing homes and are concerned about the quality of the care we may get. Unlike heterosexual women, though, we have more stress related to lack of family support, are less likely to have children, are more likely to live in poverty, and fear how caregivers may treat us, based on their attitudes about lesbian and bisexual women (Ashbrook, Gerald, & Eliason, 2011).

But there are also positive ways that lesbian and bisexual women might differ from heterosexual women as we age. These ways include:

- We are usually more independent before getting older, because many of us recognized that we would lead lives without husbands or other men to help us, so we learned to take care of the car, the yard, the household repairs, and so on. We are more prepared for aging in some ways.
- We are less concerned with meeting societal beauty standards of young and thin than are heterosexual women, so we might not be as worried about wrinkles, gray hair, and carrying a little more weight. If we partner with other women, we know that they are more tolerant of a wide variety of ages, body sizes, shapes, and ability levels. We are more likely to like, if not love, our bodies.
- We are less likely to define ourselves predominantly as mothers, so menopause and loss of reproductive capacity is not as traumatic or challenging for many of us.
- We have had practice with difficult transitions already. We came out to ourselves and others and learned to cope with sexism and heterosexism, and these coping skills may help us with the changes associated with aging.

Even though we might be better equipped than some heterosexual women, aging comes with lots of challenges and very few resources that recognize us as lesbian and bisexual women. Our social networks may change, but will we be welcomed into social groups of mostly older heterosexual women and men? LGBTQ communities tend to be youth-oriented, and aging services tend to be heterosexist, leaving us to "do it ourselves" yet again. If we lose a partner, will the grief group at the local hospital be welcoming? One recent study found that LGBT people traveled seven times the distance to a congregate meals program than heterosexual people---they needed to go further to find safe and inclusive programs (Porter, Keary, VanWagenen, & Bradford, 2014).

Many older lesbian/bisexual women are creating their own communities to age within, such as land communes or collectives and co-housing units. There are a handful of LGBT senior housing options in the U.S that those with more financial means might be able to consider. But most of us have to face aging without a physical community. That is why a lesbian/bisexual women's health movement is so important. We have an opportunity to create new community linkages that focus on supporting each other in achieving better health, particularly as we age. Thus far, agencies and institutions focused on aging have largely ignored us, so as always, we have to "do it for ourselves."

This chapter deals with several common concerns that lesbian/bisexual women have with the aging process: dealing with ageism, menopause and other biological aspects of aging, dealing with healthcare providers and systems of care, aging in relationship and community, and housing issues.

WHAT IS AGEISM?

Unlike some other aspects of diversity that are relatively stable across our lifetimes, everyone who survives their youth gets older. We start to age the minute we are born. Aging is the biological process of maturation, the passage of time from birth to death. The problem is not aging; aging is the natural process for all life on earth. The problem is ageism.

Ageism is the equivalent of sexism, racism, heterosexism, ableism, and other forms of oppression based on stereotypes, but differs from the other forms of oppression in one significant way. Most people who engage in ageist thoughts or behaviors will one day themselves be old. Ageist beliefs when younger can become internalized and create a self-fulfilling prophesy that endangers one's health and wellbeing in older adulthood. In this regard, we all discriminate against our future selves when we accept ageist stereotypes as true. Ageism is discrimination against people based on their age. Robert Butler, the medical doctor who coined the term, defined it as:

> "A deep-seated uneasiness on the part of the young and middle-aged---a personal revulsion to and distaste for growing old, disease, disability; and the fear of powerlessness, uselessness, and death" (Butler, 1969, p. 243).

Ageism stems from stereotypes about people based on the age group to which they belong, so ageism can affect people at any age. However, we tend to have the most negative attitudes about people who are older. The negative attitudes also have greater impact, because older adults generally need more health care services than younger adults. Some experts have explored more complex definitions of ageism. For example, Butler thought it had at least three components:

- Individual prejudice. This can lead to neglect or poor behavior of older adults, such as physical, emotional, verbal, financial or sexual abuse.
- Discriminatory practices. These can include marketing and media that perpetuates stereotypes about older adults, target old people for financial scams, and deny job training based on age.
- Institutional policies. This is the idea that age discrimination is built into the systems of society, and includes policies such as mandatory retirement, exclusion from clinical trials, limiting access to certain medical procedures solely based on age.

Some researchers have distinguished between two types of prejudice: Benevolent prejudice stems from pity and considering the older person as incompetent, such as treating the older adult as an infant or invalid, speaking at a slower rate with a demeaning tone (patronizing), or making decisions for older adults who are competent to make their own choices. Hostile prejudice stems from fear, aversion, or threat, such as limiting access to health resources, and may involve denying certain privileges or resources to older adults, such as organ transplants. Both forms of prejudice can result in contempt and neglect of older adults. The National Council on Aging (2002) conducted a survey about stereotypes of aging, and found that most respondents, young and old, thought that people over the age of 65 were more likely to have problems with finances, health, loneliness, and be victims of crime. The respondents who were over 65 themselves largely did not report these problems. We rarely think that stereotypes apply to us personally, but apply them to other people.

Causes of Ageism

Ageism is a relatively new phenomenon in human history. In earlier hunter/gatherer and agricultural communities, older adults were valued for their experience and knowledge and had important roles in passing down knowledge to younger generations. The rise of industrialization and move to cities in the western world eroded the authority of elders, and made older adults invisible. During the great depression in the U.S., older adults were disproportionately affected, and eventually led to the start of Social Security in 1940 when society as a whole felt it was unacceptable for older adults to be suffering in poverty after their years of contributions to society.

The media is a powerful conveyer of stereotypes (Weir, 2004);

o   Snow White syndrome: think of all the Disney movies with a beautiful innocent young woman and an ugly, wicked older woman. Children's books and TV programming also rarely address older adults in a positive way.
o   Anti-aging industry: Grew from 2004 as a 45.5 billion dollar industry to 72 billion in 2009. Anti-aging ads start to target individuals at age 35. What effect does this have on people who show signs of aging?
o   Advertising in general, particularly when women are depicted in ads. What effect does the emphasis on youth in advertising have on older adults?
o   How are older lesbian and bisexual women depicted in the media?

Why have we become an ageist society? Some theories about why ageism exists are:

•   Fear of death and dying—older people remind younger people of death. Medicalization of death removed the experience of dying from everyday life, creating greater taboo and fear;
•   A change in value systems. Currently societal emphasis on productivity is valued over the qualities of being and personhood, so once out of the workforce, a person is considered less worthy;
•   Competition for limited resources. The current economic system (neoliberalism) has made health care and other resources into limited commodities for which generations feel they must compete.

In health care settings, some experts have labeled the type of ageism that exists as "gerontophobia." This refers to a dislike or fear of caring for older patients, a preference to work in other settings, not older-patient specific settings, and avoidance of older patients. Weir (2004) proposed that this fear is related to unresolved fears of one's own aging and death that are not addressed in health care training, combined with the power of health care providers to make life and death decisions, as well as a feeling of powerlessness over chronic illness and death. Later, we will consider what happens when a healthcare provider is both ageist and homophobic.

Ageism manifests differently in lesbian/bisexual women's communities than in gay/bisexual men or transgender communities, where a focus on youth and beauty are much more in line with societal norms than among lesbian/bisexual women's communities. Chapter 5 addresses community norms about the body, but the bottom line is that ageism is not as intense, although the lesbian/bisexual women's community is not exempt from its effects.

Effects of Ageism

Stereotype Embodiment is an idea proposed by psychologist Becca Levy (2009) that suggests how ageism affects health. First, there are the negative stereotypes in society that affect individual attitudes as well the practices and policies of institutions and government agencies. We are exposed to these from the moment we are born, and continually through-out our lives. The stereotypes are perpetuated in subgroups where age segregation is common. Second, when we reach the age that our society designates as "old," we begin to identify with the label and think of ourselves as old. We already have internalized the stereotypes about what it means to be old, so we apply them to our own experiences.

Levy noted: "unlike those who have been stigmatized since birth and subsequently may acquire coping strategies from their subgroup, individuals tend to enter old age unprepared to resist negative age stereotypes" (Levy, 2009, p. 334). Here is one area where we as lesbian and bisexual women might have an advantage, because we have already developed coping skills for homophobia and heterosexism. Some of us may be able to generalize these coping skills to aging.

Negative stereotypes about aging may create a self-fulfilling prophesy. Many research studies have confirmed that older people with negative stereotypes about aging suffer more declines and disorder than adults with more positive attitudes in at least three areas:

1) Psychological functioning ("senility," memory, depression)
2) Behavioral aspects (if they believe that diseases are caused by old age, they may be less likely to engage in health-promoting activities such as exercise, diet, taking medications, stimulating their minds, etc.)
3) Physiological characteristics (those with greater negative stereotypes about age exhibit an increased cardiovascular response to stress than those with more positive attitudes about aging. Over time, this cardiovascular response contributes to greater heart disease).

In one longitudinal study, (Levy et al, 2002), older people who had positive perceptions of aging lived 7.6 years longer than people with negative attitudes about aging.

Examples of How Ageism Manifests in Health Care Settings (most from Butler, 2006):

- 35% of doctors think that increase in blood pressure is a normal aspect of aging (it's not!)
- Of adults over the age of 65, 60% do not receive recommended preventative services, and 40% are not vaccinated for flu and pneumonia. Only 10% get appropriate screening tests for bone density, colorectal and prostate cancer, and glaucoma.
- Of clinical trials to test prescription drugs, 40% exclude people over the age of 75; older adults are even more underrepresented in clinical treatment trials for all types of cancer.
- In 2005, the U.S. Congress eliminated all funding for geriatric education and training, meaning even fewer health care providers are educated about the needs of older adults.
- Emergency services often neglect older individuals: 60% of victims of Hurricane Katrina were age 61 or older. Within 24 hours of 9/11 terrorist attacks, animal advocates were rescuing pets, but older and disabled people were abandoned in their apartments for up to 7 days before rescue.
- Elderly people are less likely than younger people to be screened for cancers and therefore, less likely to be diagnosed at early stages of their conditions.
- After being diagnosed with a disease that may be potentially curable, older patients are less likely than younger patients to receive all the necessary treatments.

Laws in the United States

The federal government's Age Discrimination in Employment Act of 1967 (ADEA) prohibited employment discrimination based on age with respect to employees 40 years of age or older. The ADEA also addresses the difficulty older workers face in obtaining new employment after being displaced from their jobs, and arbitrary age limits. A study of workers over the age of 45 in 2002 reported that 67% had observed age discrimination at work (and those who were African American or Latino reported even higher levels: 72%). We know that women face more employment challenges in male-dominated careers, making the combination of sexism, ageism, and heterosexism a potent one for many women.

BIOLOGICAL ASPECTS OF AGING

Primary versus Secondary Aging

Aging is an inevitable process of decline to death, but when and how does the decline begin? Some researchers have divided the process into primary factors, the hard-wired processes in the body that lead to aging and death; and secondary aging, the environmental factors that contribute to disease. The longer we live, the more likely we are exposed to environmental toxins, stresses, viruses, injuries, and other factors that speed up the aging process. These are the secondary factors and are preventable or reducible whereas primary aging is not. Experts have estimated that if we had no secondary aging factors, maximum life expectancy would be about 115. The average life expectancy in the U.S. is 78.7 (CDC, 2014). If we did a better job of health promotion and prevention, we could extend life expectancy and quality of life significantly.

Common secondary aging factors that reduce life span are smoking, alcohol and drug use, unhealthy foods (particularly inflammation producers), lack of exercise, stress, and exposure to viruses and toxins that weaken our immune systems and create cancer and other diseases. Many of the other secondary aging factors are social determinants of health beyond the control of the individual, such as the health and safety of the neighborhood one lives in, the access to healthy foods, the quality of health care services, and state and federal laws governing health and communities. The social determinants require changes in laws and policies.

Theories about Aging

When does old age begin? There is no consensus and no biological marker for the entrance into the older age category. In the U.S., retirement and social security were set initially at age 65, but senior discounts may apply at 60 or even 55. One can belong to the American Association of Retired Persons (AARP) at 50. The answer about when a person is "old" depends on who you ask. One national survey that asked when women became old found that 20 year olds reported the onset of old age at about 50, whereas people in their 50s and 60s put it at 65 (men) or 70 (women) (Albert et al, 2002). In some cultures, aging is considered as "three acts:" 0 to 30 is youth, 31-60 is adulthood, and 61 and older is the third act, or old age. The third act is considered the time when we come into our wisdom years. In contemporary U.S. society, however, old adults are dismissed as useless, and not valued for the wisdom from accumulated years of experience.

There are multiple scientific theories about aging, and probably the true process is some combination of many of these. These are just a few of the theories (from Moody, 2002):

1. Aging is imbedded in our genes (like a clock that sets in motion different processes like puberty, menopause, and death).
2. Aging is caused by a gradual accumulation of mutations to our genes from radiation and other environmental exposures.
3. Aging is caused by wear and tear on body parts.
4. The evolutionary urge to reproduce uses up body resources early in life, leaving us vulnerable to disease later on.

Menopause

Menopause is one big marker of aging for women. There is very little research on how lesbian and bisexual women respond to the process of menopause. There is no reason to think the biological symptoms might be different, but there are psychological and cultural attitudes associated with menopause that might vary. Some authors suggest that lesbian and bisexual women have a more positive outlook about menopause because of less emphasis on youth and societal standards of beauty. Others suggest that female partners are more supportive and understanding about menopause than male partners. There are also potential challenges that arise when both women in a relationship are going through menopause.

A woman is said to reach menopause when she has gone 12 months in a row without a menstrual period. The average age of menopause is 51, but the range is 40 to 60, and it's a process rather than an event. When you are in the process, it's called peri-menopause. Over the course of several years, the hormones associated with human reproduction begin to change. Estrogen and progesterone decrease, and follicle-stimulating and luteinizing hormones increase. The main signs of this change are:

- In early peri-menopause, the menstrual cycle may actually get shorter so a woman may experience more frequent periods, sometimes with heavier flow.
- In later phases, the menstrual periods become irregular and hot flashes may occur. Some women also have cold flashes and night sweats. Hot flashes may continue for a very long time after menopause (about 15% of women have them for years after).

Other symptoms of menopause include vaginal drying (easy to treat with a little lube), weight gain (metabolism slows down even more), and bone loss. Some women at menopause age first show signs of metabolic syndrome (see Chapter 6 for more detail on metabolic syndrome). But the symptoms that most women report to be the biggest challenge of menopause are the hot flashes. Three-fourths of women have hot flashes and some are frequent and severe enough to require some treatment, because they can disrupt sleep. And when we don't get enough sleep, we get irritable, have trouble remembering things, and are just plain unpleasant to be around! Hot flashes are made worse by smoking, feeling anxious, alcohol, and caffeine. So the best bet is to try to eliminate the causes. Some women try herbal products to reduce hot flashes, but most of them do not work very well (soy, evening primrose, dong quai, gingseng, wild yams). The only one that seems to be effective for some women is black cohosh, but it can affect the liver, so take with caution. If the hot flashes are disrupting your life, talk to a health care provider about the use of low doses of estrogen. The decision to use hormones is a complicated one, so you must talk to a healthcare provider about your personal risk factors before making any decision. Menopause is a major transition time for women and signals the end of the reproductive years. For some women, there are major body image issues associated with this change that is a highly visible marker of aging.

Aging and Changes in Metabolism
There are several ways that the body changes with aging that affect how we metabolize alcohol, drugs, and even food. Some of these changes include:

- **Slower time to break down food/drugs/alcohol**. The liver and kidneys are not as efficient and take longer to break down things we eat or drink. We have less stomach acid, too. That means that alcohol circulates in the blood stream longer and so do drugs (prescription, over-the-counter, and recreational). Those substances will exert effects on our bodies for a longer period of time than when we were younger. This concept is called "half-life," and refers to the amount of time it takes for a substance to get out of your system. One of the major problems it poses is increasing the likelihood of drug-to-drug or drug/alcohol interactions. For example, if you have a couple of drinks with dinner, when you were younger, the alcohol was metabolized by the time you took a sleeping pill before bed. Now, however, you may still have some alcohol in your system which will affect how the sleeping pill affects you. You may need lower doses of drugs now and need to pay closer attention to the timing of doses of drugs that might interact.

- **Increase in body fat stores.** Some substances are stored in fat cells and then are released slowly or in irregular patterns. Anything that is "fat-soluble" will have different effects on your body if your fat stores increase. After menopause, when our estrogen levels decline, we tend to build less muscle mass and the fat stores increase. We can get some of this back via strength-training. Like slower metabolism, this factor increases the possibility of drug-drug and drug-alcohol interactions.

- **Decrease in body water**. Our blood tends to become more concentrated as we age. Less water in the blood means that alcohol, drugs, and some foods circulate in our systems in higher concentrations and may have more pronounced effects than when we were younger.

These changes in metabolism are very important. More older adults are hospitalized for drug interactions than for heart attacks, showing how often they happen, and how severe they can be.

Health Problems Related to Aging

The leading causes of death among persons aged 65 and older in the U.S. (2010 data) are:

- Heart Disease (33% of deaths)
- Cancer (20% of deaths)
- Stroke (8% of deaths)

These three account for 61% of all deaths each year, and they are all preventable to some extent. Diabetes is the third or fourth leading cause of death for American Indians, African Americans, Pacific Islanders, and Latinos in the U.S. (6th for White Americans). Death rates from disease declined in the past ten years, with lower rates of death from heart disease the most significant, but death rates from unintentional falls have increased. There is no data about mortality rates for lesbian and bisexual women, so we do not know if the causes of death are exactly the same as for heterosexuals. In the lesbian/bisexual women's health literature, there has been a lot of emphasis placed on the elevated risk factors for breast cancer. This will be discussed in a later chapter, but it is important to know that heart disease is the biggest killer of women.

Rates of Alzheimer Disease have increased with rising life expectancy, and affect mostly the oldest subgroup of elders with women more likely to be affected than men, mainly because women live longer. The table below shows the death rates from Alzheimer's per 100,000 people in the population. Fears about Alzheimer's disease as "rampant" among the older population are over-estimated. On the other hand, lesbian/bisexual women, especially those who live alone and do not have children, may have more concerns about developing Alzheimer Disease and fear the potentially hostile or violent reactions if caregivers are homophobic. Most care for people with dementia comes from children or partners, so lesbian/bisexual women who are more likely to live alone and be without children, have to worry about strangers caring for them.

Figure 2.1. Death rates from Alzheimers (from CDC data)

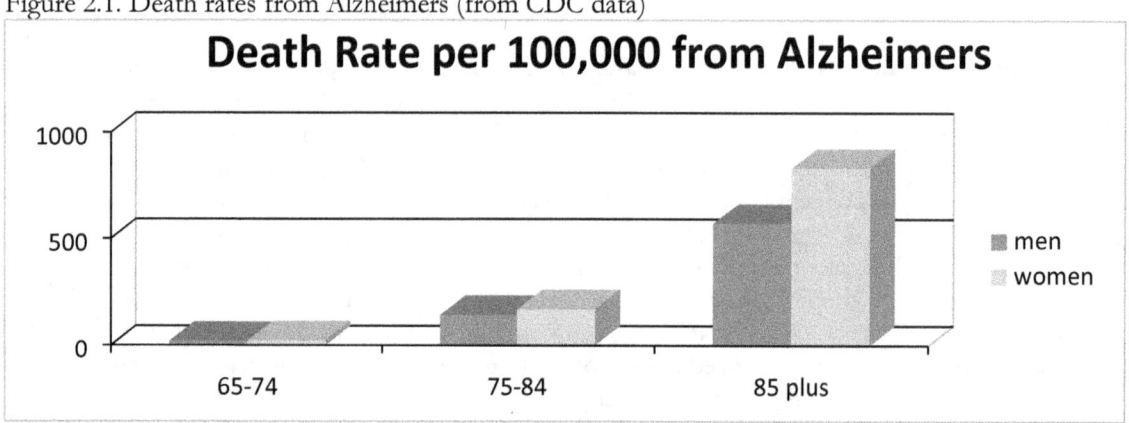

AGING IN A DIVERSE SOCIETY

There are many "cultures of aging," reflecting the diversity experienced by older adults by socioeconomic class, race, ethnicity, national or geographic origin, sexual orientation, sex, gender identity, and other human differences that result in variations in cultural beliefs, and risk for poverty, harassment, discrimination, and violence. The next section focuses on three categories: race/ethnicity, gender, and sexual orientation/gender identity. These sources of oppression can affect income level, standard of living, what neighborhoods we live in, cultural beliefs, perceptions about the world as well as health and illness, how we behave (in health-promoting or health-damaging ways), and whether we have access to quality health care services (Mehrota & Wagner, 2009). Unfortunately, most research divides up people on the basis of one of these, and does not look at the combinations, so we have little information about subgroups such as Latina lesbians over 50. An intersectional approach in the future would be much more helpful in understanding the influences on aging.

Some earlier researchers proposed that income level is one of the biggest determinants of healthy aging and proposed that poor people were "ill-derly" and wealthier people were "well-derly" (Moody, 2002), but the reality is more complicated than that. Every older person has a combination of individual factors and social determinants that contributes to health and well-being as they age.

Racial/Ethnic Diversity

The United States is experiencing major population shifts from being a predominantly white society to a multicultural nation. The Latino elder population is projected to grow at the fastest rate in the U.S. overall, but Asian/Pacific Islander growth is also substantial. There are differences in life expectancy based on race, as shown below.

Figure 2.2. Life expectancy by race in the U.S. (from CDC, 2012)

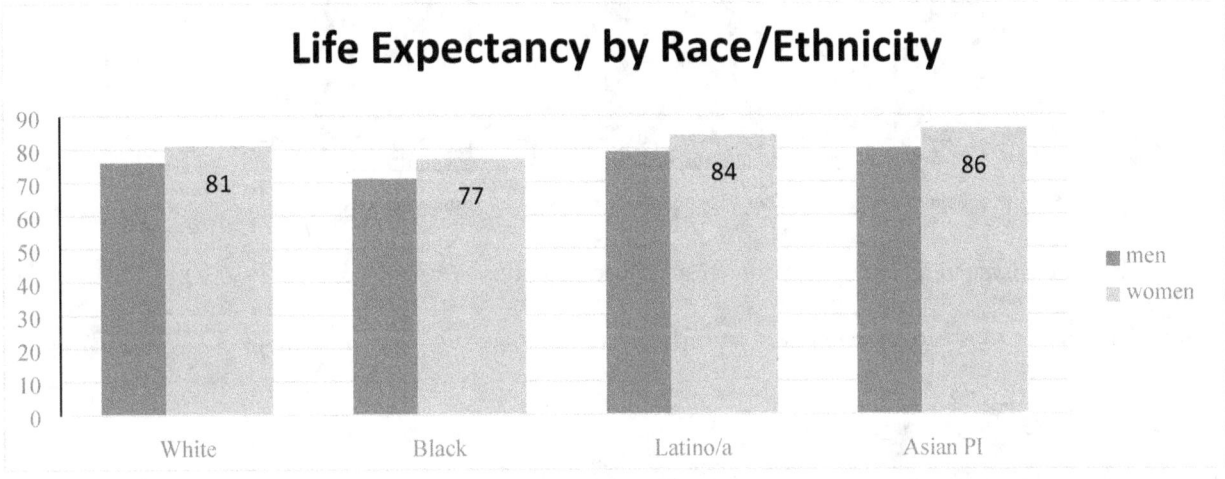

Most of the differences in health and life expectancy by race/ethnicity are related to income level differences. Other factors that influence health and aging include:

1. Differences in religious involvement: people who have strong supportive religious communities tend to be healthier (and some ethnicities are associated with greater religious involvement).
2. Greater intergenerational contact. In cultures with greater contact and connection, older adults are less likely to be placed in nursing homes, and are cared for at home.
3. Language barriers: health care access may be limited by lack of translators and health education options in a person's own language.
4. Immigration status is also a key factor in access to health care services, as well as a contributor to differing belief systems about health and illness.

Sex/Gender Diversity

Women live longer than men, on average about five years, thus make up a majority of the older population. Women have higher rates of debilitating chronic disorders such as rheumatoid arthritis and other auto-immune disorders, thyroid conditions, arthritis, and other conditions that impact quality of life in those extra years. Some of the consequences of ageism and sexism are (from Moody, 2002):

- The greater emphasis on looking young for women than men.
- The greater caregiver expectation and burden placed on older women.
- The higher chance of living in poverty because women's salaries through-out the lifetime are lower than men's and they are less likely to have benefits.
- Greater chance of living alone.

Sexual Orientation and Gender Identity Diversity (LGBT)

Approximately 10% of the older population is lesbian, gay, bisexual or transgender, and they are as diverse as other elders in terms of race/ethnicity, socioeconomic status, religion, national origin, and other personal factors (Witten & Eyler, 2012). Heterosexist oppression impacts a person's ability to make a decent living, and more LGBT elders live in poverty than other-sex couples, as shown below:

Figure 2.3. Poverty rates in same-sex couples over 50 compared to heterosexual couples (from Goldberg, 2009)

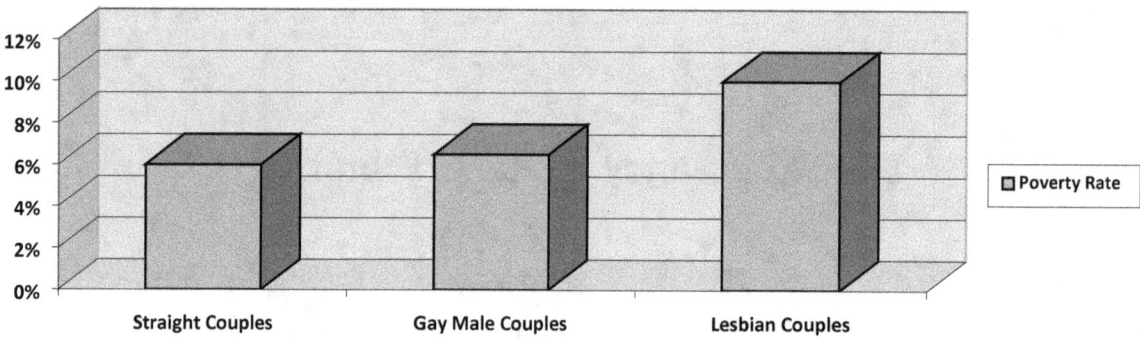

This is also demonstrated by data about annual social security income rates.

Figure 2.4. Social security income in elders from same-sex and heterosexual relationships (Goldberg, 2009)

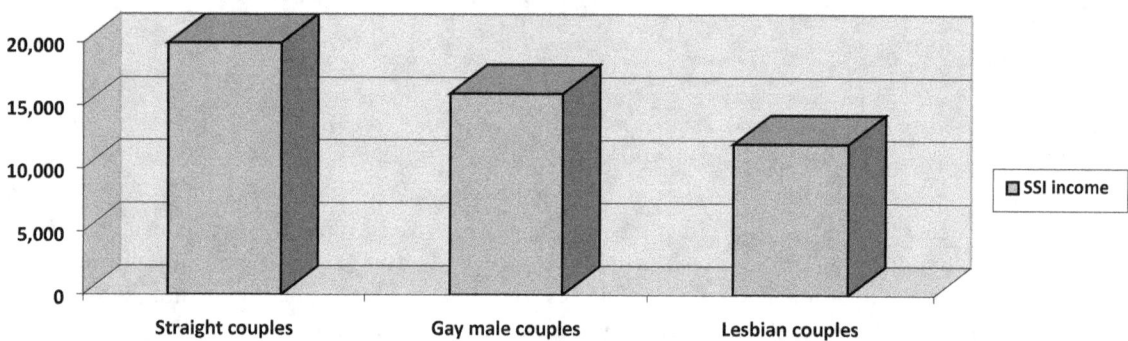

Lesbian and bisexual elders of color are more likely to have children than white lesbian/bisexual women, so may have greater sources of family support, but are even more likely to be poor and have even greater suspicion of health care systems because of the combinations of racism, sexism, ageism, and heterosexism (MetLife, 2006). A definite advantage of lesbian/bisexual women's communities that is not true of gay/bisexual men's communities, is that we are less ageist and more accepting of women at older ages and with a wide variety of body types and sizes and functions. We consider women to be sexual through-out their lifespan. That means lesbian/bisexual women are never considered too old for dating and new relationships. But there are few resources that understand our needs as we age. Most services and resources in LGBT communities are youth-oriented, small, poorly funded and precarious organizations in cities. Rural areas have few if any LGBT services, and few mainstream health or aging services are LGBT culturally sensitive.

DEVELOPMENTAL TASKS OF AGING

Cross-cultural anthropologist Angeles Arrien (2005) suggested that all elders (starting at age 50, the "youth of old age") must deal with three transitions for healthy aging. The first involves a shift from prioritizing ambition, to valuing meaning. We seek relationships that feed our hearts, not that are advantageous or help us with our career or social status. We search for activities that have deeper meaning for us, rather than superficial activities. Second, we have to integrate our inner and outer worlds. Arrien calls this the dual process of descent and ascent. Descent means delving into unresolved issues from the past and retrieving parts of ourselves that we have given away over the years, and befriending the parts of ourselves that we don't much like. That might include parts of the physical body as well as behaviors or habits that we wish we did not have. Ascent is looking beyond our identities and egos to our authentic self and transcending our physical bodies. Finally, the third shift involves giving up dualities, or black and white thinking. We finally see the complexity of life and its many, many facets. Nothing is simply yes or no, wrong or right. We learn to be more comfortable with the paradoxes and unexplainable events of life. This means that we may finally come to some level of peace with families, estranged friends, and systems, because we recognize the complexity of their responses to us.

Other mainstream aging researchers, like Erik Erikson, thought that the major tasks of mid-life and old age were generativity, or giving back something for the generations to come, and ego integrity, or achieving some peace about death and dying. Many heterosexual women satisfy the need for generativity through parenting and later grand-parenting. For lesbian and bisexual women who chose not to have children, generativity may come through creative activities, work, and/or mentoring. We really do not know much about how lesbian and bisexual women deal with challenges to their own mortality. In Chapter 9, we address spiritual health and touch on some issues that may impact this developmental task.

Retirement

Retirement is one of the main tasks of aging for which there is much research in the mainstream literature, but very little about how lesbian/bisexual women experience retirement. Because of higher rates of poverty, some lesbian/bisexual women may not have the luxury of retiring and need to continue to work for as long as health permits. Worries about finances are a major stressor for most lesbian/bisexual women as they age. One study found 57% of older lesbian/bisexual women worried about having enough money to live on as they age (Espinoza, 2014). In addition, lesbian/bisexual women were more likely to have continuous careers than heterosexual women, thus retiring from a job or career may be somewhat more stressful, particularly if the woman's identity comes primarily from an occupation.

Aging, Relationships, and Caregiving

As we age, our relationships also evolve. Partners and social networks age along with us. Age segregation in society may have pushed us into relationships primarily with those of similar age, so that our networks are not diverse in terms of age. We may be experiencing losses of mobility, increases in fears for safety, and losses as a community, increasing the possibility of isolation and loneliness. Often partners or close friends become caregivers for those in need, and there has been little research to uncover how those relationships change with the caregiver role.

Another unexplored area is the role of pets as companions and "chosen family" for older lesbian/bisexual women (Putney, 2014). Anecdotally, many lesbian/bisexual women seem unusually close to pets, but there has been little attention to paid to this in the research literature. The stresses of caring for a pet may increase for some older women who are physically or emotionally unable to deal with the needs of the pet, but on the other hand, Putney (2014) found that pets provide unconditional love, a mirroring that brings out the best in the owner, and help relieve loneliness. In addition, they may encourage physical activity for women who must walk their dogs or care for a pet, be a welcome interruption to other stressors, give life a daily structure, and give some women a reason to live.

INSTUTITIONAL STRESSES

Healthcare Providers and Systems

When younger (and presumably healthier), it was easier to avoid or delay healthcare for fear of encountering homophobic or ignorant healthcare providers. As we age, we tend to develop more serious problems that require interacting with healthcare services, disability services, and elder care. So many of us had bad experiences in the past, or had partners or close friends with bad experiences, that we may go into healthcare encounters with negative expectations and much anxiety. Chapter 16 discusses coming out to healthcare providers as a stress reducer, and also provides some information about health literacy. Many older women in our DIFO groups reported feeling a lack of confidence in their abilities to find and understand health information, forge a partnership with healthcare providers, and come out and demand to be treated with respect as lesbian/bisexual women. Chapter 13 deals more with the healthcare system, and Chapter 16 gives suggestions for coming out to providers. The more information you have about health, the easier it is to communicate with providers. But there is no doubt that accessing healthcare, even when you have a supportive provider, is stressful.

Concerns about Finances

Rising costs in housing and healthcare may disproportionately affect lesbian and bisexual women. As noted earlier, we are more likely to live in poverty and have limited means as we age because of the combination of sexism (unequal distribution of pay and benefits by sex) and heterosexism (a tendency of lesbian and bisexual women to choose careers where it is safer to be out, and those careers are often in community non-profits and health and human services that pay less). Because of financial stresses, some women are forced to move to less expensive, more rural communities where there is less visible lesbian community and few LGBT resources.

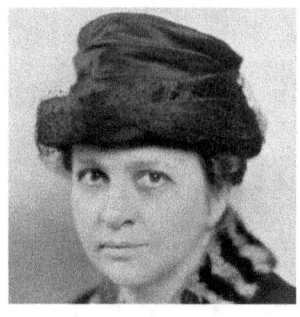

Frances Perkins

First female cabinet member as Secretary of Labor under FDR, and probably lesbian or bisexual, is largely responsible for developing the social security system.

Concerns about Housing

The ideal situation for most of us is to "age in place" or be able to live independently in one's own familiar living space for as long as possible. The factors that determine whether one is able to do that include:

- Are there family or close friends who can help out and check in on you?
- Is there social support available so you don't feel isolated?
- Is transportation available for appointments, getting groceries, etc?
- Is it safe?

When these conditions cannot be met, sometimes decisions have to be made about other kinds of housing, such as residential placements (board and care, assisted living or nursing homes) or home care. In any out of home placement, lesbian and bisexual women often fear that the caregivers may be homophobic or have other prejudices that will interfere with the quality of the care they provide, or even make the situation physically or emotionally unsafe. There is also concern that other residents of care facilities may have negative attitudes (Donaldson, Asta, & Vacha-Haase, 2014). Some lesbian/bisexual women fear that they may need to go back into the closet if they must live in a residential unit of some kind, or fear that if out, they will not be accepted by others.

Non-Medical Housing Options

We have a growing number of options for housing as we age. Here are a few of them:

- Women's land communes. Some communities have created living spaces for lesbian/bisexual women. At this point in time, many of these are lesbian separatist communities and are mostly white.
- LGBT Housing. There are a growing number of LGBT housing communities across the U.S. Check with www.gayretirementguide.com for a list of them. Unfortunately, many of these are fairly expensive. Some women who have been mostly in women's communities through-out their lives, are resistant to living with gay/bisexual men and transgender people, but for those with wider LGBT community ties, this may be an attractive option.
- Co-Housing Arrangements. Some people create housing options by buying condominiums, mobile homes, or houses that are close together physically to have both privacy and community. They create ways to build social support and help for those who need it. For ideas about how to create co-housing, see http://www.cohousing.org/what_is_cohousing. This is not strictly about LGBT or lesbian/bisexual women, but provides guidance on how to do this.
- Intentional Communities. Some women are developing arrangements with friends and family to live close by, even if not in the same building or block, but to develop strong communities of support and social life together. These are communities of women that watch out for each other.

In conclusion, lesbian and bisexual women face some unique challenges as we age, related to the stigmas of our sexual orientation, but also share many issues with heterosexual women related to the biological aspects of aging and the social consequences of ageism. We need a political and advocacy movement to help improve the conditions of the society into which we are aging.

Resources

- Old Lesbians Organizing Change (OLOC): www.oloc.org. An organization of activist lesbians over 60. Many are separatists.
- Gray Panthers: www.graypanthers.org. This is a predominantly heterosexual group dedicated to activism around aging.
- National Center for LGBT Aging: www.lgbtagingcenter.org/. A clearinghouse for information about LGBT aging issues such as housing and health care. They offer trainings for staff members in elder care agencies.
- National Center for Lesbian Rights: www.nclr.org. They have many resources for taking care of legal issues related to health, such as power of attorney and wills.
- Openhouse: http://openhouse-sf.org/. An agency in San Francisco dedicated to helping LGBT people over 55 with housing and other services.
- SAGE. http://www.sageusa.org/. Services and Advocacy for GLBT Elders.
- www.gayretirementguide.com

REFERENCES

Albert, S.M., O'Neill, M., Muller, C., & Butler, R. (2002). *When does old age begin? Results from a national survey.* NY: International Longevity Center.

Arrien, A. (2005). *The second half of life.* Boulder, CO: Sounds True.

Ashbrook, D., Gerald, G., & Eliason, M.J. (2011). LGBT Elder Needs Assessment Project, San Francisco, CA.

Butler, R.N. (2006). Ageism in America. Columbia University: National Center for Longevity.

Cronin, A., & King, A., (2010). Power, inequality, and identification: Exploring diversity and intersectionality amongst older LGB adults. *Sociology, 44(5)*, 876-892.

D'Augelli, A. & Grossman, A. (2001). Disclosure of sexual orientation, victimization, and mental health among lesbian, gay, and bisexual older adults. *Journal of Interpersonal Violence, 16*(10), 1008-1027.

Donaldson, W.V., Asta, E., & Vacha-Haase, T. (2014). Attitudes of heterosexual assisted living residents toward gay and lesbian peers. *Clinical Gerontologist, 37*, 167-189.

Espinoza, R. (2014). Out & Visible: The Experiences and Attitudes of Lesbian, Gay, Bisexual and Transgender Older Adults, Ages 45-75," Services and Advocacy for GLBT Elders, 2014, accessed February 20, 2015, http://www.sageusa.org/files/LGBT_OAMarketResearch_Rpt.pdf.

Goldberg, A. (2009). The impact of inequality for same-sex partners in employer-sponsored retirement plans. UCLA: The Williams Institute, May.

National Council on Aging (2002)

Levy, B. (2009). Stereotype embodiment: A psychosocial approach to aging. *Current Directions in Psychological Science, 18(6),* 332-336.

Levy, B., Slade, M., Kunkel, S., & Kasl, S. (2002). Longevity increased by positive self-perceptions of aging. *Journal of Personality and Social Psychology, 83,* 261-270.

Mehrota, C. & Wagner, L. (2009). *Aging and Diversity,* 2nd edition, New York: Taylor and Francis.

MetLife (2006). *Out and aging: The MetLife study of lesbian and gay baby boomers.* Westport, CT: MetLife Mature Market Institute.

Moody, H.R. (2002). *Aging: Concepts and Controversies.* 4th Edition, Thousand Oaks, CA: Pine Forge Press.

Palmore, E.B. (1990). *Ageism: Negative and Positive.* NY: Springer Press.

Porter, K., Keary, S., VanWagenen, A., & Bradford, J. (2014). Social network and nutritional value of congregate meal programs: Differences by sexual orientation. *Journal of Applied Gerontology,* doi: 073346481456042.

Putney, J.M. (2014). Older lesbian adults' psychological well-being: The significance of pets. *Journal of Gay and Lesbian Social Services, 26,* 1-17.

U.S. Census (2010). www.factfinder2.gov.

Weir, E.C. (2004). Identifying and preventing ageism among health-care professionals. *International Journal of Therapy and Rehabilitation, 11(2),* 56-63.

Witten, T. & Eyler, A.E. (2012). *Gay, lesbian, bisexual, and transgender aging: Challenges in research, practice, and policy.* Baltimore, MD: Johns Hopkins Press.

Chapter 3. Mental Health and Stress

One of the most reliable research findings that emerges when studies compare women by sexual orientation, is that lesbian and bisexual women are more likely to have symptoms of depression and anxiety than heterosexual women. This is true for current symptoms and lifetime diagnoses of mental health problems. But the research headlines might be a little misleading—being lesbian or bisexual by itself does not cause mental health problems. Most of this research suggests that the stress related to the stigma of sexual orientation is what accounts for this difference. The stress and anxiety associated with keeping a secret about one's sexuality, coming out to family and friends, wondering how one's boss or teachers might respond, and fearing discrimination in healthcare settings or in public places takes a toll and may result in symptoms of sadness, hopelessness, and anxiety.

Another set of research is finding that lesbian and bisexual women are more likely to report that they were abused as children than heterosexual women (Aaron & Hughes, 2007; Alvy, Hughes, Kristjanson, & Wilsnack, 2013; Austin et al, 2008; Balsam et al, 2005; Corliss, et al, 2002; Hughes et al, 2010; Lehavot et al., 2012; Stoddard et al, 2009). Childhood abuse is also a major predictor of mood disorders in adulthood (and substance use and abuse as well). Sometimes this abuse is linked to one's gender or sexuality, as when male family members or classmates abuse a girl who is a "tomboy" or does not conform to stereotypes about what girls/women are supposed to look like or act like. There is very little research on how/whether lesbian and bisexual women deal with the aftermath of sexual abuse differently than heterosexual women. Most women who have experienced sexual abuse find counseling to be helpful, and sometimes need couples counseling to resolve issues with sexual functioning and/or intimacy.

Other mental health problems that result from genetic or more physiologically-based causes like bipolar illness and schizophrenia seem to occur at about the same rates as among heterosexual women, lending support to the theory that the excess in mental health disorders is related to stress, not any hard-wired brain or genetic differences.

STRESS AND MENTAL HEALTH

What Stresses You?

Everyone experiences stress to some degree and at some times. It is part of the human condition, but as older lesbian and bisexual women, we have extra added challenges, known in the research literature as minority stress. Older lesbian and bisexual women have higher rates of depression, anxiety, suicidal behaviors, alcohol and drug abuse, smoking and certain physical health problems than heterosexual women (Fredriksen-Goldsen et al., 2012). Researchers have concluded that sexual orientation and gender identity are not the cause of the health problems, but rather the stress of living with the effects of oppression is the culprit. Minority stress is the stress that is on top of the concerns that are common to humans in general, such as worry about money, work-related concerns, relationship conflicts, family strife, and living with chronic illnesses (Meyer, 2003). Minority stress can come from any oppressed minority identity, related to ethnicity, age, sexual identity and many others. Most people have a combination of identities, so stress may come from many different sources. Minority stress has two major components:

- Stress from the outside world
- Stress turned inward (internalized).

External Stress. **External homophobia** includes experiences of rejection, exclusion, harassment, feeling invisible or invalidated, discrimination and violence, based on one's actual or perceived sexual orientation or gender presentation. Many lesbian and bisexual women have lost jobs, lost custody of children, experienced family rejection, had their partners excluded from family or work events, received poor treatment from a health care provider, and many other experiences that make us more paranoid and suspicious of the world around us (Lehavot & Simoni, 2011). **Biphobia** is prevalent in heterosexual populations, and among some lesbians, and can lead to bisexual women feeling excluded from community support and resources. Gender normativity is the idea that everyone born with a female body will develop feminine traits and expressions and be attracted only to men, and that there are two and only two genders. **Transphobia** can also be found in both heterosexual and lesbian communities, and can lead to transgender women and men feeling unsafe and left out.

Internalized Minority Stress. When we are exposed to external stress over a long period of time, negative attitudes about one's own sexuality or gender can be internalized (Szymanski & Chung, 2003). That is, we sometimes start to believe that we are inferior to heterosexuals, and our same-sex desires can be experienced with shame, guilt, or fear. Or we wrongly believe that our gender expression is a form of deviance. Or we absorb the messages about how women are supposed to look and behave, and then we feel inferior or flawed. Those negative emotions are the precursors to depression, anxiety, substance abuse, and suicide thoughts or attempts. Nearly every LGBT person has some degree of internalized homophobia, biphobia, and transphobia because we are exposed to the negative stereotypes and damning messages from a very early age (Szymanski & Chung, 2003). It takes many years of conscious effort to unlearn those stereotypes. The strongest, out-est, and most proud among us may still experience moments of shame, guilt, or doubt about our sexuality and gender. Some of us have also internalized messages about race, ability status, age, weight, and social class.

Some researchers are exploring the impact of the daily sources of stress--the relatively smaller events that happen often, such as being stared at in public, ignored by a store clerk, or awkward pauses in conversations with co-workers (Nadal, 2013). Every time we go to a new healthcare provider and have to fill out forms about our relationship status, we have to consider whether to come out or not. When we order an ice cream cone and someone stares at us as if to say, no wonder you are fat. When we point out sexism, we might be told, "Women are equal now. Sexism is a thing of the past." Or we are told, "Gay people can get married now, so there is no more homophobia." That's a denial of our reality. These events are called micro-aggressions, and added up over time, can create a great deal of stress that might affect one's health. We get used to these things on a conscious level and take them for granted, but our bodies react to them every time they happen.

Varieties of Minority Stress
As women, we also experience external and internalized sexism, as we absorb messages from the media, family, religion, schools, and communities about how women should look and behave. As older women, we face the stigma attached to aging. Many of us also have stress related to having a disability, being of a different race or ethnicity, religion, or having a working class background or life experience. Within the "lesbian community," many may experience transphobia, racism, sexism, ageism, classism, and other forms of oppression, because our bonding together as lesbian and bisexual women does not come automatically with greater social consciousness about other forms of oppression. Women with larger bodies are judged constantly. The pressures of all of these stressors can add up to physical and mental health problems.

Antidote to Minority Stress: Pride and Resilience
The concept of "pride" was developed to counteract those internalized messages. Instead of feeling bad for being different, we can reframe our thinking into pride for having survived homophobic families, churches, and schools; pride for having the courage to be who we really are; pride for having survived to our current age. This applies to our physical appearance as well as our sexual and gender identities. We can take pride in embracing our bodies and challenge all the forces in our environment that try to shame us. When someone says, "You don't look your age," respond that you are proud to be whatever age you are. We need to challenge fatphobia, heterosexism, ableism, racism, and other shaming forces whenever we can (and forgive ourselves if we just don't have the energy or strength to do it every time). Resilience, or the capacity to bounce back after being stressed, is a protective factor for both mental and physical health disorders. Stress can underlie many mental health disorders or cause symptoms of mental health problems whether they are diagnosable or not.

Fredriksen-Goldsen and colleagues (2014) outlined a "resilience framework" for understanding quality of life issues in LGB people over the age of 60. This resiliency model has five components. Consider whether you are satisfied with your experience of each one:

- Social Risks: This refers to the lifetime history of discrimination and victimization: if you have many traumatic experiences in your past, have you dealt with them? Resolved them or done forgiveness work?
- Identity Management Resources: Do you feel comfortable with your own sexuality? Are you out to most people? How do you feel when you have to come out to somebody new?
- Social Resources: This refers to whether you have a supportive partner, a good social network of close friends and also acquaintances, whether you engage in religious or spiritual activities, whether you feel strongly connected to a community.
- Health-promoting Behaviors: These include getting adequate physical activity, having leisure activities or hobbies, getting routine check-ups, eating healthy, and limiting alcohol, drug, and tobacco use.
- Socioeconomic Resources: This category includes having an adequate income, having health benefits/insurance, being employed, being educated, and having adequate housing.

If you have resources in all of these areas, you have a much greater likelihood of being resilient and being more satisfied with your own aging process. These categories are all associated with better quality of life as one ages.

MENTAL HEALTH DISORDERS

The following sections on mental health disorders includes information on symptoms, frequency of the disorders among lesbian and bisexual women, and treatment options, including the most commonly used medications. This is not to be considered an endorsement of any particular treatment because treatment decisions are highly individual and must be made in consultation with your healthcare providers. However, it is useful to know what the most common treatments are as a starting point. Some lesbian and bisexual women are suspicious of biomedical disease classifications and treatments, for good reason. But there is little research on the effectiveness or safety of alternative treatments, so they are not covered here.

Mood Disorders

The most commonly diagnosed mental health problems of lesbian and bisexual women are in the category called mood disorders, and include depression and anxiety problems. The figure below shows the percentage of women who ever had a mood disorder in their lifetimes. As you can see, between 40 and 50% of lesbian/bisexual women have experienced depression or an anxiety disorder (and many had both), and the rates are higher for lesbians and bisexual women than for heterosexual women. We will discuss depression and anxiety disorders (including post-traumatic stress disorder separately) in this section. Remember that most of us have some symptoms of these disorders in response to stress, loss, and grief experiences. They only become a disorder when they last a long time and interfere with our daily lives, such as affecting employment, relationships, or cause us significant pain over an extended period of time.

Figure 3.1. Lifetime experiences of mood disorders in women by sexual identity (from Bostwick and colleagues, 2009)

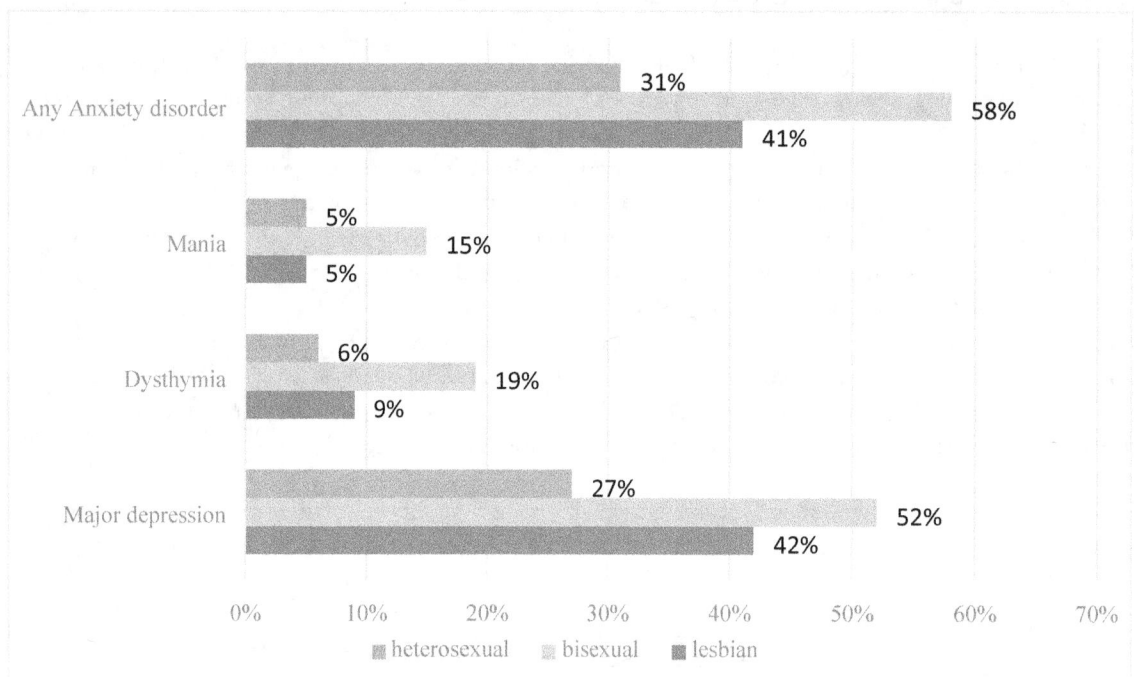

Depression

Depression is a mental health diagnosis that includes symptoms of sadness and loss of pleasure in life that interfere with the ability to cope or engage in daily functioning activities such as work and maintaining relationships. Everyone feels sad sometimes and experiences losses in life, but depression is a condition that lasts longer than typical grief reactions, and sometimes occurs without a trigger.

Types of Depression

Major depressive disorder, or major depression, is characterized by a combination of symptoms that interfere with a person's ability to work, sleep, study, eat, and enjoy once-pleasurable activities. Major depression is disabling and prevents a person from functioning normally. Some people may experience only a single episode within their lifetime, but more often a person will have multiple episodes.

Dysthymic disorder, or dysthymia, is characterized by long-term (2 years or longer) symptoms that may not be severe enough to cause a disability, but can prevent normal functioning or feeling well at times. People with dysthymia may also experience one or more episodes of major depression during their lifetimes.

Minor depression is diagnosed when symptoms last for 2 weeks or longer, but that do not meet full criteria for major depression. Without treatment, some people with minor depression are at higher risk for developing major depressive disorder.

Some forms of depression are slightly different, or they may develop under unique circumstances. *Postpartum depression* occurs in 10-15% of women after the birth of a child, and is more serious than the "baby blues" that some women experience when hormonal and physical changes and the new responsibility of caring for a newborn feel overwhelming. About 10 to 15% of women experience postpartum depression. *Seasonal affective disorder* (SAD), is when depression occurs only during the winter months, when there is less natural sunlight. The depression generally lifts during spring and summer. SAD may be treated with light therapy, but nearly half of those with SAD do not get better with light therapy alone. Antidepressant medication and psychotherapy can reduce SAD symptoms, either alone or in combination with light therapy. *Bipolar disorder*, also called manic-depressive illness, is not as common as major depression or dysthymia.

Bipolar disorder is diagnosed when mood changes, from extreme highs (e.g., mania) to extreme lows (e.g., depression), often very rapidly.

Causes

Depression is caused by a combination of genetic, biological, environmental, and psychological factors. Depressive illnesses are disorders of the brain, but are sensitive to the stressors in our lives. Brain-imaging technologies have shown that the parts of the brain involved in mood, thinking, sleep, appetite, and behavior look different in people with depression than those without depression. The brain differences are probably the consequence, not the cause of the depression.

Some types of depression tend to run in families, but depression can occur in people without family histories. Depression probably results from the influence of several genes acting together with environmental or other factors such as trauma, loss of a loved one, a difficult relationship, or any stressful situation, such as fearing being exposed as a lesbian or bisexual woman, or experiencing harassment or discrimination. Depressive episodes may occur with or without an obvious trigger.

Among lesbian/bisexual women, additional causes may be related to minority stress: the stress of living with actual or potential discrimination, harassment, violence and the internalizing of the negative attitudes of society about one's sexuality and/or gender. Some women internalize messages from religion or family that create shame and guilt about one's body or sexual desires. Long-term exposure to minority stresses can affect the brain. Finally, the greater history of childhood traumas among lesbian and bisexual women is probably a major factor in the greater likelihood of developing depression.

Diagnosing Major Depressive Episodes

This information is taken from the Diagnostic and Statistical Manual, 5th Edition, the book used to make diagnoses in mental health care in the U.S. This classification system is controversial, but it is widely used, and if you go to a mainstream psychologist or psychiatrist, they will use these criteria. A major depressive episode is diagnosed if you currently have 5 or more of these symptoms for at least 2 weeks:

☐ (1) depressed mood most of the day, nearly every day, as indicated by either subjective report (e.g., feels sad or empty) or observation made by others (e.g., appears tearful

☐ (2) noticeable loss of interest or pleasure in all, or almost all, activities most of the day, nearly every day

☐ (3) significant weight loss when not dieting or weight gain (e.g., a change of more than 5% of body weight in a month), or decrease or increase in appetite nearly every day.

☐ (4) insomnia or hypersomnia (sleeping a lot more than usual) nearly every day

☐ (5) psychomotor agitation or retardation nearly every day (observable by others, not merely subjective feelings of restlessness or being slowed down)

☐ (6) fatigue or loss of energy nearly every day

☐ (7) feelings of worthlessness or excessive or inappropriate guilt (which may be delusional) nearly every day (not merely self-reproach or guilt about being sick)

☐ (8) impaired ability to think or concentrate, or indecisiveness, nearly every day (either by subjective account or as observed by others)

☐ (9) recurrent thoughts of death (not just fear of dying), recurrent suicidal ideation without a specific plan, or a suicide attempt or a specific plan for committing suicide

Diagnosing Bipolar Disorder

In bipolar illness, the symptoms of depression above alternate with signs of mania. Mania includes excessive happiness, excitement, irritability, restlessness, increased energy, less need for sleep, racing thoughts, high sex drive, and a tendency to make grand and unattainable plans. Many people have mild mood swings, depending on events of the day. Bipolar disorder involves extremes of mood cycling.

Co-Occurring Disorders

Anxiety disorders, such as post-traumatic stress disorder (PTSD), obsessive-compulsive disorder, panic disorder, social phobia, and generalized anxiety disorder, often accompany depression. PTSD can occur after a frightening event or ordeal, such as child abuse, a violent assault, a natural disaster, an accident, terrorism, or military combat. People experiencing PTSD are especially prone to having co-existing depression. LGBT people may have PTSD that results from experiences of discrimination and trauma, such as a hate crime or losing custody of children.

Depression also may occur with alcohol and drug problems as well as other serious medical illnesses such as heart disease, stroke, cancer, HIV/AIDS, diabetes, and Parkinson's disease. People who have depression along with another medical illness or substance abuse pattern tend to have more severe symptoms of both depression and the other illness, more difficulty adapting to their medical condition, and more medical costs than those who do not have co-existing depression. Treating the depression can also help improve the outcome of treating the co-occurring illness.

Lesbian and bisexual women may also have co-occurring internalized lesbian or biphobia, which consists of feelings of shame, guilt, self-doubt, and fear about one's sexual orientation or sexual desires. This may stem from religious upbringing or negative attitudes from one's family of origin. Internalized racism, ageism, and other forms of oppression may also contribute to depression or anxiety symptoms. Internalized homophobia (as well as sexism, ageism, and other isms) makes us question our self-worth.

Treatments

The most common treatments are medication and psychotherapy, however, there are a growing number of alternative and complementary practices that may help for mild depression, or in combination with other treatments, be effective for moderate to severe depression. For example, exercise has been found to be as effective or even more effective than most medications for some forms of mild depression. Some lesbian and bisexual women are suspicious of using medications. This is an individual decision and requires much discussion with healthcare providers. The following section gives some general information about the types of medications that are currently available. DIFO does not endorse or recommend any particular forms of treatment. This section is meant for informational purposes only.

Medications

Antidepressants work on brain chemicals called neurotransmitters, especially serotonin, norepinephrine and dopamine. The latest information on approved medications for treating depression is available on the U.S. Food and Drug Administration (FDA) website. Some of the newest and most popular antidepressants are called selective serotonin reuptake inhibitors (SSRIs). Fluoxetine (Prozac), sertraline (Zoloft), escitalopram (Lexapro), paroxetine (Paxil), and citalopram (Celexa) are some of the most commonly prescribed SSRIs for depression. Most are available in generic versions. Serotonin and norepinephrine reuptake inhibitors (SNRIs) are similar to SSRIs and include venlafaxine (Effexor) and duloxetine (Cymbalta). SSRIs and SNRIs tend to have fewer side effects than older antidepressants, but they sometimes produce headaches, nausea, jitters, or insomnia when people first start to take them. These symptoms tend to fade with time. Some people also experience sexual problems with SSRIs or SNRIs, which may be helped by adjusting the dosage or switching to another medication. One popular antidepressant that works on dopamine is bupropion (Wellbutrin). Bupropion tends to have similar side effects as SSRIs and SNRIs, but it is less likely to cause sexual side effects. However, it can increase a person's risk for seizures. Bupropion is also used for tobacco cessation, because it decreases craving for tobacco for some people.

Tricyclics are older antidepressants; they are not used as much today because their potential side effects are more serious. They may affect the heart in people with heart conditions. They sometimes cause dizziness, especially in older adults. They also may cause drowsiness, dry mouth, and weight gain. These side effects can usually be corrected by changing the dosage or switching to another medication. However, tricyclics may be especially dangerous if taken in overdose. Tricyclics include imipramine and nortriptyline.

Monoamine oxidase inhibitors (MAOIs) are the oldest class of antidepressant medications. They can be especially effective in cases of "atypical" depression, such as when a person experiences increased appetite

36

and the need for more sleep rather than decreased appetite and sleep. They also may help with anxious feelings or panic symptoms. People who take MAOIs must avoid certain foods and beverages (including cheese and red wine) that contain a substance called tyramine. Certain medications, including some types of birth control pills, prescription pain relievers, cold and allergy medications, and herbal supplements, also should be avoided while taking an MAOI. These substances can interact with MAOIs to cause dangerous increases in blood pressure. If you are taking an MAOI, your doctor should give you a complete list of foods, medicines, and substances to avoid. MAOIs can also react with SSRIs to produce a serious condition called "serotonin syndrome," which can cause confusion, hallucinations, increased sweating, muscle stiffness, seizures, changes in blood pressure or heart rhythm, and other potentially life-threatening conditions. MAOIs should not be taken with SSRIs.

All these antidepressants must be taken for 4 to 6 weeks before they have a full effect. It is recommended that you continue to take the medication, even if you are feeling better, to prevent the depression from returning. Medication should be stopped only under a health care provider's supervision. Some medications need to be gradually stopped to give the body time to adjust. Although antidepressants are not habit-forming or addictive, suddenly ending an antidepressant can cause withdrawal symptoms or lead to a relapse of the depression. Some individuals with chronic or recurrent depression may need to stay on the medication indefinitely. Research shows that people who did not get better after taking a first medication increase their chances of reducing their depression symptoms by switching to a different medication or adding another medication to their existing one. Sometimes stimulants, anti-anxiety medications, or other medications are used together with an antidepressant, especially if a person has a co-existing illness. However, neither anti-anxiety medications nor stimulants are effective against depression when taken alone, and both should be taken only under a doctor's supervision.

FDA warning on antidepressants.
In 2004, the Food and Drug Administration (FDA) reviewed studies of antidepressants use with nearly 4,400 children and adolescents and found that 4% of those taking antidepressants thought about or attempted suicide (although no suicides occurred), compared to 2% of those receiving placebos (pills with no active medications in them). This information prompted a "black box" warning label on all antidepressant medications to alert the public about the potential increased risk of suicidal thinking or attempts in children and adolescents taking antidepressants. In 2007, the FDA proposed that makers of all antidepressant medications extend the warning to include young adults up through age 24. A "black box" warning is the most serious type of warning on prescription drug labeling. The warning emphasizes that patients of all ages taking antidepressants should be closely monitored, especially in the early weeks of treatment. Possible side effects to look for are worsening depression, suicidal thinking or behavior, or any unusual changes in behavior such as sleeplessness, agitation, or withdrawal from normal social situations.

St. John's wort?
The extract from the herb St. John's wort (Hypericum perforatum) has been used for centuries in many folk and herbal remedies. It is used extensively in Europe to treat mild to moderate depression. However, recent studies have found that St. John's wort is no more effective than placebo in treating major or minor depression. In 2000, the FDA issued a Public Health Advisory letter stating that the herb may interfere with certain medications used to treat heart disease, depression, seizures, certain cancers, and those used to prevent organ transplant rejection. The herb also may interfere with the effectiveness of oral contraceptives. Consult with your healthcare provider before taking any herbal supplement. This is true of other over-the-counter (OTC) medications as well. Many of us consider OTC drugs and herbal supplements as "harmless" when they are not. They have side effects and can interact negatively with other drugs and foods in the same way as prescription drugs.

Psychotherapy
Several types of psychotherapy can help people with depression. Cognitive-behavioral therapy (CBT) and interpersonal therapy (IPT) are the most common and seem to be effective in treating depression. CBT is

based on the idea that it is our negative thoughts that cause the pain of depression, thus it is designed to help people with depression restructure negative thought patterns to interpret their environment and interactions with others in a positive and realistic way. It may also help you recognize things that may be contributing to the depression and help you change behaviors that may be making the depression worse. IPT helps people understand and work through difficult relationships that may cause the depression or make it worse. If the depression is related to rejection from family of origin, or old dysfunctional relationship patterns, IPT may work best for you. For mild to moderate depression, psychotherapy may be the best option. However, for severe depression or for certain people, psychotherapy alone may not be enough. A study looking at depression treatment among older adults found that people who responded to initial treatment of medication and IPT were less likely to have recurring depression if they continued their combination treatment for at least 2 years. Some lesbian and bisexual women have difficulties finding therapists who are sensitive to LGBT issues (or know the differences between lesbian and bisexual women and gay/bisexual and transgender people). You may need to interview therapists to find a good fit. A homophobic therapist will likely do more harm than good. There is a referral source for LGBT-affirmative therapists at the end of this chapter.

Electroconvulsive therapy and other brain stimulation therapies

In cases where medication and/or psychotherapy does not help relieve depression and a person is suffering, electroconvulsive therapy (ECT) may be considered. ECT, formerly known as "shock therapy," has a bad reputation. But in recent years, the procedure has been greatly improved and can provide relief for people with severe depression who have not been able to feel better with any other treatments. Before ECT begins, a patient is put under brief anesthesia and given a muscle relaxant. She sleeps through the treatment and does not consciously feel the electrical impulses. Within 1 hour after the treatment session, which takes only a few minutes, the patient is awake and alert. A person typically will undergo ECT several times a week, and often will need to take an antidepressant or other medication along with the ECT treatments. Although some people will need only a few courses of ECT, others may need maintenance ECT—usually once a week at first, then gradually decreasing to monthly treatments. ECT may cause some side effects, including confusion, disorientation, and memory loss. Usually these side effects are short-term, but sometimes they can linger. Newer methods of administering the treatment have reduced the memory loss and other cognitive difficulties associated with ECT. Research has found that after 1 year of ECT treatments, most patients showed no adverse cognitive effects.

How do women experience depression?

Depression is more common among women than among men because of biological, life cycle, hormonal, and psychosocial factors. Some hormones directly affect the brain chemistry that controls emotions and mood. For example, women are especially vulnerable to developing postpartum depression after giving birth. Some women may also have a severe form of premenstrual syndrome (PMS) called premenstrual dysphoric disorder (PMDD). PMDD is associated with the hormonal changes that typically occur around ovulation and before menstruation begins. During peri-menopause, some women experience depression. In addition, osteoporosis—bone thinning or loss—may be associated with depression. Many women face the additional stresses of work and home responsibilities, caring for children and aging parents, abuse, poverty, and relationship strains. It is still unclear why some women with enormous challenges develop depression, while others with similar stress levels do not. Most research shows that chronic exposure to minority stress causes the increased rates of depression in non-heterosexual women. For example, in one study, women who reported excellent or good emotional health reported between 1 and 2 discrimination experiences in their lives, but women who reported that that their emotional health was fair or poor had about 3 or more discrimination experiences in the past (Averett and coauthors, 2013).

Anxiety Disorders

Anxiety is a normal reaction to stress and can be beneficial in some situations. For some people, however, anxiety can become excessive and negatively affect day-to-day living. Anxiety disorders are among the most common mental disorders experienced by Americans. Specific types of anxiety disorders are:

- generalized anxiety disorder (GAD)
- obsessive-compulsive disorder (OCD),
- panic disorder,
- post-traumatic stress disorder (PTSD), and
- social phobia (or social anxiety disorder).

Causes

Mental illnesses are complex and probably result from a combination of genetic, environmental, psychological, and developmental factors. Although studies of twins and families suggest that genetics play a role in the development of some anxiety disorders, problems such as PTSD are triggered by trauma. Genetic studies may help explain why some people exposed to trauma develop PTSD and others do not. Several parts of the brain are key actors in the production of fear and anxiety. Using brain imaging technology and neurochemical techniques, scientists have discovered that the amygdala and the hippocampus play significant roles in most anxiety disorders. The amygdala is an almond-shaped structure deep in the brain that is believed to be a communications hub between the parts of the brain that process incoming sensory signals and the parts that interpret these signals. It can alert the rest of the brain that a threat is present and trigger a fear or anxiety response. The emotional memories stored in the central part of the amygdala may play a role in anxiety disorders involving very distinct fears, such as fears of dogs, spiders, or flying. The hippocampus is the part of the brain that codes threatening events into memories. The hippocampus appears to be smaller in some people who were victims of child abuse or who served in military combat.

Signs & Symptoms

Unlike the relatively mild, brief anxiety caused by a stressful event (such as speaking in public or a first date), anxiety disorders last at least 6 months and can get worse if they are not treated. Each anxiety disorder has different symptoms, but all the symptoms cluster around excessive, irrational fear and dread. Anxiety disorders commonly occur along with other mental or physical illnesses, including alcohol or substance abuse, which may mask anxiety symptoms or make them worse. In some cases, these other illnesses need to be treated before a person will respond to treatment for the anxiety disorder.

Who Is At Risk?

Anxiety disorders affect about 18% of people in the U.S. in any given year, causing feelings of fearfulness and uncertainty. Women are 60% more likely than men to experience an anxiety disorder over their lifetime. Non-Hispanic blacks are 20% less likely, and Latinos are 30% less likely, than non-Hispanic whites to experience an anxiety disorder during their lifetime.

Lesbian/Bisexual Women and Anxiety Disorders

As noted at the beginning of this chapter, lesbian/bisexual women in many studies have shown higher rates of anxiety disorders. There are several possible reasons for this: higher rates of self-reported child abuse among lesbian/bisexual women, greater experiences of discrimination, harassment, and rejection because of sexual identity, and greater daily stress from the smaller, but persistent sexist, racist, and heterosexist biases of daily life (micro-aggressions). Some lesbian and bisexual women have experienced hate crimes.

Diagnosis

A healthcare provider must conduct a careful diagnostic evaluation to determine whether a person's symptoms are caused by an anxiety disorder or a physical problem. If an anxiety disorder is diagnosed, the type of disorder or the combination of disorders that are present must be identified, as well as any coexisting conditions, such as depression or substance abuse. Sometimes alcoholism, depression, or other coexisting conditions have such a strong effect on the individual that treating the anxiety disorder must wait until the coexisting conditions are brought under control.

Treatments

In general, anxiety disorders are treated with medication, specific types of psychotherapy, or both. Treatment choices depend on the problem and the person's preference. Often people believe that they have "failed" at treatment or that the treatment didn't work for them when, in fact, it was not given for an adequate length of time or was administered incorrectly. Sometimes people must try several different treatments or combinations of treatment before they find the one that works for them.

Medication

Medication will not cure anxiety disorders, but it can keep them under control while the person receives psychotherapy. Medication must be prescribed and monitored by healthcare professionals who can either offer psychotherapy themselves or work as a team with psychologists, social workers, or counselors who provide psychotherapy. The principal medications used for anxiety disorders are antidepressants, anti-anxiety drugs, and beta-blockers to control some of the physical symptoms. Antidepressants were developed to treat depression but are also effective for anxiety disorders. Although these medications begin to alter brain chemistry after the very first dose, their full effect are not felt until about 4 to 6 weeks. It is important to continue taking these medications long enough to let them work. See the section under depression to learn more about different types of antidepressants.

Anti-Anxiety Drugs

High-potency benzodiazepines combat anxiety and have few side effects other than drowsiness. People can get used to them (develop tolerance and/or addiction) and may need higher and higher doses to get the same effect, so benzodiazepines are generally prescribed for short periods of time, especially for people who have abused drugs or alcohol and who become dependent on medication easily. One exception to this rule is people with panic disorder, who can take benzodiazepines for up to a year without harm.

Clonazepam (Klonopin®) is used for social phobia and GAD, lorazepam (Ativan®) is helpful for panic disorder, and alprazolam (Xanax®) is useful for both panic disorder and GAD. Some people experience withdrawal symptoms if they stop taking benzodiazepines abruptly instead of tapering off, and anxiety can return once the medication is stopped. These potential problems have led some physicians to shy away from using these drugs or to use them in inadequate doses. Buspirone (Buspar®), an azapirone, is a newer anti-anxiety medication used to treat GAD. Possible side effects include dizziness, headaches, and nausea. Unlike benzodiazepines, buspirone must be taken consistently for at least 2 weeks to achieve an anti-anxiety effect.

Beta-Blockers

Beta-blockers, such as propranolol (Inderal®), which is used to treat heart conditions, can prevent the physical symptoms that accompany certain anxiety disorders, particularly social phobia. When a feared situation can be predicted (such as giving a speech), a doctor may prescribe a beta-blocker to keep physical symptoms of anxiety under control.

Taking Medications

Before taking medication for an anxiety disorder:

- Ask your healthcare provider to tell you about the effects and side effects of the drug, and report any alternative therapies or over-the-counter medications you are using.
- Ask your healthcare provider when and how the medication should be stopped. Some drugs must be tapered off slowly under a doctor's supervision.
- Be aware that some medications are effective only if they are taken regularly and that symptoms may recur if the medication is stopped.

Psychotherapy

Psychotherapy involves talking with a trained mental health professional, such as a psychiatrist, psychologist, social worker, or counselor, to discover what caused an anxiety disorder and how to deal with its symptoms. Cognitive-behavioral therapy (CBT) is very useful in treating anxiety disorders. The cognitive part helps people change the thinking patterns that support their fears, and the behavioral part helps people change the way they react to anxiety-provoking situations. For example, CBT can help people with panic disorder learn that their panic attacks are not really heart attacks and help people with social phobia learn how to overcome the belief that others are always watching and judging them. When people are ready to confront their fears, they are shown how to use exposure techniques to desensitize themselves to situations that trigger their anxieties.

People with OCD who fear dirt and germs are encouraged to get their hands dirty and wait increasing amounts of time before washing them. The therapist helps the person cope with the anxiety that waiting produces; after the exercise has been repeated a number of times, the anxiety diminishes. People with social phobia may be encouraged to spend time in feared social situations without giving in to the temptation to flee and to make small social blunders and observe how people respond to them. Since the response is usually far less harsh than the person fears, these anxieties are lessened. People with PTSD may be supported through recalling their traumatic event in a safe situation, which helps reduce the fear it produces. CBT therapists also teach deep breathing and other types of exercises to relieve anxiety and encourage relaxation.

Exposure-based behavioral therapy has been used for many years to treat specific phobias. The person gradually encounters the object or situation that is feared, perhaps at first only through pictures or tapes, then later face-to-face. Often the therapist will accompany the person to a feared situation to provide support and guidance.

CBT or behavioral therapy often lasts about 12 weeks. It may be conducted individually or with a group of people who have similar problems. Group therapy is particularly effective for social phobia. Often "homework" is assigned for participants to complete between sessions. There is some evidence that the benefits of CBT last longer than those of medication for people with panic disorder, and the same may be true for OCD, PTSD, and social phobia. If a disorder recurs at a later date, the same therapy can be used to treat it successfully a second time. Medication can be combined with psychotherapy for specific anxiety disorders, and this is the best treatment approach for some people.

Ways to Make Treatment More Effective

Many people with anxiety disorders benefit from joining a self-help or support group and sharing their problems and achievements with others. Internet chat rooms can also be useful but any advice received over the Internet should be used with caution, as Internet acquaintances have usually never seen each other and false identities are common. Talking with a trusted friend or member of the clergy can also provide support, but it is not a substitute for care from a mental health professional.

Stress management techniques and meditation can help people with anxiety disorders calm themselves and may enhance the effects of therapy. There is evidence that aerobic exercise may have a calming effect. Since caffeine, certain illicit drugs, and even some over-the-counter cold medications can aggravate the symptoms of anxiety disorders, they should be avoided. Check with your physician or pharmacist before taking any additional medications.

The family can be important in the recovery of a person with an anxiety disorder. Ideally, family members should be supportive but not help perpetuate their loved one's symptoms. Family members should not trivialize the disorder or demand improvement without treatment. For some lesbian/bisexual women, family of origin are or were, the major source of stress and anxiety, and support needs to come from families of choice.

Lesbian and bisexual women may be uneasy about group therapies with heterosexual strangers. It is difficult to be part of a therapy group without talking about significant others and the stresses that arise from being part of a minority group based on one's sexual orientation. Not knowing if the group might contain homophobic members is yet another source of stress and anxiety. If you are considering a therapy group, ask the therapist or group facilitator how she or he deals with group members who exhibit homophobic behavior or language. If the therapist cannot answer this question, consider finding another therapist or group!

Post-Traumatic Stress Disorder (PTSD)

PTSD is a prolonged response to experiencing trauma in one's life. It was first described as "combat fatigue" in military personnel, but soon researchers recognized that the same symptoms could arise from natural disasters, accidents or injuries, or assaults and abuse. In a research study, lesbian and bisexual women were more likely to report a diagnosis of PTSD than heterosexual women, and these stemmed from all sorts of traumas. Almost 9 out of 10 lesbians had been exposed to some kind of trauma, but only 18% of them developed PTSD (Roberts et al., 2010). Bisexual women had the highest rate of PTSD at 26% of those exposed to any trauma.

Figure 3.2. PTSD in women by sexual orientation: Prevalence of lifetime PTSD (from Roberts et al., 2010)

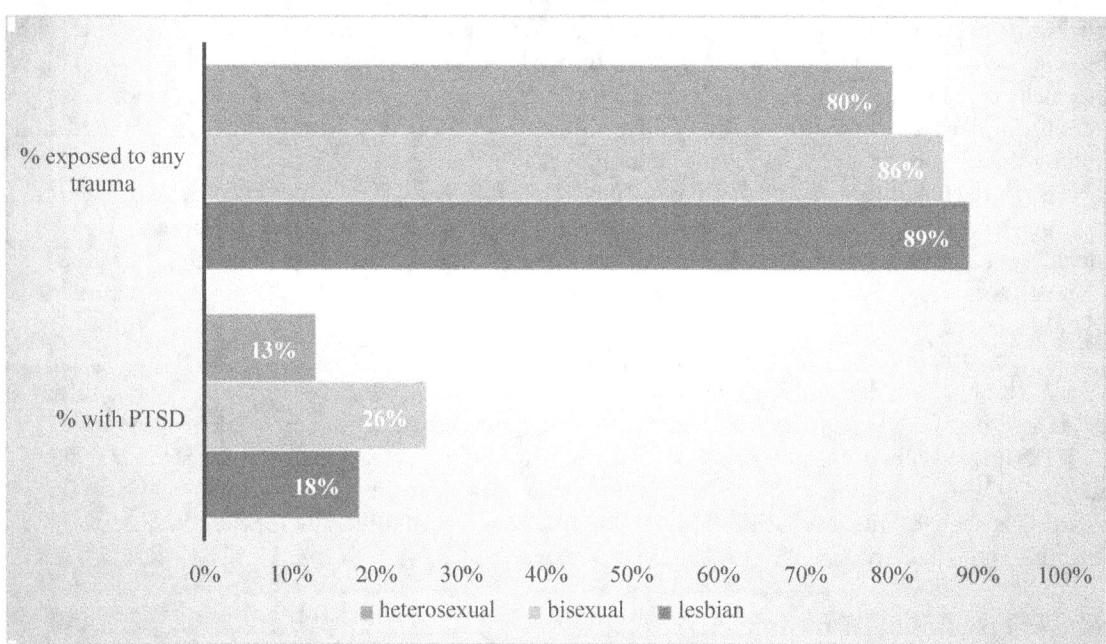

How does PTSD develop?

Most people who experience trauma have some negative symptoms at the beginning. Only some will develop PTSD over time. Whether or not you get PTSD depends on many things:

- How intense the trauma was or how long it lasted
- If you were injured or lost someone important to you
- How close you were to the event
- How strong your reaction was
- How much you felt in control of events
- How much help and support you got after the event

What are the symptoms of PTSD?

PTSD symptoms usually start fairly soon after the traumatic event, but sometimes they may not appear until months or even years later. They also may come and go over many years. If the symptoms last longer than 4 weeks, cause you great distress, or interfere with your work or home life, you might have PTSD. There are four main symptoms of PTSD:

1. Reliving the event (also called re-experiencing symptoms). You may have bad memories or nightmares. You even may feel like you're going through the event again. This is called a flashback.
2. Avoiding situations that remind you of the event. You may try to avoid situations or people that trigger memories of the traumatic event. You may even avoid talking or thinking about the event.

3. **Negative changes in beliefs and feelings.** The way you think about yourself and others may change because of the trauma. You may feel fear, guilt, or shame. You may not be interested in activities you used to enjoy. This is another way to avoid memories.
4. **Feeling keyed up (also called hyperarousal).** You may be jittery, always alert and on the lookout for danger, or have trouble concentrating or sleeping.

People with PTSD may also have other problems that tend to go along with PTSD. These can include:
- Feelings of hopelessness, shame, or despair
- Depression or anxiety
- Drinking or drug problems (to self-medicate the emotional pain)
- Physical symptoms or chronic pain
- Employment problems (because of concentration problems)
- Relationship problems, including divorce

What treatments are available?
There are two main types of treatment: psychotherapy (counseling) and medication. Sometimes people combine psychotherapy and medication.

Psychotherapy for PTSD: There are different types of psychotherapy:
- **Cognitive behavioral therapy (CBT)** is the most often-studied treatment for PTSD. There are different types of CBT such as cognitive therapy and exposure therapy.
  Cognitive Processing Therapy (CPT) is where you learn to understand how trauma changed your thoughts and feelings.
  Prolonged Exposure (PE) therapy is where you talk about your trauma repeatedly in a safe environment until memories are no longer upsetting. You also go to places that are safe, but that you have been staying away from because they are related to the trauma.
- **Eye movement desensitization and reprocessing (EMDR)**. This therapy involves focusing on sounds or hand movements while you talk about the trauma.

Medications for PTSD: Selective serotonin reuptake inhibitors (SSRI), which are also used for depression, are effective for PTSD. Another medication called Prazosin has been found to be helpful in decreasing nightmares related to the trauma.

IMPORTANT: Benzodiazepines and atypical antipsychotics should generally be avoided for PTSD treatment because they do not treat the core PTSD symptoms.

Another issue to consider that is different for lesbian/bisexual women than heterosexual women is that sometimes the treatment providers or law enforcement personnel downplay the traumas that we experience. They don't believe that being abused by a same-sex partner who is also female could be traumatizing, or they do not recognize how terrifying a hate crime may be. Some LGBT people have reported feeling victimized again by the law enforcement or treatment providers who may have questioned whether the victim did something to bring on the attack (being too blatant, being openly lesbian, etc) or who created a hostile environment.

SUICIDE
Another area where, unfortunately, lesbian and bisexual women have more problems than heterosexual women, includes suicide behaviors. We don't know much about completed suicide, because death records usually don't record sexual orientation, but lesbian and bisexual women have higher rates of suicidal thoughts, making a suicide plan, and attempting suicide, than heterosexual women (Haas, et al., 2011). The graph below shows recent data from a representative population of U.S. women on suicide attempts.

One study of youth found that first suicide attempts often corresponded with the recognition that one was lesbian, gay, or bisexual (Meyer, Teylan, & Schwartz, 2014). In that study, seeking help from a religious or spiritual advisor was associated with more suicide attempts. Most of the research has focused on youth and that highly stressful time of coming out. We do not know if older lesbian/bisexual women have elevated rates of suicide thinking or attempts compared to heterosexual women, but the increased financial concerns and greater likelihood of living alone might increase risks for older lesbian/bisexual women.

Figure 3.3. Lifetime suicide attempts in women (Bolton & Sareen, 2011)

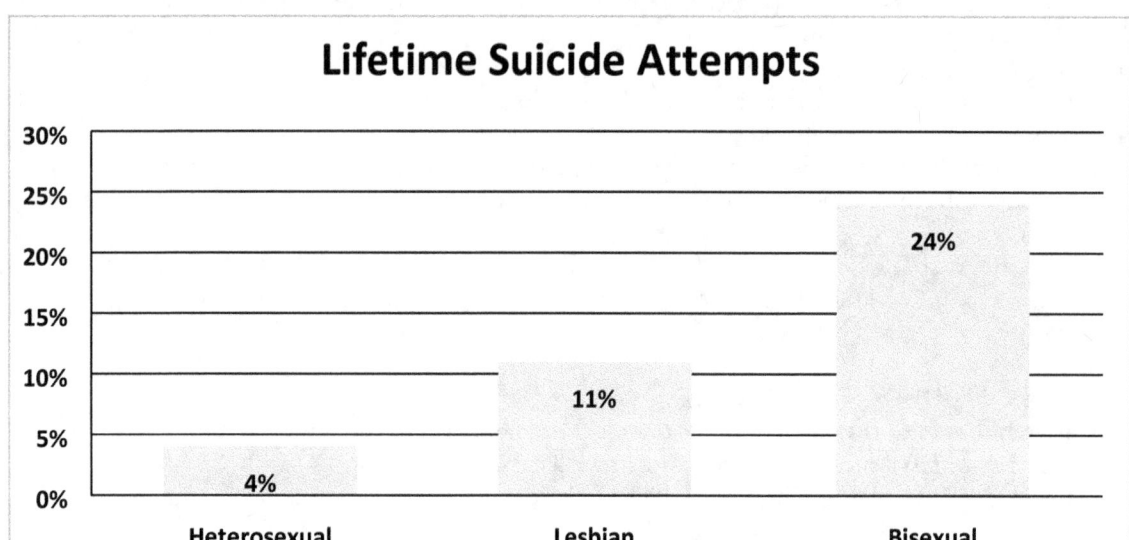

Some warning signs of suicide in an older woman might include:

- She is socially isolating herself
- She talks about death in conversations
- She has a recently diagnosed chronic illness or disability
- She has a relapse of severe depression or other mental health problem

Resources

If you feel suicidal or know someone who is, we recommend talking to a professional or trusted person. LGBT hotlines or gay-affirmative counselors are available in many locations. There is a myth that people who talk about suicide will not make an attempt; that is a myth. Take any talk of suicide seriously. One resource is the Trevor hotline (1-866-488-7386). This is a 24 hour service, geared to LGBT youth, but if you need an LGBT-friendly voice in the middle of the night, someone is always there. Monday-Friday there is a GLBT National Help Center (1-888-843-4564) that addresses all ages.

- Finding a therapist or primary care provider that is LGBT sensitive: www.glma.org (national); or Gaylesta.org (San Francisco Bay Area).
- GLBT National Help Center (1-888-843-4564)
- Local LGBT Centers (to find one, check: Center Link: http://www.lgbtcenters.org/)
- Healthcare Guild: referrals for medical and psychological resources (http://healthcareguild.com/)

In conclusion, this chapter has focused on the effects of stress, and the most common mental health problems found in lesbian and bisexual women. Some studies have pointed to the higher rates of stress from being a woman, lesbian/bisexual, and older as factors in the development of mental health symptoms. Information about biomedical and western psychological therapies was provided but no recommendations are made about how individual women should address such symptoms. Choices to use medications, psychotherapy, or other treatment options must be made carefully and each individual is different. If therapy is chosen, it is critical to find a therapist who understands how oppression works and is comfortable working with lesbian and bisexual women.

REFERENCES:

Aaron, D. & Hughes, T. (2007). Association of childhood sexual abuse with obesity in a community sample of lesbians. *Obesity, 15*, 1023-1028.

Alvy, L.M., Hughes, T.L., Kristjanson, A., & Wilsnack, S. (2013). Sexual identity group differences in child abuse and neglect. *Journal of Interpersonal Violence, 28*, 2088-2111,

Austin, S.B., Jun, H.J., Jackson, B., Spiegelman, D., Rick-Edwards, J., Corliss, H., et al. (2008). Disparities in child abuse victimization in lesbian, bisexual, and heterosexual women in the Nurses' Health Study II. *Journal of Women's Health, 17*, 595-606.

Averett, P., Yoon, I., & Jenkins, C.L. (2013). Older lesbian experiences of homophobia and ageism. *Journal of Social Service Research, 39*, 3-15.

Balsam, K.F., Lehavot, K., Beadnell, B., & Circo, E. (2010). Childhood abuse and mental health indicators among ethnically diverse lesbian, gay, and bisexual adults. *Journal of Consulting and Clinical Psychology, 78*(4), 459-468.

Bolton, S-L., & Sareen, J. (2011). Sexual orientation and its relation to mental disorders and suicide attempts: Findings from a nationally representative sample. *Canadian Journal of Psychiatry, 56*(1), 35-43.

Bostwick, W.B., Boyd, C.J., Hughes, T.L., & McCabe, S.E. (2010). Dimensions of sexual orientation and the prevalence of mood and anxiety disorders in the United States. *American Journal of Public Health, 100*(3), 468-475.

Corliss, H., Cochran, S.D., & Mays, V.M. (2002). Reports of parental maltreatment during childhood in a U.S. population-based survey of homosexual, bisexual, and heterosexual adults. *Child Abuse and Neglect, 26*, 1165-1178.

Fredriksen-Goldsen, K., Emlet, C. A., Kim, H., Muraco, A., Erosheva, E. A., Goldsen, J. et al. (2012). The physical and mental health of LGB older adults: The role of key health indicators and risk and protective factors. *The Gerontologist, 53*, 664–675.

Haas, A., Eliason, M.J., Mays, V.M., et al. (2011). Suicide and suicide risk in lesbian, gay, bisexual, and transgender populations: Review and recommendations. *Journal of Homosexuality, 58*, 10-51.

Lehavot, K., Molina, Y., & Simoni, J.M. (2012). Childhood trauma, adult sexual assault, and adult gender expression among lesbian and bisexual women. *Sex Roles, 67*, 272-284.

Meyer, I. (2013). Prejudice, social stress and mental health in lesbian, gay, and bisexual populations: conceptual issues and research evidence. *Psychology of Sexual Orientation and Gender Diversity, 1(S)*, 3-26.

Meyer, I., Teylan, M., & Schwartz, S. (2014). The role of help-seeking in preventing suicide attempts among lesbians, gay men, and bisexuals. Suicide and Life-Threatening Behavior, DOI: 10.1111/sltb12104.

Nadal, K. (2013). *That's so gay! Microaggressions and LGBT community*. Washington, DC:APA Press.

Roberts, A.L., Austin, S.B., Corliss, H.L., Vandemorris, A.K., & Koenen, K.C. (2010). Pervasive trauma exposure among U.S. sexual orientation minority adults and risk of PTSD. *American Journal of Public Health, 100*, 2433-2441.

Stoddard, J.P., Dibble, S.L., & Fineman, N. (2009). Sexual and physical abuse: A comparison between lesbians and their heterosexual sisters. *Journal of Homosexuality, 56*, 407-420.

Chapter 4. Substance Use/Abuse

Many substances have mood-altering aspects that make them desirable stress-reducers. These can include alcohol, recreational drugs, tobacco, and food. Some suggest that certain behaviors can also be stress-reducers and addictive, such as sex, shopping, gambling, and surfing the internet. This chapter focuses on alcohol, drugs, and tobacco, since there is very little research on any of the other potentially addictive behaviors among lesbian and bisexual women. We raise the possibility that some types of food may be addictive at the end of this chapter.

DRUGS AND ALCOHOL

There is considerable research showing that lesbian and bisexual women use and abuse alcohol and other drugs more often than heterosexual women, and some develop serious consequences from their substance use. The figure below shows some recent data from a national survey on the use and abuse patterns of women by sexual orientation (Bostwick and colleagues, 2009). In nearly every category, bisexual women report higher rates of use and abuse of substances, but both lesbian and bisexual women exceed the use patterns of heterosexual women by a considerable margin. Most of the research has been consistent, showing that lesbian and bisexual women are more likely to report that they currently or in the past, had a problem with alcohol abuse. Fewer lesbian/bisexual women are non-drinkers than heterosexual women, and more lesbian and bisexual women report that they are in recovery from alcohol problems. However, it is important to keep in mind that most lesbian/bisexual women do not have substance abuse problems.

Figure 4.1. National data on substance use in the U.S. women's population by sexual orientation (from Bostwick et al, 2009)

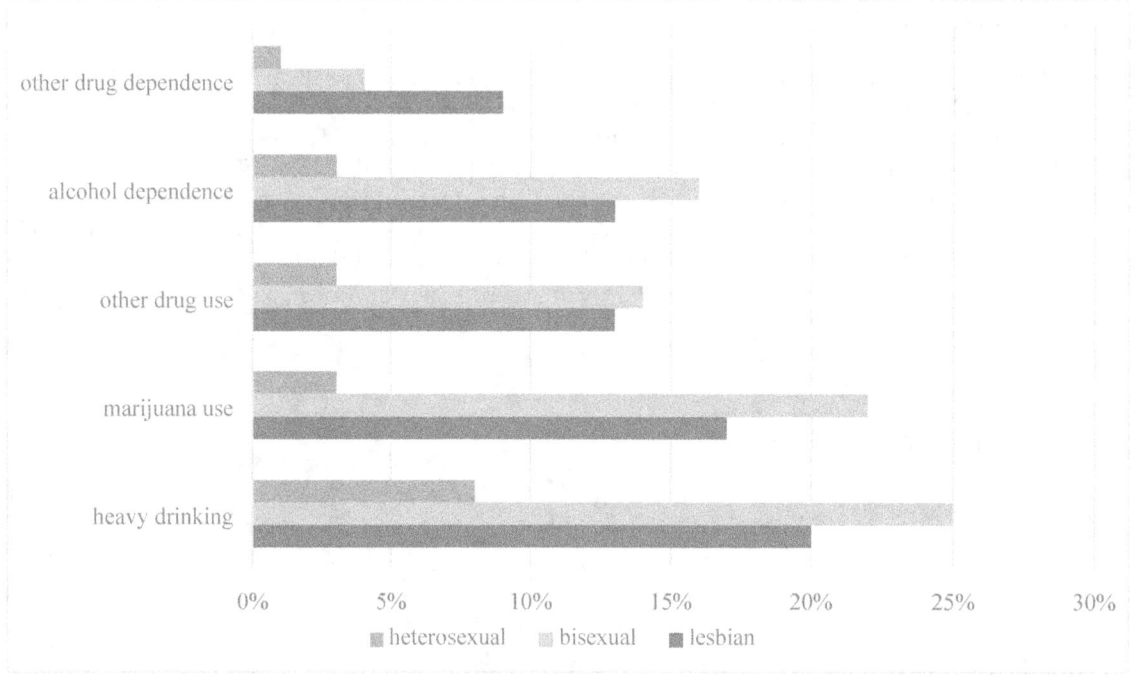

There is some data about how women of color differ from their heterosexual counterparts in terms of substance use. Vickie Mays from UCLA led a team of researchers in a study of women in Los Angeles from three ethnic groups: African American, Latina, and Asian American (Mays, Yancey, et al, 2002). The graph below shows the percent that reported drinking three or more drinks on an occasion when they drink (this is the definition of binge drinking for older women). In all cases, lesbian/bisexual women drank more than heterosexual counterparts of the same ethnicity. Obviously, being lesbian or bisexual increases the daily level of stress for ethnic minority women.

Figure 4.2. Drinking patterns by sexual orientation and race (from Mays et al., 2002)

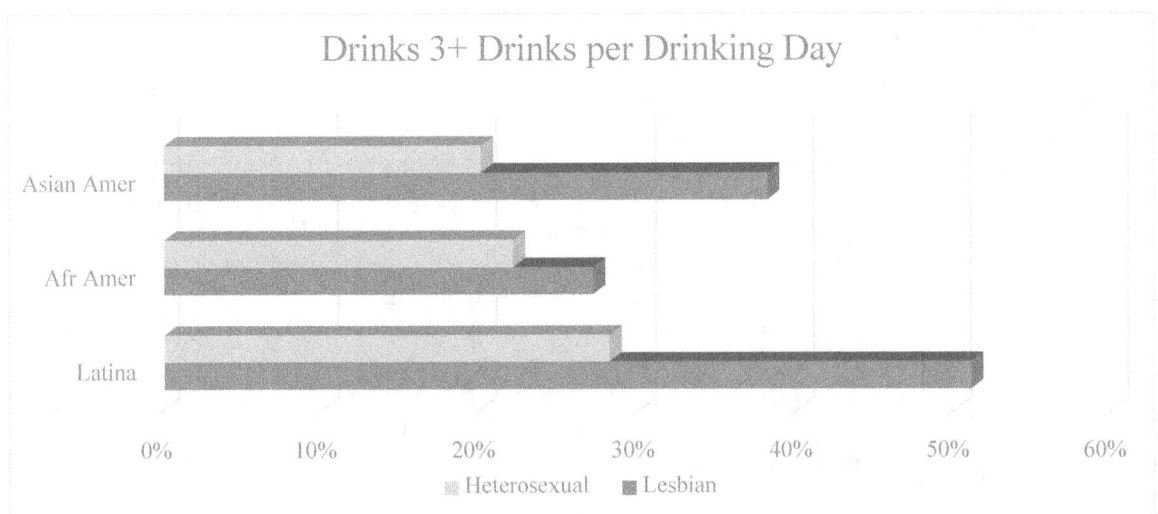

Why Higher Rates?

Alcohol and Drug Norms: In the past, there were very few places where lesbian and bisexual women could feel safe and accepted except for a gay bar. Gay bars have served as LGBT community centers in many areas that lack LGBT resources. Unfortunately, when social life revolves around a bar, women are likely to meet partners and good friends there, increasing the likelihood of being in a heavy drinking social network. A bar mindset also alters one's perception of community norms. When everyone in your social network is a heavy drinker or recreational drug user, it "normalizes" the experience (Gruskin et al., 2006). In addition, alcohol companies target ads in our magazines and sponsor LGBT events. LGBT people tend to be loyal to brands that advertise in our communities, because so few industries even acknowledge us.

Minority Stress: Some authors suggest that minority stress is one of the factors that cause the higher rates of drug and alcohol problems. Lesbian and bisexual women turn to substances to medicate the emotional pain that is associated with being rejected, harassed, or discriminated against because of their ethnicity, social class, sexual identities or other factors.

Higher Rates of Mood Disorders: We know that many people with depression and anxiety disorders feel a great deal of emotional pain and distress and turn to substances to relieve those uncomfortable feelings. Unfortunately, in the long run, the drug/alcohol use makes the depression and anxiety symptoms worse, and may develop into addiction.

Childhood Traumas: There is quite of bit of research showing that experiencing abuse as a child is a major risk factor for later substance abuse (and several other negative consequences like depression and weight gain). Several studies have found higher rates of childhood abuse among lesbian and bisexual women. One study from a national substance abuse treatment survey showed rates of childhood sexual abuse to be higher for lesbian and bisexual women (35%) compared to heterosexual women (10%) (Hughes, McCabe, Wilsnack, West & Boyd, 2010). It is never too late to seek help for childhood abuse issues because they can continue to cause serious problems in adulthood if unaddressed. Child abuse has been linked to such problems in adulthood as depression, anxiety, substance abuse, and larger body weight.

Do I have a problem with alcohol? Here is a commonly used screening test called the CAGE:
- o   Have you ever felt you should cut down on your drinking?
- o   Have people annoyed you by criticizing your drinking?

- Have you ever felt bad or guilty about your drinking?
- Have you ever had a drink first thing in the morning to steady your nerves or to get rid of a hangover (eye opener)?

Scoring: If you said yes to 2 or more questions, you <u>may</u> have a problem with alcohol. It would be good to discuss your answers with a professional.

Controversies over red wine. The media is full of praise for red wine as a protective factor for heart disease, but the research is not totally clear yet whether the effect is as strong for women as for men or even whether there is a protective factor at all. In recent studies, people who drank grape juice from red-wine grapes had similar effects. The alcohol is not necessary, and may be the source of risk for many women. For older women, drinking at the level of even one glass of wine per day increases the risk for breast cancer and mental health problems, and may cancel out the positive effect on the heart. The medical research community does not recommend alcohol as a means of prevention of heart disease. In addition, wine, like other forms of alcoholic beverages, provides empty calories with lots of sugar and no nutrients. A glass of wine can have from 80 to 180 (in dessert wines like port) calories, mostly from sugar. Finally, as we age, there is a much higher chance of drug and alcohol interactions which can lead to falls or other serious health outcomes.

Treatment Issues for Lesbian/Bisexual Women

Availability of LGBT or Sexual Minority Women-Specific Treatment
Substance use disorder treatment systems generally do not have programs and services that are responsive to the treatment needs of lesbian and bisexual women. Cochran, Peavy and Robohm (2007) contacted 911 U.S. substance abuse treatment programs about specialized services for LGBT populations, and found only 7% provided LGBT-specific services, 4% said that their agencies were accepting of sexual minorities, and 9.3% stated that they did not have separate groups, but that they did not discriminate.

The study did not consider the possibility that lesbian and bisexual women might have different treatment needs than sexual minority men, thus did not assess for the availability of women-specific services that might be appealing to women, such as women-only treatment groups, parenting help, and reproductive health services. So far, no one has surveyed women-specific treatment programs to determine if they are welcoming to lesbian and bisexual women. There are a handful of LGBT-specific treatment programs in the U.S., but there is no indication as to whether they have gender-sensitive treatment options. The few studies that have examined specific treatment modalities for sexual minority clients have generally focused on men who have sex with men (MSM), because of the link between substance abuse and HIV/AIDS in MSM populations.

Getting Treatment
The good news is that lesbian and bisexual women do often seek help if they have drug and alcohol problems. In fact, in some studies lesbian and bisexual women seem to be more likely than heterosexual women to participate in treatment services and to seek help for alcohol and drug related problems (Cochran, et al., 2000). Lesbian and bisexual women respondents in the National Alcohol Survey were also more likely to report ever having sought help for alcohol problems compared to heterosexual women (Drabble, et al., 2005). Even regional studies that found few differences in alcohol consumption between heterosexual and lesbian/bisexual women, found that lesbian and bisexual women were more likely to report being in recovery or having been in treatment in the past than their heterosexual counterparts (Bloomfield, 1993; Hughes, 2003; Hughes, Haas, Razzano, Cassidy, & Matthews, 2000; Hughes, et al., 2006).

Grella and colleagues (2009) examined treatment seeking in California, and found lesbian and bisexual women were more likely to have received treatment for substance use and mental health problems than heterosexual women. The authors noted that lesbian and bisexual women sought treatment even when they had no diagnosable disorders. It may be that lesbian/bisexual women have more positive attitudes about mental health services and/or they seek help to cope with discrimination, violence or other stressors (Grella, Greenwell, Mays, & Cochran, 2009).

Most states do not collect data on sexual orientation in their statewide substance abuse treatment data reporting systems, but the few exceptions are providing valuable information. A study in the state of Washington found that LGB clients entered treatment with more severe problems (a higher level of both alcohol and drug use and therefore more negative consequences) and more mental health problems (Cochran & Cauce, 2006) than heterosexuals. In fact, Lipsky and colleagues (2012) found almost double the rates of co-occurring mental health and substance use disorders (COD) among LGB participants than heterosexuals. COD was a predictor of doing poorly in treatment. This is not surprising given what we know about the high rates of depression and anxiety in lesbian and bisexual women. What we don't know is whether some women are depressed/anxious because of substance use, whether some women start drinking or using drugs to relieve the negative feelings of depression/anxiety, or whether psychological distress about sexual orientation or childhood sexual abuse cause both substance abuse and mental health problems. Probably the last one is true for many lesbian/bisexual women.

Experiences In Treatment

Treatment counselors in urban and rural settings often lack understanding of specific issues of lesbian and bisexual clients, such as internalized homophobia, legal documents such as power of attorney, or concerns about family of origin (Eliason, 2000; Eliason & Hughes, 2004). In one study, half of counselors in both urban and rural areas had negative or ambivalent attitudes toward LGBT clients, and had more negative attitudes about bisexual women than lesbians (Eliason & Hughes, 2004). Senreich (2010) found that client openness about sexual orientation was positively correlated with treatment completion, treatment satisfaction, and feeling connected to the program. A few studies have reported that some lesbian and bisexual women have philosophical difficulties with mainstream recovery options, such as Alcoholics Anonymous groups that may replicate the sexism, racism, ageism, and heterosexism of mainstream society (Eliason, Amodia, and Cano, 2006; Hall, 1996). Some women resist the concept of powerlessness, because of a lifetime of being made to feel powerless by the sexism, heterosexism, racism, and so on, of society. They often seek more empowering types of treatment.

Agency Level Policies and Procedures.

The checklist at the end of this chapter can be used to screen healthcare provider agencies such as clinics, community mental health centers, or hospitals, to find out how welcoming and inclusive they are for lesbian and bisexual women. One thing to look for in addition to LGBT inclusive services, is to see if the agency is trauma-informed. A significant number of lesbian and bisexual women, as well as others regardless of their gender or sexual orientation, have experienced traumatic experiences in their childhood, adolescence, or adulthood related to military experiences, sexual abuse, chronic oppressive situations, or other traumas and would benefit from a trauma-informed perspective. Trauma-informed treatment agencies make an assumption that any client entering the door may be a trauma survivor, and create safety and education before initiating substance abuse treatment. This includes trauma screening, treating participants as active members of the treatment team and giving them control/autonomy over aspects of their treatment (Harris & Fallot, 2001). Trauma-informed agencies are likely to be safer and more humane than non-trauma informed services.

Treatment Interventions

Immediate Treatment Needs. There is very little research so far on whether lesbian and bisexual women respond to the typical drug and alcohol treatment modalities (Twelve step, cognitive behavioral, motivational interviewing) in the same way as heterosexual women. Lesbian and bisexual women in treatment have to decide whether to disclose their sexuality to staff and/or to other clients in treatment, usually after testing the climate of the program to determine whether disclosure is safe. If clients do not disclose, counselors may develop a treatment plan that does not include the most critical issues, such as 1) coming out to family, 2) internalized oppressions that led to shame, guilt, fear, body image concerns, and suicide thoughts, 3) coping with past and current experiences with harassment, discrimination, and violence, 4) partner and family issues, 5) the role of religion. Many lesbian and bisexual women need assistance with parenting and partner relationships, dealing with gender stereotypes and biases, and/or have women's health issues related to reproduction, menopause, breast and cervical cancer screening, and others.

Sobriety offers a new opportunity to explore one's sexuality, and some women come out during their recovery process. For women who used alcohol or drugs to self-medicate the anxiety provoked by same-sex desires, or to overcome deep religious, familial, or societal stigma about same-sex attraction, facing those attractions while sober will be challenging. Some women have never or rarely had sex when sober, and must resolve the shame and guilt issues that triggered substance use before initiating relationships again.

The most common mental health problems among lesbian and bisexual women that may go along with substance abuse include depression, anxiety, PTSD, and suicide risk (IOM, 2011) as well as internalized oppression and external homophobia (that combine to create minority stress; Meyer, 2013). If the woman has experienced trauma of any sort, the substance abuse and trauma must be treated at the same (Morrisey, Jackson, Ellis et al., 2005). There is no research to indicate whether sexual minority women respond to treatment for abuse experiences any differently than heterosexual women. It is possible that the dynamics of relationships could differ enough to make the impact on relationships somewhat different for female same-sex couples than for those in other-sex relationships. That is, female partners may respond differently to the symptoms of abuse in their significant others than do male partners. We really need research on this topic because so many lesbian and bisexual women have experienced sexual abuse in their past.

Aftercare Planning Needs. When lesbian and bisexual women finish the initial treatment experience, the next step is to consider how to avoid or reduce triggers for relapse. If they spent time in gay bars or heavy –drinking social networks, they may need to find different social outlets. Because there are fewer resources available for lesbian and bisexual women in communities, bars and social groups may have greater significance in coping with everyday life, and the advice to find "new playmates and playgrounds" can prove to be nearly impossible. If possible, women in recovery need to be linked up with clean and sober groups in LGBT communities to find lesbian/bisexual role models and sponsors. Some communities have LGBT social services, support groups and recovery groups. Some lesbian and bisexual women were alienated from their communities because of behaviors related to their substance use, and need help finding ways to boost their social capital and develop more social support. More information about treatment considerations can be found in Finnegan and McNally (2002), and SAMHSA (2001).

One way that sexual minority women seem to differ from many men and heterosexual women is a greater acceptance of alternative health options such as meditation, acupuncture, herbal products, chiropracty and so on (Dillworth, Kaysen, Montoya, & Larimer, 2009; Matthews, et al., 2005). This may increase the options for resources in the community and provide alternatives to western medicine that has often been neglectful of or discriminatory to lesbian and bisexual women.

SMOKING

Smoking cigarettes is a classic example of an unhealthy stress reducing behavior. Cigarettes are legal, highly portable, and its relatively easy to get a "hit" almost anytime of the day or night. The trouble is that it does not actually reduce stress; lots of research shows it makes it worse. And it's highly addictive. Tobacco is equal to crack cocaine in the power of the addiction and difficulty quitting. Lesbian and bisexual women may start smoking because of a sense of rebellion against norms that "good girls" don't smoke, to relieve stress, to join in at the bar when everyone else is smoking, to look "cool" to peers, or a host of other reasons.

There is ample evidence that lesbian/bisexual women smoke at higher rates than heterosexual women across a wide variety of study methodologies from convenience samples to population-based surveys such as statewide health surveillance tools; and across most age groups, racial/ethnic groups, educational levels, and socioeconomic classes (e.g. Aaron, Markovic, Danielson, et al., 2001; Gruskin, Hart, Gordon, et al., 2001; Sanchez, Meacher, & Beil, 2005; Skinner & Otis, 1996; Tang, Greenwood, Cowling, et al, 2004; Valanis, Bowen, Bassford, et al, 2000). More lesbian and bisexual women are former smokers than heterosexual women, and at most age groups, they are also more likely to be current smokers. The chart below shows the most recent data on current smoking from a national study of health behaviors.

In addition to being a smoker, lesbian and bisexual women may be exposed to tobacco smoke more often than heterosexual women. One study (Cochran, Bandiera, & Mays, 2013) of a national sample of women, showed that lesbian women were more likely to be exposed to smoking at the workplace (21% of lesbians; 7% of bisexual women; 8% of heterosexual women). Bisexual women were more likely to be exposed to smoking at home (17% of bisexual women; 3% of lesbians, and 5% of heterosexual women). Smoking and/or secondhand exposure to smoke, may underlie some of the greater physical health burden reported by lesbians, and may be linked to higher rates of cancer and asthma, although this has not been directly studied.

Figure 4.3. Current smoking rates in women by sexual orientation (from Ward et al., 2014)

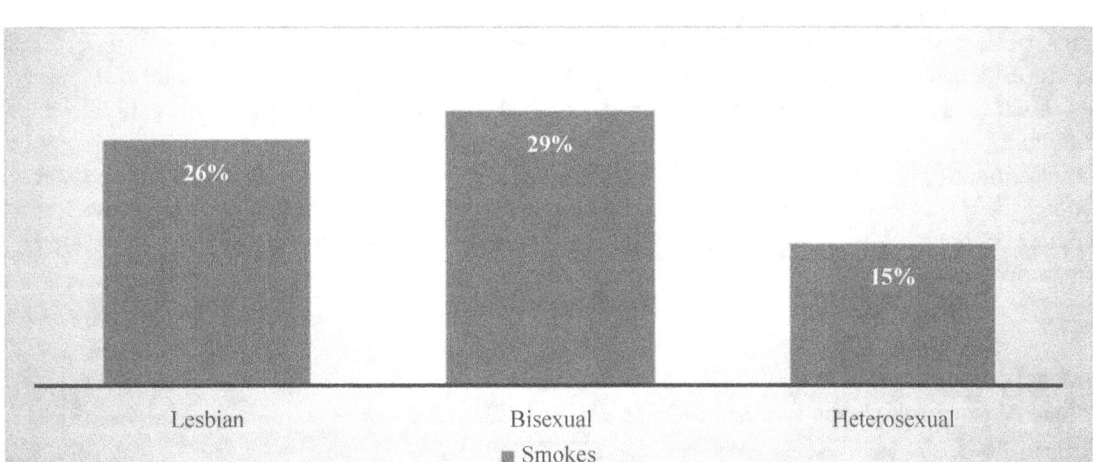

A few studies have considered quit attempts in lesbian/bisexual women smokers. Bye, Gruskin, Greenwood, et al (2005) studied Californian LGBT individuals' use of cessation interventions and their attitudes and found that 63% of the smokers had made a quit attempt in the past year, with women more likely than men to make a quit attempt. One-fourth of those attempts involved use of a nicotine replacement therapy, which is higher than the general population (16%), suggesting that lesbians might be more amenable to this approach. In the general population, 57% of smokers had been advised to quit by a health care professional, but only 40% of the lesbians had been so advised.

In one of the few studies to evaluate a smoking cessation intervention, Eliason, Dibble, Gordon, and Soliz (2012) examined the outcomes for 233 participants of *The Last Drag*. *The Last Drag* is a program designed specifically for LGBT community members who want to quit, and is based on the American Cancer Society's successful program of 7 sessions to support individuals during a quit attempt. Of the 233 who participated, fewer than 30% were lesbian or bisexual women. *The Last Drag* has an impressive success rate, and using even the most conservative estimates, nearly 40% were still smoke-free six months after the intervention. Although they had similar success rates to men in the intervention, women were consistently under-represented in the program. This raises the question of why women are less likely to seek out and participate in this highly successful, free, LGBT-specific smoking cessation intervention; one that is facilitated by an openly lesbian woman.

CAN FOOD BE ADDICTIVE?

The concept behind groups like Over-Eaters Anonymous is that some people get addicted to over-eating, and they describe binge-eating as a compulsive behavior (out of control) with periods of guilt and remorse afterwards. One study suggested that about 5% of the population fits the label of "food addict" and describe it as a type of eating disorder. Obviously, not all food is addictive. How often do we want to binge on broccoli or not be able to stop eating squash? The most likely culprit that triggers overeating, and possibly addiction, is sugar. Some studies find changes in the brain from sugar consumption that look a lot like what alcohol and drugs do to the brain. For those science nerds who want to know how it works, a high dose of sugar reduces the production of a chemical in the brain called Brain-Derived Neurotrophic Factors (BDNF), a substance that helps us form new memories and contributes to insulin resistance. There is also a link between BDNF and depression and dementia.

In addition, chronic overconsumption of sugar interferes with the brains mechanism that tell us to stop eating (it reduces production of oxytocin) so you constantly feel hungry and crave more sugar. The news program 60 Minutes did a good piece on this in 2012 if you want more information (www.cbsnews.com/videos/is-sugar-toxic/). Other experts think that combination of high sugar, high fat, high salt foods, as is the case with many highly processed sweets, is the deadly combination that causes addiction. These highly processed items should not really even be called "food!"

Thus far, there is no research to indicate whether lesbian and bisexual women are more likely to have food addictions, or be more likely than any other persons in our culture to consume high rates of these processed foods or high sugar items. But these foods are often in the category of "comfort food" and readily available to us, so in times of stress, which we as lesbian/bisexual women experience more of the time, we might be more tempted to eat these products.

In conclusion, this chapter has addressed the addictions---to alcohol, drugs, tobacco, and maybe even food—that affect the quality of life of many lesbian and bisexual women. When we seek help for these problems, we may encounter further stigma and discrimination, or find that treatment providers and systems know nothing about our needs.

Resources

- National Institute of Mental Health   www.nimh.gov
- National Alliance for Mental Illness (NAMI) www.nami.org
- American Psychological Association   www.apa.org
- LGBTQ Healthcare Guild   http://healthcareguild.com/contact.html
- Pride Institute (www.pride-institute.com) is one of the few LGBT-specific substance abuse treatment programs in the U.S.
- NIAAA module on LGBT substance abuse: http://pubs.niaaa.nih.gov/publications/Social/Module10GSexualOrientation/Module10G.html
- Providers guide of LGBT substance abuse: Free resource from Substance Abuse and Mental Health Services Administration (SAMHSA): http://store.samhsa.gov/product/A-Provider-s-Introduction-to-Substance-Abuse-Treatment-for-Lesbian-Gay-Bisexual-and-Transgender-Individuals/SMA12-4104
- Smoking Cessation Program for LGBT People: The Last Drag. **http://www.lastdrag.org/**
- Gaylesta: www. gaylesta.org. To locate an LGBTQ friendly provider in Northern California

REFERENCES

Averett, P., Yoon, I., & Jenkins, C.L. (2013). Older lesbian experiences of homophobia and ageism. *Journal of Social Service Research, 39,* 3-15.

Bloomfield, K. (1993). A comparison of alcohol consumption between lesbians and heterosexual women in an urban population. *Drug and Alcohol Dependence, 33,* 257-269.

Bostwick, W., Boyd, C.J., Hughes, T. & McCabe, S. (2009). Dimensions of sexual orientation and the prevalence of mood and anxiety disorders in the United States. *American Journal of Public Health, 99,* 1-10.

Bye, L., Gruskin, E., Greenwood, G., Albright, V., & Kriotki, K. (2005). *California lesbians, gays, bisexuals, and transgender (LGBT) tobacco use survey—2004.* Sacramento, CA: CA Department of Health Services.

Cochran, B. N., & Cauce, A. M. (2006). Characteristics of lesbian, gay, bisexual, and transgender individuals entering substance abuse treatment. *Journal of Substance Abuse Treatment, 30,* 135-146.

Cochran, B. N., Peavy, K. M., & Cauce, A. M. (2007). Substance abuse treatment providers' explicit and implicit attitudes regarding sexual minorities. *Journal of Homosexuality, 53*(3), 181-207.

Cochran, B. N., Peavy, K. M., & Robohm, J. S. (2007). Do specialized services exist for LGBT individuals seeking treatment for substance misuse? A study of available treatment programs. *Substance Use & Misuse, 42*(161-176).

Cochran, S. D., Ackerman, D., Mays, V. M., & Ross, M. W. (2004). Prevalence of non-medical drug use and dependence among homosexually active men and women in the US population. *Addiction, 99*, 989-998.

Cochran, S. D., Keenan, C., Schober, C., & Mays, V. M. (2000). Estimates of alcohol use and clinical treatment needs among homosexually active men and women in the U.S. population. *Journal of Consulting and Clinical Psychology, 68*(6), 1062-1071.

Cochran, S. D., Mays, V. M., Ortega, A. N., Alegria, M., & Takeuchi, D. (2007). Mental health and substance abuse disorders among Latino and Asian American lesbian, gay, and bisexual adults. *Journal of Consulting and Clinical Psychology, 75*(5), 785-794.

Drabble, L., & Trocki, K. (2005). Alcohol consumption, alcohol-related problems, and other substance use among lesbian and bisexual women. *Journal of Lesbian Studies, 9*(3), 19-30.

Drabble, L. & Eliason, M.J. (2012). Sexual minority women and treatment for substance use disorders: A review of literature. *Journal of LGBT Counseling: Special Issue on Addictions in LGBTQ Communities, 6*(4), 274-292.

Dillworth, T. M., Kaysen, D., Montoya, H. D., & Larimer, M. E. (2009). Identification with mainstream culture and preference for alternative alcohol treatment approaches in a community sample. *Behavior Therapy, 40*(1), 72-81.

Eliason, M.J., Amodia, D.S., & Cano, C. (2006). Spirituality and substance abuse treatment: The role of culture. *Alcoholism Treatment Quarterly. 24(3),* 121-141.

Eliason, M. J. (2000). Substance abuse counselors' attitudes regarding lesbian, gay, bisexual and transgender clients. *Journal of Substance Abuse, 12*, 311-328.

Eliason, M. J., & Hughes, T. L. (2004). Treatment counselor's attitudes regarding lesbian, gay, bisexual, and transgendered clients: Urban vs. rural settings. *Substance Use & Misuse, 39*, 625-644.

Finnegan, D.G., & McNally, E.B. (2002). *Counseling LGBT substance abusers: Dual identities.* New York: Haworth.

Grella, C. E., Greenwell, L., Mays, V. M., & Cochran, S. D. (2009). Influence of gender, sexual orientation, and need on treatment utilization for substance use and mental disorders: Findings from the California Quality of Life Survey. *BMC Psychiatry, 9*, 52-61.

Gruskin, E., Byrne, K., Kools, S., & Altschuler, A. (2006). Consequences of frequenting the lesbian bar. *Women and Health, 44*, 103-120.

Gruskin, E.P., Byrne, K.M., Altschuler, A., & Dibble, S.L. (2008). Smoking it all away: Influences of stress, negative emotions and stigma on lesbian tobacco use. *Journal of LGBT Health Research, 4(4),* 167-179.

Gruskin, E., Hart, S., Gordon, N., et al. (2001). Patterns of cigarette smoking and alcohol use among lesbians and bisexual women enrolled in a large HMO. *American Journal of Public Health, 91(6),* 976-979.

Hall, J. M. (1996). Lesbians' participation in Alcoholics Anonymous: experiences of social, personal, and political tensions. *Contemporary Drug Problems, 23*, 113-138.

Harris, M. & Fallot, R.D. (2001). *Using trauma theory to design service systems.* San Francisco: Jossey-Bass.

Hughes, T. L. (2003). Lesbians' drinking patterns: Beyond the data. *Substance Use & Misuse, 38*(11-13), 1739-1758.

Hughes, T.L. (2011). Alcohol use and alcohol-related problems among sexual minority women. *Alcoholism Treatment Quarterly, 29*, 403-435.

Hughes, T. L., Haas, A. P., Razzano, L., Cassidy, R., & Matthews, A. (2000). Comparing lesbians' and heterosexual women's mental health: A multi-site survey. *Journal of Gay & Lesbian Social Services, 11*(1), 57-76.

Hughes, T. L., Welsnack, S. C., Szalacha, L. A., Johnson, T., Bostwick, W. B., Seymour, R., et al. (2006). Age and racial/ethnic differences in drinking and drinking-related problems in a community sample of lesbians. *Journal of Studies on Alcohol, 67*(4), 579.

Lipsky, S., Kupski, A. Roy-Byrne, P., Huber, A., Lucenko, B.A., & Mancuso, D. (2012). Impact of sexual orientation and co-occurring disorders on chemical dependency treatment outcomes. *Journal of Studies on Alcohol and Drugs, 73*, 401-412.

Matthews, A. K., Hughes, T. L., Osterman, G. P., & Kodl, M. M. (2005). Complementary medicine practices in a community-based sample of lesbian and heterosexual women. *Health Care for Women International, 26*(5): 430-47.

Morrissey, J.P., Jackson, E.W., Ellis, A.R., Amaro, H., Brown ,V.B., & Najavits, L.M. (2005). Twelve-month outcomes of trauma-informed interventions for women with co-occurring disorders, *Psychiatric Services, 56(10),* 1213-1222.

Sanchez, J., Meacher, P., & Beil, R. (2005). Cigarette smoking and lesbian and bisexual women in the Bronx. *Journal of Community Health, 30(1),* 23-37.

Tang, H., Greenwood, G., Cowling, D., et al. (2004). Cigarette smoking among lesbians, gays, and bisexuals: how serious a problem? *Cancer Causes and Control*, 15, 797-803.

Chapter 5: Body Size/Shape/Satisfaction

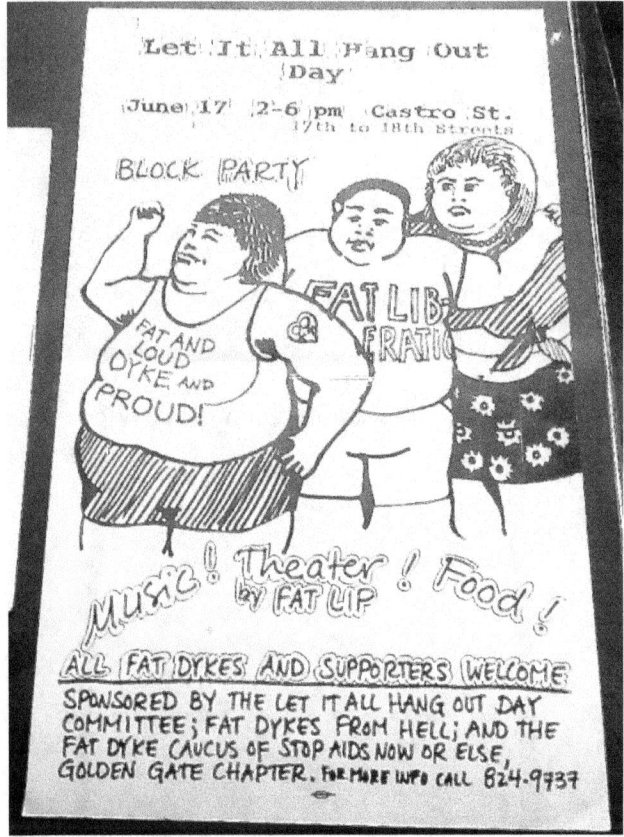

This poster was on display at the GLBT Historical Museum in San Francisco, showing the long history of fat activism in lesbian communities in the bay area. How do you feel about taking on fat as an identity?

"…I'm bad because I'm a fat woman and I'm bad because I'm a lesbian and I'm bad because I'm a woman…" (respondent in Roberts, Stuart-Shor & Oppenheimer, 2010, p. 1989)

Harvard scientist (and lesbian) Nancy Krieger (2005) noted that the body tells stories about people's social conditions; often stories that individuals cannot tell in public discourses because of their relatively powerless position in the power structure of society. For lesbian and bisexual women, the multiple forms of oppressions might be reflected in the greater body mass and in certain disorders or limitations. This chapter explores issues of body size, acceptance and body image and eating disorders as these are definitely important to our health. How we feel about own bodies is linked to overall self-esteem and self-confidence, and to how we care for our bodies. Are we fighting against an enemy within and punishing our bodies, or embracing our physical containers, no matter whether they fit some societal expectations or not? How much of the poor treatment we get in society is because of our sexual identity, our gender or gender expression, our age, or our body size and ability levels? The chapter concludes with a discussion of fat positive movements and the efforts to reduce or eliminate weight stigma.

BODY SIZE

Are lesbian/bisexual women heavier than heterosexual women?

As part of the federal initiative that funded DIFO, we reviewed all the studies that reported on weight differences by sexual identity (Eliason, Ingraham, Fogel, et al., 2015). The majority of these that found a difference, reported that lesbian and bisexual women were heavier than heterosexual women. These studies are surprisingly consistent even across different methodologies (random population studies versus convenience samples, across age groups, geographic differences, and other differences). These studies found that the weight difference is usually present in late adolescence and is fairly consistent across the age span, although at least one study found that heterosexual women slowly gain weight over time and catch up to lesbian/bisexual women at some point past middle age. Although the studies are statistically significant, the differences are often not really very large—maybe 5 to 10 pounds difference between groups, as shown in the graphs below.

Looking at the Weight Difference More Closely

The figure below shows studies done in the U.S. that assessed what percentage of women in the study had a BMI of 30 or higher, the level considered by the biomedical community as "obese." The studies are in order of age of the participants, with first study by Everett of young adults (where there was little difference in BMI) and the last study (Frederiksen2) of women over 50. This data looks like lesbians are quite a bit heavier than heterosexual women. Only 4 of the studies looked at lesbians and bisexual women separately, and in those cases, bisexual women showed mixed results—sometimes heavier than heterosexual women and sometimes lighter (see Eliason et al., 2015 for the citations for these studies).

Figure 5.1. Percent of women who are obese by sexual orientation (from Eliason, et al., 2015)

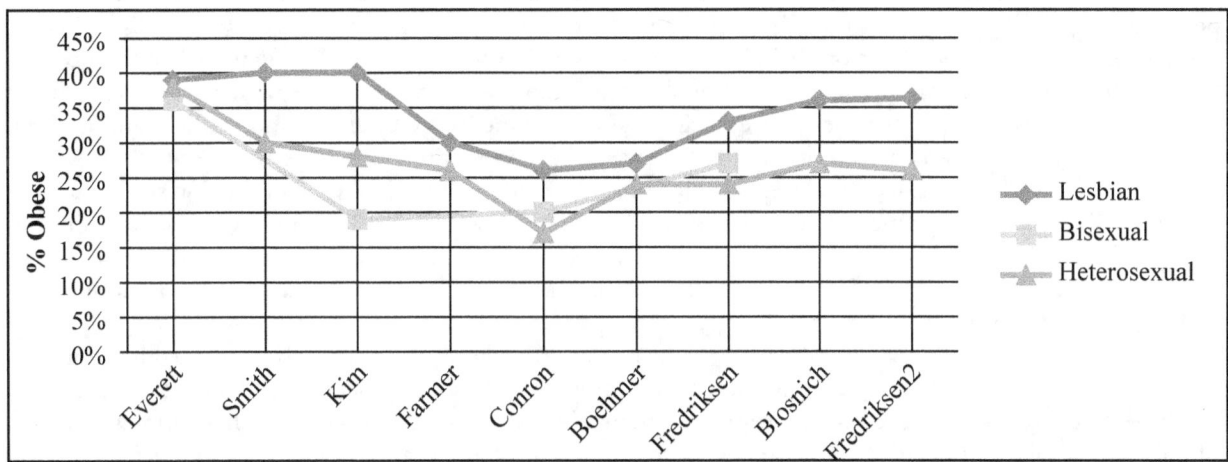

The next chart looks at the average BMI and the differences between lesbians and heterosexual women (there was not enough data to show bisexual women here) look smaller. The names on the left are the first author of the research papers. In reality, the differences are probably not enough to account for more health problems strictly because of weight. Societal stigma and discrimination are probably much bigger risk factors for health problems in lesbian and bisexual women than weight. Keep in mind that weight and BMI are not good measures of health, so all we are looking at is whether lesbian and bisexual women are bigger than heterosexual women. This is important, because a growing number of authors are recommending that weight loss programs be developed for lesbian and bisexual women. To make sense of the chart below, a BMI of 25 to 30 is considered to be in the "overweight" category, and BMI of 30 and higher to be "obese." The chart reports averages by group, so you would expect that about half of the women would be over that average number and half would be under it. In every case, lesbian/bisexual women had slightly higher average BMI.

Figure 5.2. Average BMI by sexual orientation for women (From Eliason et al., 2015)

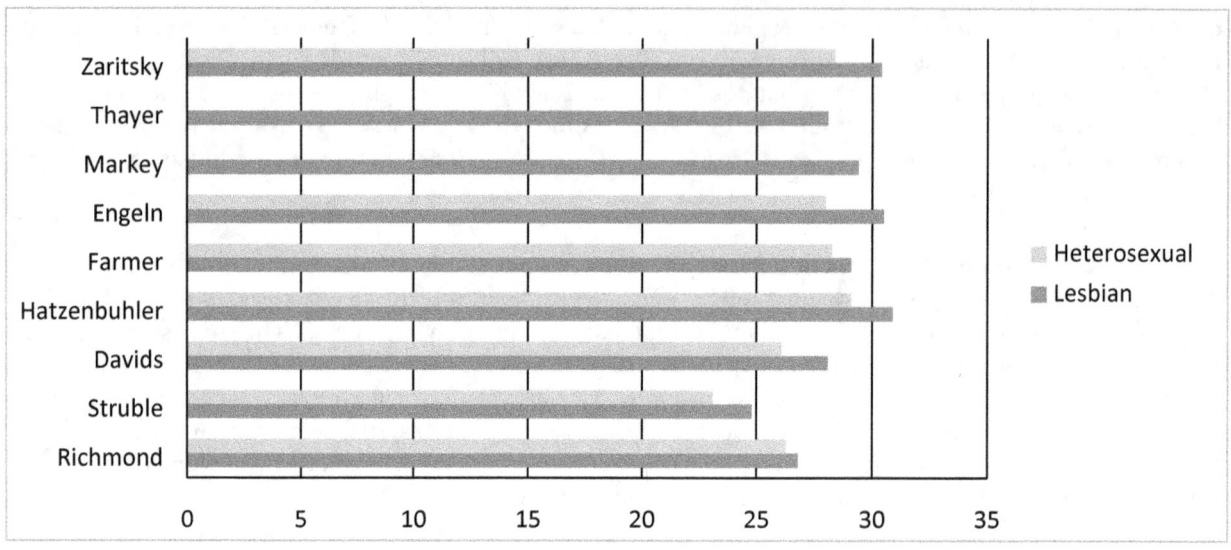

The studies reported in the two charts above are at one point in time. It is more useful to know how a person's weight changes by measuring them over an extended period of time (called a longitudinal study). Jun and colleagues (2012) used data from the Nurses' Health Study to follow women's weight over time, and reported that lesbian/bisexual women were more likely to show the more dangerous rapid weight gain pattern whereas heterosexual women showed slower weight gain over time. But they also found that lesbian/bisexual women were more likely to be in the group that lost weight from one time to the next.

Few studies have looked at subsets of the lesbian/bisexual population. One of the few studies to examine lesbian/bisexual women of color, (Dibble, Eliason, & Crawford, 2012) found that 85% of a sample of 123 African American lesbian and bisexual women were "overweight," with 13% having a BMI over 40 or higher (considered in the bio-med literature as "morbidly obese"), and Mays and colleagues (2002) found higher rates of overweight and obesity in lesbians of color compared to heterosexual women of color.

In the biomedical fields and the press, there is a strong belief that being obese (and maybe being overweight) is associated with higher rates of diabetes, heart disease, some cancers, high blood pressure, and other health disorders. The next chapter explores whether lesbian/bisexual women have higher rates of any of these, and challenges the idea that weight is a good predictor of any health problem. However, it is safe to conclude that as a group, lesbian and bisexual women tend to be larger than heterosexual women.

The Obesity Paradox

Before going on, we should discuss the limitations of the concept of BMI or body mass index, and the problems with research on weight. First, BMI is based on a calculation of weight to height ratio, and was first described in the late 1800s. Insurance companies started using it as a predictor of who might die early—insurance companies don't usually go out and measure people, so they used the most convenient measure of BMI and explored different formulas of calculating it. The current measurement came from a 1972 study of 7400 men that compared many different ways to come up with a score, and they selected this one, which now got named BMI. So it was based on data from only men! Because the measure was cheap and easy, it started to be used in hundreds of research studies and in doctor's offices around the world. But if you look at that 1972 paper, the author (Ancel Keys) clearly said that this measurement was for group data and should never be applied to individuals. Lots of research shows that your waist circumference is a better indicator of health than BMI, because abdominal fat is more problematic than fat around the hips or the legs for example. Robert Lustig (2012) noted that many thin people have excess abdominal fat and he calls them TOFIs—thin on the outside, fat on the inside. If you have a lot of muscle tissue, you will have a greater BMI because muscle weighs more than fat. If you have more dense bones, your BMI will be higher. Some critiques have called the BMI "mathematical snake oil" or "the Baloney Mass Index." So the message is to be very cautious in putting much stock in a BMI (or a number on a scale, for that matter).

Another issue to consider is that the research linking weight to health problems has been flawed. A growing number of biomedical researchers are challenging the assumption that fat is unhealthy. They point to studies that show that some degree of extra body fat is actually good. Fat people recover from some illnesses and surgeries faster than thin people because they have more reserves. Fat people are less likely to break bones when they fall. In a few studies of mortality rates, thin and "normal" weight people died earlier than overweight or even some people labeled as "obese." All of these studies suggest that older studies have been too simplistic and that weight and BMI are not good predictors of health. Yet multi-billion dollar campaigns to coerce people into losing weight, usually with unhealthy or ineffective methods, have sprung up and they maintain the myth that fat is unhealthy to keep people buying their products and services. All this research on the weight or BMI of lesbian and bisexual women misses a critical point. Why should we worry about weight unless we know that higher weight is associated with a poor health outcome? Fat may not be the direct cause of health problems, but weight stigma and the societal pressures put on people to look a certain way certain do affect us all, and one of the areas that is affected is our body satisfaction.

BODY SATISFACTION

An important factor in wellbeing and health is body acceptance or satisfaction. Women who are not satisfied with their bodies are more likely to engage in health-damaging practices such as calorie restriction diets, diet pills, surgeries, and other behaviors that are hard on the body. They may also experience depression and anxiety about their bodies, and this negativity about the body can affect relationships. Concerns about weight are certainly not limited to those that society labels as overweight. In one study of adolescents (of all sexualities), 64% who had a "healthy weight" were concerned about their weight and 13% of those considered "obese" were not concerned about weight (Woodruff et al., 2008). Women at any size can be pressured by societal expectations for how women should look.

Some research shows that lesbian and bisexual women are more satisfied with their bodies than are heterosexual women, but it appears that the findings are complicated. In one study, butch lesbians were satisfied with their bodies at a higher weight and femme lesbians were more likely to be dissatisfied with their bodies. The more one rejects feminine beauty standards, the more likely she is to embrace her body at any size. Some studies find an increase in body acceptance and satisfaction shortly after coming out as lesbian or bisexual, when the woman recognizes that other women do not expect supermodel bodies on the women they date. Finally, the newly out woman feels attractive and expresses herself in diverse ways, not just through rigid societal beauty standards.

Another study looked at the influence of romantic relationships on lesbian body satisfaction. One theory suggests that if one partner is thinner, the larger partner may feel more threatened and have more body concerns than women who are about the same size as their partners. Charlotte and Patrick Markey (2013) studied 72 female same-sex couples. Some (43%) were in the same weight category, and the rest were in different categories. They found the same pattern of worries that they found in earlier studies with heterosexual women. Women who were larger than their partners had significantly more weight concerns than women who were similar to, or smaller, than their partners. In general, however, the greater the BMI of a woman, the more likely that she would experience weight concerns, regardless of the size of the partner. So partner size is just one factor in a world that stigmatizes larger bodies.

But even though lesbians and bisexual women are relatively more satisfied with their bodies than heterosexual women, many are not accepting of their size, shape, or ability levels. Feminism has tried to address this body dissatisfaction and through media literacy and other means, educate women to be more comfortable in their own bodies. Some of these movements in feminism are political, so we need to discuss the politics of fat. The media and other discourses in society, particularly biomedicine, has created pressures on all women that are hard to escape and affect our attitudes toward our own bodies.

Other Factors in Body Satisfaction
Our society also pressures women to fit white beauty standards: straight hair, certain facial features, light-skin, all factors that women of color may not meet. Much has been written about the dismissal of women of color

with natural hair styles from public jobs, like newscasters, and the need for lesbian and bisexual women in the media to meet some degree of feminine standards. Rarely do butch lesbians achieve celebrity status. We tend to glamorize the extraordinarily physically fit, who got that way from much hard work and the luck of the draw related to genes and lack of illness/injury. We cannot all look like lesbian Diana Nyad who was the first person to swim from Cuba to Florida. We have diverse body types, sizes, and shapes. Dawn Atkins' (1999) edited book on body image in LGBT people was one of the first to explore the various experiences that people with diverse sexual and gender identities have with their own bodies and considers the intersections between sex/gender, sexuality, race, gender expressions, and many other factors.

Thin Privilege

The following list came from a blogger Shannon Ridgway, on Jezebel (Nov 30, 2012). Ridgway suggested that we get bombarded with mass-media messages that "normal" size is actually thin. The assumption that you need to be thin in order to be acceptable in society leads to much harassment of larger bodied people. People who have been thin most of their lives may never have thought of the benefits of being thin. Sizeism is one of the acceptable "isms" in society. Thin privilege may underlie most of the body dissatisfaction of women in our culture.

Examples of Thin Privilege:
- You are not assumed to be unhealthy just because of your size.
- Your size is not the first thing people notice about you.
- When you are grocery shopping, people do not try to be "helpful" by commenting on the food selection in your cart.
- Your health insurance rates are not higher than everyone else's.
- You can expect to pay reasonable prices for your clothing.
- You can expect to find your clothing size sold locally.
- You can expect to find clothing in the latest styles and colors instead of colorless, shapeless and outdated styles meant to hide your body.
- You don't receive suggestions from your friends and family to join Weight Watchers or any other weight-loss program.
- When you go to the doctor, they don't suspect diabetes (or high blood pressure, high cholesterol, or other "weight-related" diagnoses) as the first/most likely diagnosis.
- You don't get told, "You have such a pretty/handsome face" (implying: if only you'd lose weight you could be even more attractive).
- People do not assume that you are lazy, based solely on your size.
- You're not the brunt of jokes for countless numbers of comedians.
- Airlines won't charge you extra to fly.
- You are not perceived as looking sloppy or unprofessional based on your size.
- You can eat what you want, when you want in public and not have others judge you for it or make assumptions about your eating habits.
- You can walk out of a gas station with a box of doughnuts and not have people yell at you to "Lay off them doughnuts, fatty!"
- People don't ask your partners what it's like to have sex with you because of your size.
  Your body type isn't sexually fetishized.
- You're more likely to get a raise or promotion at work than someone who is fat.
  Friends don't describe you to others using a qualifier (e.g. "She's kind of heavy, but REALLY nice, though").
- The media doesn't describe your body shape as part of an "epidemic".
- You can choose to not be preoccupied with your size and shape.

EATING DISORDERS

The most common types of eating disorders are anorexia, a form of self-starvation and extreme deprivation; bulimia, a pattern of binge eating followed by purging through vomiting, laxatives, or extreme exercise; and binge eating, a lack of control over eating. Recently, researchers reviewed the academic literature for studies about eating disorders among lesbian and bisexual women (Bankoff & Pantalone, 2014). Gay and bisexual men have received more attention in regards to disordered eating. The earlier research proposed that being lesbian was a protective factor against eating disorders for many of the same reasons we discussed in the body satisfaction section—that lesbians do not buy into societal standards of thinness, thus do not diet. Dieting is a risk factor for developing eating disorders. More recent studies, though, suggest that lesbian and bisexual women are quite varied in their body satisfaction and desire to fit into societal standards for appearance, and that certain types of eating disorder, particularly binge eating, is at least as common, or maybe even more common in lesbian/bisexual women than heterosexual women. A few studies of youth find higher rates of bulimia among young women who identify as bisexual or not completely heterosexual and one study found twice the rate of a past or present eating disorder among bisexual women than lesbians (Koh & Ross, 2006). These newer studies find no differences in rates of anorexia and bulimia by sexual orientation, and no differences in the numbers in each group who are concerned about their weight. Within lesbian/bisexual communities, there may be differences based on gender expression, with more feminine women having greater drive for thinness, thus more risk for eating disorders, but there is not enough research yet to support this. Age may also be a factor, because older women may care less about what others think of them.

THE POLITICS OF FAT

Reclaiming Fat

Some authors propose that we take the stigma out of the word fat by using it as a descriptor of body size—there are thin people and fat people, tall and short. They propose that we not use the medicalized terms of overweight and obese, because they imply that the mere fact of being fat is unhealthy. Esther Rothblum (2015) proposed that lesbians should be the ones to lead women to greater fat acceptance and body satisfaction. We have examined societal beauty standards and have found that they don't have to apply to us. Another thing that we can do as lesbian and bisexual women, is to examine the parallels and intersections of fat oppression and oppression based on our sexuality and gender. There are similarities, as shown in the chart below. If fat is a form of oppression, then it operates like other oppressions. Fat people are considered to have a set of characteristics (lazy, not as smart, unmotivated, gluttonous, sloppy, and other stereotypes), and thin is the privileged position given extra favors in society. This corresponds to being a lesbian or bisexual woman in a world where heterosexuality is the privileged position.

Myth	Being Fat	Having Same Sex Desires
It's a choice	Probably a combination of genes and environment. Who chooses to be fat? No one sets out with a goal to be fat.	Probably a combination of genes and environment. Who would choose to be gay? No one sets out to be gay.
You could change if you tried hard enough	Diet and exercise only work in the short term under extreme conditions of self-monitoring. No matter how motivated, the body's natural processes overcome and 95% of people put the weight back on.	One can repress or deny same-sex feelings for short periods of time, but rarely do people change their underlying attraction patterns through religion, therapy, or willpower. The body's natural desires win.
Its sinful or immoral	The person is thought to be indulging in the sins of gluttony and sloth (laziness). But fat people are no more likely to be lazy or greedy than thin people.	The person is thought to be indulging in the sin of sodomy or unnatural desires. LGBT people are no more likely to be "immoral" or "unethical" than heterosexual people.

Myth	Being Fat	Having Same Sex Desires
It's a new thing	The "obesity epidemic" has been labeled in the past 20 years, but there have been fat people thru-out recorded history.	Sexual orientation was named and labeled around 1900, but same-sex desires have been around thru-out recorded history.
It's unhealthy	Being large itself is not unhealthy; but unnatural foods, lack of exercise and being treated badly increase stress which increases illness.	Having same-sex desires are not unhealthy; but being treated badly and rejected by family, society can increase stress which increases illness.
It's a burden on society	Do fat people use more health resources or cost the government more? People with diabetes, heart disease, cancer, etc. use more services, but not people who are merely fat. If fat people were not stigmatized, they would be healthier.	Do gay people demand special rights? Is same-sex marriage leading to the destruction of the family? So far, there is no evidence that gay people add any burden to society, and if not stigmatized, they would be healthier.

Note: This is not to say that being fat and having same-sex desires are exactly the same, because they are not. However, they are similar in at least these six ways because of societal stigma and stereotypes (myth).

The Fat Positive or Fat Liberation Movement

In early 1970s, the Fat Underground was formed in Los Angeles, stemming from feminist challenges to the societal messages women get about their bodies, and especially the body shaming that was occurring not only in the media, but in medicine, schools, the law, and other institutions of society, as well as in public spaces. Lesbian Judy Freespirit was one of the authors of the following piece:

Fat Liberation Manifesto

1. WE believe that fat people are fully entitled to human respect and recognition.

2. WE are angry at mistreatment by commercial and sexist interests. These have exploited our bodies as objects of ridicule, thereby creating an immensely profitable market selling the false promise of avoidance of, or relief from, that ridicule.

3. WE see our struggle as allied with the struggles of other oppressed groups against classism, racism, sexism, ageism, financial exploitation, imperialism and the like.

4. WE demand equal rights for fat people in all aspects of life, as promised in the Constitution of the United States. We demand equal access to goods and services in the public domain, and an end to discrimination against us in the areas of employment, education, public facilities and health services.

5. WE single out as our special enemies the so-called "reducing" industries. These include diet clubs, reducing salons, fat farms, diet doctors, diet books, diet foods and food supplements, surgical procedures, appetite suppressants, drugs and gadgetry such as wraps and "reducing machines".

WE demand that they take responsibility for their false claims acknowledge that their products are harmful to the public health, and publish long-term studies proving any statistical efficacy of their products. We make this demand knowing that over 99% of all weight loss programs, when evaluated over a five-year period, fail utterly, and also knowing the extreme proven harmfulness of frequent large changes in weight.

6. WE repudiate the mystified "science" which falsely claims that we are unfit. It has both caused and upheld discrimination against us, in collusion with the financial interests of insurance companies, the fashion and garment industries, reducing industries, the food and drug industries, and the medical and psychiatric establishment.

7. WE refuse to be subjugated to the interests of our enemies. We fully intend to reclaim power over our bodies and our lives. We commit ourselves to pursue these goals together.

FAT PEOPLE OF THE WORLD, UNITE! YOU HAVE NOTHING TO LOSE ....

By Judy Freespirit and Aldebaran, November, 1973

Fat Positive movements in the U.S. have challenged the idea that to be large is to be of less value, less healthy, or less attractive, and show that through-out recorded history, there has been a wide diversity of body sizes and shapes. There is no ideal size. Yet, we have stigmatized people for their weight or if their bodies function differently than the majority. Fat positive movements have been mostly grass-roots, feminist or other liberation movements, and have had limited impact on biomedical practices or weight stigma in healthcare settings. However, they have been very useful in helping some women accept their bodies and feel better about themselves. Many liberation movements have had success because they find a middle ground between the two polarized opposite viewpoints like the differences between fat positive feminists and biomedical researchers. Health at Every Size (HAES) is a bridge model between traditional biomedical assumptions about larger bodies, and fat positive movements. HAES is based in science, so has greater appeal to biomedical practitioners, and more potential to impact health care professionals. This DIFO book goes into much detail in Chapter 17 about intuitive eating, the nutritional program that is endorsed by the Health at Every Size model, but HAES is about reducing weight stigma and body acceptance as well. There is also a national advocacy group, the National Association to Advance Fat Acceptance (NAAFA), that attempts to reduce weight discrimination in society. When asked about experiences of discrimination in our DIFO program, more women felt they had been treated differently by others because of their weight than because of their sexual orientation or sex. Weight discrimination may be an important contributor to stress for many lesbian and bisexual women of size.

Conclusion

In summary, lesbian and bisexual women, as a group, are larger than heterosexual women, and some are more satisfied with their bodies and less focused on fitting traditional beauty standards, including being thin. However, many other lesbian and bisexual women feel pressured to look a certain way; sometimes that way is the societal beauty standards and sometimes the pressure is to "look like a lesbian." Either type of pressure can create anxiety, depression, body dissatisfaction, and eating disorders. Little is known about how lesbian/bisexual women's body image changes with aging.

Resources

Health At Every Size website: www.haescommunity.org
NAAFA website: http://naafaonline.com/dev2/
There are now dozens of fat positive blogs and websites, as well as more generic body positive sites. A great resource for developing body positivity is a new book by Linda Bacon and Lucy Aphamor (2014) called Body Respect published by BenBella Books in Texas.

REFERENCES

Atkins, D. (1999). *Looking queer: Body image in LGBT communities*. New York: Haworth Press.
Bankoff, S.M. & Pantalone, D.W. (2014). Patterns of disordered eating behavior in women by sexual orientation: A review of the literature. *Eating Disorders, 22*, 261-274.
Eliason, M.J., Ingraham, N., Fogel, S., McElroy, J., Lorvick, J., & Mauery, R. (2015). A systematic review of weight in sexual minority women. *Women's Health Issues,*
Dibble, S. L., Eliason, M. J., & Crawford, B. (2012). Correlates of wellbeing among African American lesbians. *Journal of Homosexuality, 59*, 820–838.
Jun, H. J., Corliss, H. L., Nichols, L. P., Pazaris, M., Spiegelman, D., & Austin, S. B. (2012). Adult body mass index trajectories and sexual orientation: The Nurses' Health Study II. *American Journal of Preventive Medicine, 42*, 348–354.
Krieger, N. (2005). Embodiment: a conceptual glossary for epidemiology. *Journal of Epidemiology and Community Health, 59*, 350-355.
Koh, A. & Ross, L.K. (2006). Mental health issues: A comparison of lesbian, bisexual, and heterosexual women. *Journal of Homosexuality, 51*, 33-57.
Markey, C., & Markey, P. M. (2013). Weight disparities between female same-sex romantic partners and weight concerns: Examining partner comparison. *Psychology of Women Quarterly*, doi: 10.1177/0361684313484128

Mays, V.M., Yancey, A.K., Cochran, S.D., Weber, M. & Fielding, J.E. (2002). Heterogeneity of health disparities among African American, Hispanic, and Asian American women: Unrecognized influences of sexual orientation. *American Journal of Public Health, 92*(4), 632-639.

Rothblum, E. (2014). Commentary: Lesbians should take the lead in removing the stigma that has long been associated with body weight. *Psychology of Sexual Orientation and Gender Diversity,* doi:.org/10.1037/sgd0000065.

Woodruff, S.J., Hanning, R.M., Lambraki, I., Storey, K.E., & McCargar, L. (2008). Healthy Eating Index-C is compromised among adolescents with body weight concerns, weight loss dieting, and meal skipping, *Body Image, 5*(4), 404-408.

Chapter 6: Chronic Physical Health Disorders

How do the years of stress of being lesbian or bisexual women affect the physical body? Do lesbian and bisexual women have more chronic health problems than heterosexual women? There is no straightforward answer to this. Most of the large scale health surveys used to track illness and disease in the population have not included questions about sexual identity, although some are starting to gather this information. There are many reasons why we might suspect that lesbian/bisexual women would have higher rates of chronic physical health disorders. From the research that is available, it appears that:

- Mental health problems associated with stress are found more often among lesbian and bisexual women. This includes depression and anxiety disorders. For example, recent national mental health data showed that major depression was found in 42% of lesbians and 52% of bisexual women compared to 27% of heterosexual women. See Chapter 3. Physical health problems are elevated in women with mental health problems.

- Child abuse is associated with increased chronic health problems in adulthood, and lesbian and bisexual women report higher rates of childhood sexual and physical abuse than do heterosexual women.

- Lesbian/bisexual women are more likely than heterosexual women to smoke, have problem drinking patterns, and use recreational drugs, especially marijuana. For example, recent data from a drug abuse survey shows past year alcohol dependence in 13% of lesbians, 16% of bisexual women, and less than 3% of heterosexual women. Marijuana use in the past year was reported by 17% of lesbians, 22% of bisexual women, and less than 3% of heterosexual women (Chapter 4 describes this). Substance abuse can cause a lot of physical health problems over time.

- Lesbian/bisexual women are heavier than heterosexual women. They have a higher BMI (body mass index) as a group and a higher percentage of women who qualify as "obese" by biomedical classifications. We do not know yet whether this heavier weight is associated with health problems, but it is related to more exposure to discrimination and harassment because of fat phobia (discussed in Chapter 5). Whether because of weight itself, or weight stigma, most researchers assume that the BMI of lesbian/bisexual women as a group might lead to more health problems.

- Finally, minority stress affects opportunities in life. Lesbian and bisexual women are more likely to live in poverty, lack access to quality healthcare, and be uninsured than heterosexual women. When lesbian/bisexual women do access healthcare, they often encounter healthcare providers who are actively hostile and discriminatory, or more often, heterosexist---we are merely invisible to them and they do not even know that their care is insensitive. All of these are risk factors for physical health problems. And if we avoid or delay getting care, we might have conditions that are undetected and untreated until they are far advanced and have caused a lot of damage to our bodies.

Because of these risk factors, theoretically, lesbian/bisexual women are at higher risk for diabetes, heart disease, asthma, some cancers, and a host of other physical health disorders. Many of these disorders are also associated with aging and with other forms of oppression besides sexual identity, so many women will experience one or more of these disorders. There is no evidence that lesbian and bisexual women have a shortened life span because of any physical health problems (Cochran & Mays, 2014).

All of these elevated risk factors and disorders/illnesses are related to the stress of living in a world that is homophobic, biphobic, sexist, ageist, racist, ableist, and so on. Chronic stress can produce disease and disorder if we do not have enough protective factors to combat stress, like healthy coping strategies, supportive communities, and loving relationships. There is also research to show that racial discrimination, age discrimination, and other forms of oppression have similar effects on health: chronic stress produces vulnerability to illness and fear of discrimination creates avoidance or delay in seeking healthcare. We begin this chapter with discussion of one general problem that cuts across many chronic illnesses and disorders: Pain. Then we discuss some of the most common chronic health problems that affect older populations.

PHYSICAL PAIN

Pain can come from many sources, including injuries and chronic physical health ailments. Cochran and Mays (2007) studied California women's reports of some conditions that can result in pain and found differences by sexual orientation as shown in the chart below. Lesbian and bisexual women reported more disability, arthritis, chronic pain, chronic fatigue, and back pain than heterosexual women. Bisexual women had more headaches and asthma.

Figure 6.1. Causes of pain among women by sexual orientation (from Cochran & Mays, 2007)

Disorder	Heterosexual	Lesbian	Bisexual
Migraines/headaches	19%	18%	26%
Asthma	9%	13%	19%
Arthritis	21%	34%	18%
Back problems	14%	23%	27%
Functional health limitations	21%	31%	38%
Chronic pain	12%	19%	19%
Chronic fatigue, fibromyalgia	5%	9%	12%

Pain management strategies are discussed in several of the chapters in Part III, because they are multi-faceted. Pain management can include exercise, stress reduction methods, and changing how we eat, as well as medications and medical treatments. As of yet, there is no research on lesbian/bisexual women's experiences of pain or management of pain. Pain is a major quality of life issue, particularly as we age. However, since many lesbian/bisexual women are willing to consider alternative and complementary health options, we may have more options for dealing with pain than do heterosexual women.

METABOLIC SYNDROME

Many of the chronic health disorders that are discussed below have the same or very similar causes, rooted in inflammation processes in the body. One of the reliable measures of chronic inflammation, and the body processes that underlie disease, is called metabolic syndrome. If you can monitor and reduce these lab/physical health markers, you reduce your risks for all the health problems that follow.

Metabolic syndrome is not a disease, but a cluster of health markers. Although there are several definitions of metabolic syndrome, in the United States most health care professionals use the criteria from the National Heart, Lung, and Blood Institute (NHLBI) and the American Heart Association. That definition says you must have at least three of the following five markers to be diagnosed with metabolic syndrome:

- A waist measurement of more than 35 inches around.
- A fasting blood glucose level of 100 mg/dL or higher; or already taking medication because you have high blood glucose levels.
- A triglyceride level at or above 150 mg/dL. Triglycerides are a form of fat in your blood.
- An HDL cholesterol level (the "good" cholesterol) below 50 mg/dL; or already taking medication to increase your HDL level.

- A blood pressure at or above 130 mm Hg systolic (the top number) or 85 mm Hg diastolic (the bottom number); or already taking medication to treat high blood pressure.

According to the American Heart Association, 47 million Americans have metabolic syndrome, although many may not know it. Metabolic syndrome is linked to several health conditions, particularly heart disease and diabetes. Although rates of metabolic syndrome are the same in men and women, women with a condition called polycystic ovary syndrome (PCOS) are up to 11 times more likely to have metabolic syndrome than those without PCOS. One study found an increased rate of polycystic ovary syndrome in lesbians (Agrawal et al., 2004), but two other studies did not find a difference between heterosexual women and lesbian/bisexual women (deSutter et al, 2008; Smith et al, 2011).

Additionally, rates of metabolic syndrome increase with age, occurring in about 45 percent of those aged 60 to 69. Researchers have discovered the risk of metabolic syndrome in women begins to rise around perimenopause, which seems to be related to increases in testosterone at that time.

The reason so many Americans have metabolic syndrome is related to three things: type of foods consumed, lack of exercise and genetic factors. Not everyone who is overweight has it, and many people who are "normal" weight do have it. Estimates are that about 22% of overweight and 60% of obese people have metabolic syndrome, with the risk directly related to the amount of abdominal fat. Abdominal, or visceral, fat is defined by your waist circumference. Later, we'll talk more about why this increases your risk for certain diseases.

Latina and South Asian women have a higher risk of metabolic syndrome and so do women who do not get sufficient exercise, or have a diet high in fried foods, carbohydrates and so-called "empty calories" like soda. On the other hand, a diet high in whole grains, fiber, and lots of fruits and vegetables can lower risk. The reality, however, is that any *one* of the five risk factors increases your risk of cardiovascular disease whether you have metabolic syndrome or not. So whether you have one or all five of the components, you and your health care professional need to work together to reduce your risks. We do not know if lesbian and bisexual women are more likely to have metabolic syndrome than heterosexual women.

If you have polycystic ovary syndrome, or PCOS, you should ask your health care professional to evaluate you for metabolic syndrome. PCOS affects between 7- 8% of women of childbearing age. Typical symptoms include irregular or absent menstruation, a larger body size, and hair on the face and other parts of the body where women typically don't have much hair, a condition called hirsutism. Women with PCOS also often have high levels of testosterone and often have trouble getting pregnant. Some research finds that women with PCOS are up to 11 times more likely to have metabolic syndrome. We don't know whether the components of metabolic syndrome cause the PCOS or vice versa. But women with PCOS tend to be overweight, have insulin resistance, have high levels of fasting blood glucose and, as a consequence, they have a much higher risk overall of cardiovascular disease and diabetes. One study reported that lesbians had higher rates of PCOS than heterosexual women (Agrawal et al, 2004), but two others failed to find a difference (DeSutter et al, 2008; Smith et al, 2011).

Treatment

The treatment for metabolic syndrome is improving your diet and increasing levels of physical activity. Studies find a diet high in saturated fat, simple sugars and cholesterol contributes to metabolic syndrome. Several specific dietary strategies are recommended for the treatment of metabolic syndrome, including:

- Eating foods high in fruits, vegetables, nuts, whole grains and olive oil. In one study, participants who ate the Mediterranean diet experienced greater weight loss, lower blood pressure, lower markers of inflammation and improved insulin resistance and lipid profiles than people on a standard low-fat diet.
- The D.A.S.H. diet, which includes a sodium intake of less than 2,400 mg per day and a higher dairy intake than the Mediterranean diet. When compared with a weight-reducing diet that emphasized healthy food choices, the D.A.S.H. diet resulted in greater improvements in fasting glucose, triglycerides and diastolic blood pressure, even after controlling for weight loss.

- A low-glycemic diet, which includes foods with a low glycemic index and replaces refined grains with whole grains, fruits and vegetables and eliminates high-glycemic beverages. Researchers are not sure yet if it is the low glycemic index itself or the increase in high-fiber foods (or both) that produces the beneficial effects.

The second part of the equation is physical movement. When you move your body, your cells become more receptive to insulin. Regular exercise (a 30-minute walk a day; chair dancing; lifting light weights) can make a huge difference in improving most of the risk factors for metabolic syndrome.

Health care provider may recommend medication to treat some components of metabolic syndrome, such as metformin (Glucophage), pioglitazone (Actos) and rosiglitazone (Avandia) to improve insulin resistance. Metformin may help prevent diabetes in people with prediabetes. If you have both high blood pressure and metabolic syndrome, the treatment for each may have to be changed. Large doses of some commonly prescribed blood pressure drugs, such as diuretics and beta-blockers, can make insulin resistance worse. ACE inhibitors such as enalapril (Vasotec) and benazepril (Lotensin) and angiotensin receptor blockers like losartan (Cozaar) seem to work better in patients with diabetes.

There aren't many drugs that can raise HDL cholesterol, but if LDL levels are high, statins *can* improve HDL cholesterol somewhat. Additionally, if your 10-year risk of heart disease is high, you may want to talk to your health care professional about aspirin therapy. You can learn more about your risk of heart disease at www.nhlbi.nih.gov/guidelines/cholesterol/risk_tbl.htm. Drugs may be prescribed in combination with a healthy diet to reduce high triglycerides. Prescription drugs include omega-3 fatty acids (Lovaza) and the fibrates gemfibrozil (Lopid) and clofibrate (Atromid-S). Talk to your health care provider about the risks and benefits of these drugs, based on your personal medical history. The best way to prevent metabolic syndrome is identical to the treatment: healthier food and more activity.

DIABETES

What is diabetes?

Diabetes is a disease caused by high blood glucose (sugar) levels. Most of the food we eat is turned into glucose, or sugar, for our bodies to use for energy. The pancreas, an organ near the stomach, makes a hormone called insulin to help glucose get into the cells of our bodies. With diabetes, the body either does not make enough insulin or cannot use its own insulin efficiently. This causes sugar to build up in the bloodstream. Diabetes can cause serious health complications including heart disease, blindness, kidney failure, and lower-extremity amputations. Diabetes is the sixth leading cause of death in the United States.

What are the symptoms of diabetes?
- Frequent urination
- Excessive thirst
- Unexplained weight loss
- Extreme hunger
- Sudden vision changes
- Tingling or numbness in hands or feet
- Feeling very tired much of the time
- Very dry skin
- Sores that are slow to heal
- More infections than usual.
- Nausea, vomiting, or stomach pains may accompany some of these symptoms in the abrupt onset of insulin-dependent diabetes, now called type 1 diabetes.

Diabetes is diagnosed when you consistently have a fasting blood sugar level of greater than 100. Another common test is the hemoglobin A1C test, which measures the average amount of blood sugar over about a three month period. The values for HbA1C are:

Normal:	less than 5.7%
Pre-diabetes:	5.7 to 6.4%
Diabetes:	6.5% or higher

What are the types of diabetes?

Type 1 diabetes, previously called insulin-dependent diabetes mellitus (IDDM) or juvenile-onset diabetes, accounts for 5% of all diagnosed cases of diabetes. **Type 2 diabetes**, previously called non-insulin-dependent diabetes mellitus (NIDDM) or adult-onset diabetes, accounts for 90-95% of all diagnosed cases of diabetes. **Gestational diabetes** is a type of diabetes that only pregnant women get. Gestational diabetes develops in 2-10% of pregnancies but usually disappears when a pregnancy is over.

What are the risk factors for diabetes?

Risk factors for type 2 diabetes include older age, heavier weights, family history of diabetes, prior history of gestational diabetes, impaired glucose tolerance, physical inactivity, and experiencing racism or other forms of oppression. African Americans, Hispanic/Latino Americans, American Indians, and some Asian Americans and Pacific Islanders are at high risk for type 2 diabetes. Risk factors are less well defined for type 1 diabetes than for type 2 diabetes, but autoimmune, genetic, and environmental factors are involved in developing this type of diabetes. Gestational diabetes occurs more frequently in African Americans, Hispanic/Latino Americans, American Indians, and people with a family history of diabetes than in other groups. Obesity is also associated with higher risk. Women who have had gestational diabetes have a 35- 60% chance of developing diabetes in the next 10–20 years.

Do lesbians get diabetes more often than heterosexual women?

No, it appears from several studies that the rates of diabetes are about the same in lesbian and bisexual women as in heterosexual women. Out of 12 studies (the four that divided samples into lesbian, bisexual, and heterosexual are shown below), only one found a significant difference, and in that case, heterosexual women had higher rates of diabetes (Matthews & Lee, 2014). Other factors, such as genetics, your individual diet, age, and racial/ethnic group, seem to be more important predictors of diabetes risk. However, there is research that lesbian/bisexual women are less likely to see routine, preventative health care, thus the signs of diabetes may not be caught as early as they would for women who get regular care.

Figure 6.2. Rates of diabetes among women by sexual orientation (from Eliason, 2014)

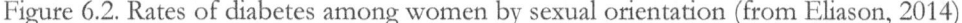

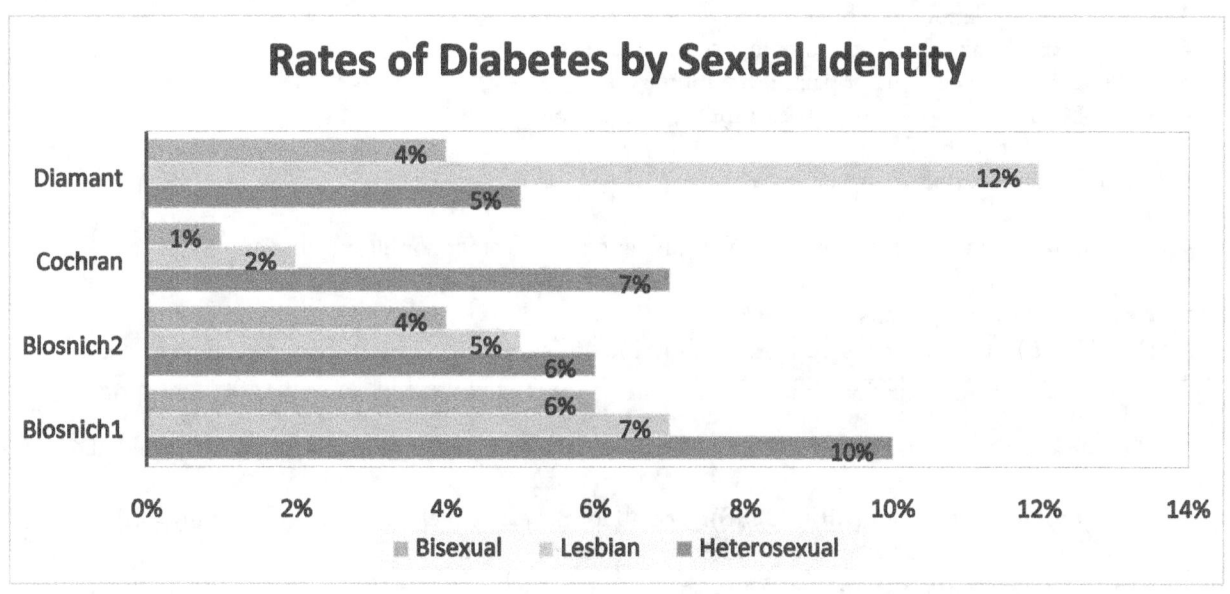

What is the treatment for diabetes?
Healthy eating, physical activity, and insulin injections are the basic therapies for type 1 diabetes. The amount of insulin taken must be balanced with food intake and daily activities. Blood glucose levels must be closely monitored through frequent blood glucose testing. Healthy eating, physical activity, and blood glucose testing are the basic therapies for type 2 diabetes. In addition, many people with type 2 diabetes require oral medication, insulin, or both to control their blood glucose levels. People with diabetes should see a health care provider to monitor their diabetes control and help them learn to manage their diabetes. In addition, people with diabetes may see endocrinologists, who may specialize in diabetes care; ophthalmologists for eye examinations; podiatrists for routine foot care; and dietitians and diabetes educators who teach the skills needed for daily diabetes management.

Can diabetes be prevented?
Researchers are making progress in identifying the exact genetics and "triggers" that predispose some individuals to develop type 1 diabetes, but prevention remains elusive. A number of studies have shown that regular physical activity can significantly reduce the risk of developing type 2 diabetes. Type 2 diabetes is associated with high amounts of belly fat, poverty, stress, diet, and many other factors. Thus far, there is no cure for diabetes.

BREAST CANCER

What is breast cancer?
Cancer is a term used for diseases in which abnormal cells divide out of control and invade other tissues. Cancer cells can spread to other parts of the body through the blood and lymph systems. Except for skin cancer, breast cancer is the most common cancer among American women. Out one out of every eight women (12%) will develop breast cancer in her lifetime.

What are the symptoms of breast cancer?
Different people have different warning signs for breast cancer. Some people do not have any signs or symptoms at all. A woman may find out they have breast cancer after a routine mammogram. Some warning signs of breast cancer are:

1. New lump in the breast or underarm (armpit).
2. Thickening or swelling of part of the breast.
3. Irritation or dimpling of breast skin.
4. Redness or flaky skin in the nipple area or the breast.
5. Pulling in of the nipple or pain in the nipple area.
6. Nipple discharge other than breast milk, including blood.
7. Any change in the size or the shape of the breast.
8. Pain in any area of the breast.

Keep in mind that some of these warning signs can happen with other conditions that are not cancer.

What are the types of breast cancer?
The kind of breast cancer depends on which cells in the breast turn into cancer. Breast cancer can begin in different parts of the breast, like the ducts or the lobes. Common kinds of breast cancer are:

Ductal carcinoma. It is most common kind of breast cancer. It begins in the cells that line the milk ducts in the breast.
- **Ductal carcinoma in situ (DCIS).** The abnormal cancer cells are only in the lining of the milk ducts, and have not spread to other tissues in the breast.
- **Invasive ductal carcinoma.** The abnormal cancer cells break through the ducts and spread into other parts of the breast tissue. Invasive cancer cells can also spread to other parts of the body.

Lobular carcinoma. In this kind of breast cancer, the cancer cells begin in the lobes, or lobules, of the breast. Lobules are the glands that make milk.

- **Lobular carcinoma in situ (LCIS).** The cancer cells are found only in the breast lobules. Lobular carcinoma in situ, or LCIS, does not spread to other tissues.
- **Invasive lobular carcinoma.** Cancer cells spread from the lobules to the breast tissues that are close by. These invasive cancer cells can also spread to other parts of the body.

One of the best discussions about types of breast cancer can be found at
http://www.mayoclinic.com/health/breast-cancer/HQ00348

What are the risk factors for breast cancer?
- **Reproductive Risk Factors**
  1. Being younger when you first had your menstrual period.
  2. Starting menopause at a later age.
  3. Being older at the birth of your first child.
  4. Never giving birth.
  5. Not breastfeeding.
  6. Long-term use of hormone-replacement therapy.
- **Other Risk Factors**
  7. Getting older.
  8. Personal history of breast cancer or some non-cancerous breast diseases.
  9. Family history of breast cancer (mother, father, sister, brother, daughter, or son).
  10. Treatment with radiation therapy to the breast/chest.
  11. Breast density by mammogram.
  12. Being overweight (increases risk for breast cancer after menopause).
  13. Having changes in the breast cancer-related genes BRCA1 or BRCA2.
  14. Drinking alcohol (more than one drink a day).
  15. Not getting regular exercise.
  16. Smoking

Having a risk factor does not mean you will get the disease. Most women have some risk factors and most women do not get breast cancer. If you have breast cancer risk factors, talk with your doctor about ways you can lower your risk and about screening for breast cancer.

Do lesbian/bisexual women get breast cancer more often than heterosexual women?
The short answer to this question is we don't know. The large cancer registries that are used to determine the number of cases of breast cancer in specific groups do not collect data about sexual orientation. Some people currently believe that lesbian and bisexual women have an increased risk of developing breast cancer, based on a "cluster of risk factors" theory.* Of the risk factors listed above, numbers 3,4,5,12,14, and 16 occur more often in lesbian/bisexual than heterosexual women. We just don't know if these risk factors taken together result in more breast cancer for lesbians. So far, only two studies have found a slightly higher risk for breast cancer in lesbian/bisexual women, and ten studies have not found differences (Eliason, 2014).

What is the treatment for breast cancer?
Breast cancer treatment depends on the kind of breast cancer and how far it has spread. Treatments include surgery, chemotherapy, hormonal therapy, biologic therapy, and radiation. People with breast cancer often get more than one kind of treatment.
1. **Surgery.** An operation where doctors cut out and remove cancer tissue.
2. **Chemotherapy.** Using special medicines, or drugs to shrink or kill the cancer. The drugs can be pills you take or medicines given through an intravenous (IV) tube, or, sometimes, both.
3. **Hormonal therapy.** Some cancers need certain hormones to grow. Hormonal treatment is used to

block cancer cells from getting the hormones they need to grow. These are usually in the form of pills.

4. **Biological therapy.** This treatment works with your body's immune system to help it fight cancer or to control side effects from other cancer treatments. These are in the form of pills or injections that boost your body's own ability to fight off the cancer. Side effects are how your body reacts to drugs or other treatments. Biological therapy is different from chemotherapy, which attacks cancer cells directly.
5. **Radiation.** The use of high-energy rays (similar to X-rays) to kill the cancer cells. The rays are aimed at the part of the body where the cancer is located.

It is common for doctors from different specialties to work together in treating breast cancer: Surgeons perform operations; Medical oncologists treat cancers with medicines; Radiation oncologists treat cancers with radiation.

Can breast cancer be prevented?

Researchers are making progress in identifying the exact genetics and "triggers" that predispose some individuals to develop breast cancer, but prevention remains elusive. Risk reduction by modifying your behavior risk profile is the best alternative at this time. But also beware of the research on environmental toxins and substances such as hormones in foods that may be factors, and advocate for a safer food supply and environment.

COLORECTAL CANCER

What is colorectal cancer?

Colorectal cancer is cancer that occurs in the colon or rectum. The colon is the large intestine or large bowel and the rectum is the passageway that connects the colon to the anus. Colorectal cancer affects men and women of all racial and ethnic groups, and is most often found in people aged 50 years or older. In the United States, it is the third most common cancer for men and women not including skin cancer. Lifetime risk for colorectal cancer is 5%.

Of cancers that affect both men and women, colorectal cancer is the second leading cancer killer in the United States, but it doesn't have to be. If everybody aged 50 or older had regular screening tests, as many as 60% of deaths from colorectal cancer could be prevented.

Colorectal cancer screening saves lives. Screening can find precancerous polyps—abnormal growths in the colon or rectum—so that they can be removed before turning into cancer. Screening also helps find colorectal cancer at an early stage, when treatment often leads to a cure. About nine out of every 10 people whose colorectal cancer is found early and treated are still alive five years later.

The symptoms of colorectal cancer

Early colorectal cancer often has no symptoms, which is why screening is so important. Most colorectal cancers begin as a polyp, a small growth in the wall of the colon. As a polyp grows, it can bleed or obstruct the intestine. See your doctor if you have any of these warning signs:

- Bleeding from the rectum
- Blood in the stool or in the toilet after having a bowel movement
- Dark-or black-colored stools
- A change in the shape of the stool
- Cramping pain in the lower stomach
- A feeling of discomfort or an urge to have a bowel movement when there is no need to have one
- New onset of constipation or diarrhea that lasts for more than a few days
- Unintentional weight loss
- Weakness or fatigue

Keep in mind that some of these warning signs can happen with other conditions that are not cancer.

Types of colorectal cancer
About 96% of colorectal cancers are adenocarcinomas, which evolve from glandular tissue. The great majority of these cancers arise from an adenomatous polyp, which is visible through a scope or on an x-ray-like image.

Risk factors for colorectal cancer
The risk of developing colorectal cancer increases with advancing age. More than 90% of cases occur in people aged 50 or older. Other risk factors include having:

1. Inflammatory bowel disease.
2. A personal or family history of colorectal cancer or colorectal polyps.
3. A genetic syndrome such as familial adenomatous polyposis (FAP) or hereditary non-polyposis colorectal cancer (Lynch syndrome).
4. Lifestyle factors that may contribute to increased risk of colorectal cancer include—
   • Lack of regular physical activity.
   • Low fruit and vegetable intake
   • A low-fiber and high-fat diet.
   • Overweight and obesity.
   • Alcohol consumption.
   • Tobacco use.

Having a risk factor does not mean you will get the disease. Most women have some risk factors and most women do not get colorectal cancer. If you have colorectal cancer risk factors, talk with your doctor about ways you can lower your risk and about screening.

Screening tests for colorectal cancer
Screening tests help your doctor find polyps or cancer before you have symptoms. Finding and removing polyps may prevent colorectal cancer. Also, treatment for colorectal cancer is more likely to be effective when the disease is found early. To find polyps or early colorectal cancer all people in their 50s and older should be screened. People who are at higher-than-average risk of colorectal cancer should talk with their doctor about whether to have screening tests before age 50, what tests to have, the benefits and risks of each test, and how often to schedule appointments. The following screening tests can be used to detect polyps, cancer, or other abnormal areas. Your doctor can explain more about each test:

• *Fecal occult blood test* (FOBT): Sometimes cancers or polyps bleed, and the FOBT can detect tiny amounts of blood in the stool. If this test detects blood, other tests are needed to find the source of the blood. Benign conditions (such as *hemorrhoids*) also can cause blood in the stool.
• *Sigmoidoscopy*: Your doctor checks inside your rectum and the lower part of the colon with a lighted tube called a *sigmoidoscope*. If polyps are found, the doctor removes them. The procedure to remove polyps is called a *polypectomy*.
• *Colonoscopy*: Your doctor examines inside the rectum and entire colon using a long, lighted tube called a *colonoscope*. Your doctor removes polyps that may be found.
• *Double-contrast barium enema*: You are given an enema with a barium solution, and air is pumped into your rectum. Several *x-ray* pictures are taken of your colon and rectum. The barium and air help your colon and rectum show up on the pictures. Polyps or tumors may show up.
• *Digital rectal exam*: A rectal exam is often part of a routine physical examination. Your doctor inserts a lubricated, gloved finger into your rectum to feel for abnormal areas.

There are pros and cons to each test. Be sure to discuss them thoroughly with your healthcare provider.

Do lesbian/bisexual women get colorectal cancer more often than heterosexual women?

The short answer to this question is we don't know. The large cancer registries that are used to determine the number of cases of colorectal cancer in specific groups do not collect data about sexual orientation. Some people currently believe that lesbians have an increased risk of developing colorectal cancer, based on a "cluster of risk factors" theory (4). Of the risk factors listed above, numbers 7, 8, 9, 10, 11, 12 occur more often in lesbians that heterosexual women. We just don't know if these risk factors taken together result in more colorectal cancer for lesbians. So far, no studies have found higher rates of colorectal cancer, but there are just not enough studies to draw any conclusions (Eliason, 2014). A recent study also found no differences in screening rates for colorectal cancer by sexual orientation (Boehmer et al, 2014).

Treatment for colorectal cancer

Colorectal cancer is treated in several ways. It depends on the type and location of colorectal cancer and how far it has spread. In addition the age and vitality of the individual is taken into account. Treatments include surgery, chemotherapy, biologic therapy, and radiation. People with colorectal cancer often get more than one kind of treatment.

- **Surgery.** An operation where doctors cut out and remove cancer tissue.
- **Chemotherapy.** Using special medicines, or drugs to shrink or kill the cancer. The drugs can be pills you take or medicines given through an intravenous (IV) tube, or, sometimes, both.
- **Biological therapy.** This treatment works to boost your body's immune system to help it fight cancer or to control side effects from other cancer treatments. Side effects are how your body reacts to drugs or other treatments. Biological therapy is different from chemotherapy, which attacks cancer cells directly.
- **Radiation.** The use of high-energy rays (similar to X-rays) to kill the cancer cells. The rays are aimed at the part of the body where the cancer is located.

Can colorectal cancer be prevented?

At least 6 out of every 10 deaths from colorectal cancer could be prevented if all people aged 50 years or older were screened routinely. Precancerous polyps (abnormal growths) can be present in the colon for years before invasive cancer develops. They may not cause any symptoms. Colorectal cancer screening can find precancerous polyps so they can be removed before they turn into cancer. In this way, colorectal cancer is prevented. Screening can also find colorectal cancer early, when there is a greater chance that treatment will be most effective and lead to a cure. Some studies suggest that people may reduce their risk of developing colorectal cancer by increasing physical activity, eating fruits and vegetables, limiting alcohol consumption, and avoiding tobacco.

HEART DISEASE

Heart disease is known by many names: cardiovascular disease, coronary heart disease, coronary artery disease, and includes problems like heart attacks (myocardial infarction), heart failure, irregular heart beats, and blocked arteries. Coronary artery disease (CAD) is the most common type and is the leading cause of heart attacks. When you have CAD, your arteries become hard and narrow. Blood has a hard time getting to the heart, so the heart does not get all the blood it needs. CAD can lead to:

- Angina (an-JEYE-nuh). Angina is chest pain or discomfort that happens when the heart does not get enough blood. It may feel like a pressing or squeezing pain, often in the chest, but sometimes the pain is in the shoulders, arms, neck, jaw, or back. It can also feel like indigestion (upset stomach). Angina is not a heart attack, but having angina means you are more likely to have a heart attack.
- Heart attack. A heart attack occurs when an artery is severely or completely blocked, and the heart does not get the blood it needs for more than 20 minutes.

- Heart failure occurs when the heart is not able to pump blood through the body as well as it should. This means that other organs, which normally get blood from the heart, do not get enough blood. It does *not* mean that the heart stops. Signs of heart failure include:
  - Shortness of breath (feeling like you can't get enough air)
  - Swelling in feet, ankles, and legs
  - Extreme tiredness
- Heart arrhythmias (uh-RITH-mee-uhz) are changes in the beat of the heart. Most people have felt dizzy, faint, out of breath or had chest pains at one time. These changes in heartbeat are harmless for most people. As you get older, you are more likely to have arrhythmias. Don't panic if you have a few flutters or if your heart races once in a while. If you have flutters *and* other symptoms such as dizziness or shortness of breath, call 911 right away.

Women and heart disease

Among all U.S. women who die each year, one in four dies of heart disease. In 2004, nearly 60 percent more women died of cardiovascular disease (both heart disease and stroke) than from all cancers combined. The older a woman gets, the more likely she is to get heart disease. But women of all ages should be concerned about heart disease. All women should take steps to prevent heart disease. Both men and women have heart attacks, but more women who have heart attacks die from them. Treatments can limit heart damage but they must be given as soon as possible after a heart attack starts. Ideally, treatment should start within one hour of the first symptoms.

Do lesbian/bisexual women have higher rates of heart disease?

We do not have an answer to this question yet. A few studies suggested a slightly higher rate of heart disease among lesbian and bisexual women (Diamant & Wold, 2003). Conron and colleagues' (2010) analysis of statewide data in Massachusetts suggested that 34% of lesbian and 41% of bisexual women were at high risk for cardiovascular disease compared to 27% of heterosexual women. This risk was based on the findings that lesbians and bisexual women were more likely to have an elevated BMI or be smokers plus have one other risk factor (i.e., lack of moderate physical activity, lifetime diabetes, high blood pressure, or high cholesterol), or have three or more other risk factors in the absence of obesity or smoking. Farmer and coauthors (2013) also predicted greater risk for CVD for sexual minority women. After controlling for other factors, sexual minority women had vascular systems that were 5.7% older than heterosexual women.

Those studies looked at risk factors, not actual presence of heart disease. The data on actual prevalence of CVD is not clear. In the Women's Health Initiative (Valanis et al, 2000), lesbians had the highest prevalence of heart attack (heterosexual = 2.0%; bisexual = 1.2%; lifetime lesbian = 3.1%; and adult lesbians = 4.3%). Five other studies did not find any difference in rates of heart disease. Three studies reported on cholesterol levels and none found a difference by sexual identity. Hypertension (high blood pressure) is one of the warning signs for heart disease, but out of 12 studies, none found higher rates of hypertension in lesbian or bisexual women (Eliason, 2014). African American and Latina women tend to have more risk factors for heart disease than white women. These risk factors include higher body mass, lack of physical activity, high blood pressure, and diabetes.

Prevention of heart disease

You can reduce your chances of getting heart disease by taking these steps:

- Know your blood pressure. Years of high blood pressure can lead to heart disease. People with high blood pressure often have no symptoms, so have your blood pressure checked every 1 to 2 years and get treatment if you need it.
- Don't smoke. If you smoke, try to quit.
- Get tested for diabetes. People with diabetes have high blood glucose (often called blood sugar). People with high blood glucose often have no symptoms, so have your blood glucose checked regularly. Having diabetes raises your chances of getting heart disease.

- Get your cholesterol and triglyceride levels tested. High blood cholesterol (koh-LESS-tur-ol) can clog your arteries and keep your heart from getting the blood it needs. This can cause a heart attack. Triglycerides (treye-GLIH-suh-ryds) are a form of fat in your blood stream. High levels of triglycerides are linked to heart disease in some people. People with high blood cholesterol or high blood triglycerides often have no symptoms, so have both levels checked regularly. If your levels are high, talk to your doctor about what you can do to lower them. You may be able to lower your both levels by eating better and exercising more. Your doctor may prescribe medication to help lower your cholesterol.
- Add more fruits, vegetables, and whole grains to your diet.
- Each week, aim to get at least 2 hours and 30 minutes of moderate physical activity, 1 hour and 15 minutes of vigorous physical activity, or a combination of moderate and vigorous activity.
- If you drink alcohol, limit it to no more than one drink (one 12 ounce beer, one 5 ounce glass of wine, or one 1.5 ounce shot of hard liquor) a day.
- Find healthy ways to cope with stress. Lower your stress level by talking to your friends, exercising, or writing in a journal.

Chapters 15-18 give suggestions for reducing all of these risk factors.

What does high blood pressure have to do with heart disease?

Blood pressure is the measure of how forcefully your blood beats against the walls of the arteries. The pressure is highest when your heart pumps blood into your arteries during the heart beats. It is lowest between heart beats, when your heart relaxes. A doctor or nurse will write down your blood pressure as the higher number over the lower number. For instance, you could have a blood pressure of 110/70 (read as "110 over 70"). A blood pressure reading below 120/80 is usually considered normal. Very low blood pressure (lower than 90/60) can sometimes be a cause of concern and should be checked out by a doctor. High blood pressure, or hypertension, is a blood pressure reading of 140/90 or higher. Years of high blood pressure can damage artery walls, causing them to become stiff and narrow. This includes the arteries carrying blood to the heart, and your heart cannot get the blood it needs to work well. This can cause a heart attack.

How can I lower my blood pressure?

If you have hypertension or prehypertension, you may be able to lower your blood pressure by:
- Getting more physical activity each week.
- Limiting alcohol to one drink per day
- Quitting smoking if you smoke
- Reducing stress
- Cutting down on salt and sodium and eating healthy foods, such as fruits, vegetables.
- If lifestyle changes do not lower your blood pressure, your doctor may prescribe medicine.

What does high cholesterol have to do with heart disease?

Cholesterol is a waxy substance found in cells in all parts of the body. Too much cholesterol in your blood can build up on the walls of your arteries and cause blood clots. Cholesterol can clog your arteries and keep your heart from getting the blood it needs. This can cause a heart attack. There are three main measures of cholesterol:
- *Low-density lipoprotein* (LDL) is often called the "bad" type of cholesterol because it can clog the arteries that carry blood to your heart. For LDL, lower numbers are better.
- *High-density lipoprotein* (HDL) is known as "good" cholesterol because it takes the bad cholesterol out of your blood and keeps it from building up in your arteries. For HDL, higher numbers are better.
- *Triglycerides* are a measure of the breakdown of carbohydrates in the body. When too high, it gets stored in the hips and belly. Some experts think that triglyceride is the best measure of the effects of sugar on the body.

All women age 20 and older should have their blood cholesterol and triglyceride levels checked at least once every 5 years.

Table 6.1. What do cholesterol numbers mean?

Total cholesterol level – Lower is better. Less than 200 mg/dL is best.

Total cholesterol level	
Less than 200 mg/dL	Desirable
200 - 239 mg/dL	Borderline high
240 mg/dL and above	High

LDL (bad) cholesterol – Lower is better. Less than 100 mg/dL is best.

LDL cholesterol level	
Less than 100 mg/dL	Optimal
100-129 mg/dL	Near optimal/above optimal
130-159 mg/dL	Borderline high
160-189 mg/dL	High
190 mg/dL and above	Very high

HDL (good) cholesterol - Higher is better. More than 60 mg/dL is best.
Triglyceride levels - Lower is better. Less than 150mg/dL is best. Very high levels of triglyceride (500 and higher) are associated with heart disease.

Lowering cholesterol
- Get more fit if you are out of shape. Eat better. Eat foods low in *trans* fats, and added sugar. Eat more:
    o Fish, poultry (chicken, turkey--breast meat or drumstick is best), and lean meats (round, sirloin, tenderloin). Broil, bake, roast, or poach foods.
    o Fruits and vegetables (try for 5 a day)
    o Cereals, breads, rice, and pasta made from whole grains (such as "whole-wheat" or "whole-grain" bread and pasta, rye bread, brown rice, and oatmeal)
- Eat less:
    o Packaged and processed foods
    o Sugar
- Get moving. Exercise can help lower LDL ("bad cholesterol") and raise HDL ("good cholesterol").
- Take your medicine. If your doctor has prescribed medicine to lower your cholesterol, take it exactly as you have been told.

How do I know if I have heart disease?

Heart disease often has no symptoms. But, there are some signs to watch for. Chest or arm pain or discomfort can be a symptom of heart disease and a warning sign of a heart attack. Shortness of breath (feeling like you can't get enough air), dizziness, nausea (feeling sick to your stomach), abnormal heartbeats, or feeling very tired also are signs. Talk with your doctor if you're having any of these symptoms. Tell your doctor that you are concerned about your heart. Your doctor will take a medical history, do a physical exam, and may order tests.

What are the signs of a heart attack?

The most common sign of a heart attack is pain or discomfort in the center of the chest. The pain or discomfort can be mild or strong. It can last more than a few minutes, or it can go away and come back. Other common signs of a heart attack include:

- Pain or discomfort in one or both arms, back, neck, jaw, or stomach
- Shortness of breath (feeling like you can't get enough air). The shortness of breath often occurs before or along with the chest pain or discomfort.
- Nausea (feeling sick to your stomach) or vomiting
- Feeling faint or woozy
- Breaking out in a cold sweat

Women are more likely than men to have these other common signs of a heart attack, particularly shortness of breath, nausea or vomiting, and pain in the back, neck, or jaw. Women are also more likely to have less common signs of a heart attack, including:

- Heartburn
- Loss of appetite
- Feeling tired or weak
- Coughing
- Heart flutters

Sometimes the signs of a heart attack happen suddenly, but they can also develop slowly, over hours, days, and even weeks before a heart attack occurs. The more heart attack signs that you have, the more likely it is that you are having a heart attack. Also, if you've already had a heart attack, your symptoms may not be the same for another one. Even if you're not sure you're having a heart attack, you should still have it checked out. If you think you, or someone else, may be having a heart attack, wait no more than a few minutes—five at most—before calling 911.

Figure 6.3. Warning signs of a heart attack

Heart Attack: Warning Signs

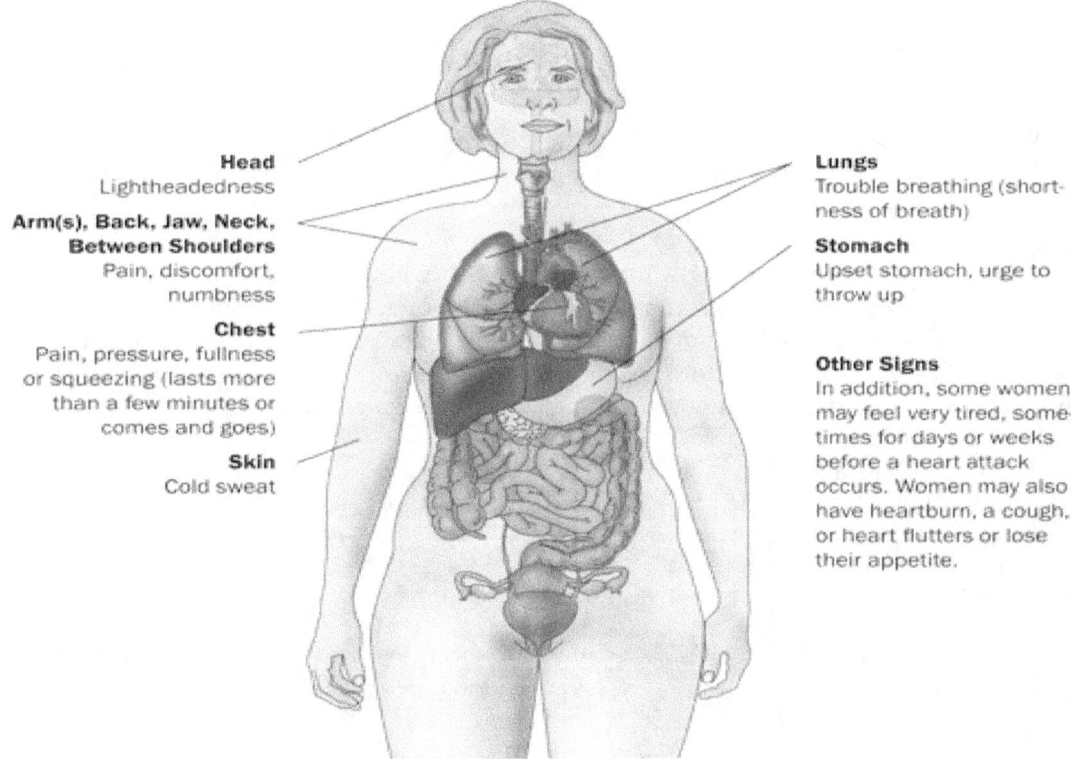

Head
Lightheadedness

Arm(s), Back, Jaw, Neck, Between Shoulders
Pain, discomfort, numbness

Chest
Pain, pressure, fullness or squeezing (lasts more than a few minutes or comes and goes)

Skin
Cold sweat

Lungs
Trouble breathing (shortness of breath)

Stomach
Upset stomach, urge to throw up

Other Signs
In addition, some women may feel very tired, sometimes for days or weeks before a heart attack occurs. Women may also have heartburn, a cough, or heart flutters or lose their appetite.

Family risk factors for heart attack

If your father or brother had a heart attack before age 55, or if your mother or sister had one before age 65, you are more likely to develop heart disease. This does not mean you will have a heart attack. It means you should take extra good care of your heart to keep it healthy.

What do changes in heart beat mean?

Most people have changes in their heartbeat from time to time. These changes in heartbeat are, for most people, harmless. As you get older, you're more likely to have heartbeats that feel different. Don't panic if you have a few flutters or if your heart races once in a while. If you have flutters *and* other symptoms such as dizziness or shortness of breath (feeling like you can't get enough air), call 911.

Should I take a daily aspirin to prevent heart attack?

Aspirin may be helpful for women at high risk, such as women who have already had a heart attack. Aspirin can have serious side effects and may be harmful when mixed with certain medicines. If you're thinking about taking aspirin, talk to your doctor first. If your doctor thinks aspirin is a good choice for you, be sure to take it exactly as your doctor tells you to.

Do birth control pills increase risk for heart disease?

Taking birth control pills is generally safe for young, healthy women if they do not smoke. But birth control pills can pose heart disease risks for some women, especially women older than 35; women with high blood pressure, diabetes, or high cholesterol; and women who smoke. Talk with your doctor if you have questions about the pill. If you're taking birth control pills, watch for signs of trouble, including:

- Eye problems such as blurred or double vision
- Pain in the upper body or arm

- Bad headaches
- Problems breathing
- Spitting up blood
- Swelling or pain in the leg
- Yellowing of the skin or eyes
- Breast lumps
- Unusual (not normal) heavy bleeding from your vagina

If you have any of these symptoms, call 911.

Does menopausal hormone therapy (MHT) increase risk for heart disease?

Menopausal hormone therapy (MHT) can help with some symptoms of menopause, including hot flashes, vaginal dryness, mood swings, and bone loss, but there are risks, too. For some women, taking hormones can increase their chances of having a heart attack or stroke. If you decide to use hormones, use them at the lowest dose that helps for the shortest time needed. Talk with your doctor if you have questions about MHT.

Table 6.2. How often to get screening tests

Recommended Schedule for Screening Tests

Recommended Screenings	How Often?	Starting when?
Blood pressure	Each regular healthcare visit or at least once every 2 years if blood pressure is less than 120/80 mm Hg	Age 20
Cholesterol ("fasting lipoprotein profile" to measure total, HDL and LDL cholesterol, and triglycerides)	Every 5 years for normal-risk people; more often if any of the following apply to you: • total cholesterol above 200 mg/dL • you are over age 50 • your HDL (good) cholesterol is less than 50 mg/dL • you have other risk factors for heart disease and stroke	Age 20
Waist circumference	As needed to help evaluate cardiovascular risk	Age 20
Blood glucose test	Every 3 years	Age 45
Discuss smoking, physical activity, diet	Each regular healthcare visit	Age 20

Reducing Risk for Stroke

Essentially, the same risk factors for heart disease are risk factors for stroke. In February of 2014, the U.S. government released new guidelines for prevention of stroke in women. They are:

- Before taking birth control pills, women should be screened for high blood pressure because of the associated increased stroke risk.
- Women who suffer from migraine headaches with aura should stop smoking to reduce stroke risk.
- Low-dose aspirin and/or calcium supplement therapy should be considered for women with a history of high blood pressure before pregnancy in order to reduce preeclampsia risk.
- Preeclampsia should be seen as a risk factor for stroke long after pregnancy, since women who have the condition have twice the risk of stroke and four times the risk of high blood pressure later in life.
- Women who have preeclampsia should be treated early for obesity, smoking and high cholesterol.
- Women over the age of 75 should be screened for atrial fibrillation because of its association with increased stroke risk.

- Pregnant women with severe high blood pressure (160/110 mmHg or above) should be treated with blood pressure medication, while expectant mothers with moderately high blood pressure (150-159 mmHg/100-109 mmHg) should be considered for treatment.

ASTHMA

Asthma is a lung disease. It is one of the most common long-term diseases of children, but adults can also have asthma that starts in childhood and persists, or has its onset in adulthood. Asthma causes wheezing, breathlessness, chest tightness, and coughing at night or early in the morning. If you have asthma, you have it all the time, but you will have asthma attacks only when something bothers your lungs. In most cases, we do not know what causes asthma or how to cure it. We know that if someone in your family has asthma you are more likely to have it. About 8% of the adult population in the U.S. has asthma.

Signs of Asthma

It can be hard to tell if someone has asthma. Having a healthcare provider check how well your lungs work and check for allergies can help you find out if you have asthma. During a checkup, the healthcare provider will ask if you cough a lot, especially at night, and whether your breathing problems are worse after physical activity or at certain times of year. Other diagnostic questions are about chest tightness, wheezing, and colds lasting more than 10 days; whether anyone in your family has or has had asthma, allergies, or other breathing problems; and conditions about your home. One test for asthma is a breathing test, called spirometry, to find out how well your lungs are working. The doctor will use a computer with a mouthpiece to test how much air you can breathe out after taking a very deep breath. The spirometer can measure airflow before and after you use asthma medicine.

Lesbian/Bisexual Women and Asthma

There is quite a bit of evidence that lesbian and bisexual women have higher rates of asthma than heterosexual women. In reviewing data from national and statewide studies, nine out of 10 studies that reported differences found lesbian/bisexual women to have higher rates of asthma, running from about 10 to 32% for lesbian/bisexual women compared to 8-17% for heterosexual women (Eliason, 2014). Reasons for this increase are not known, although lesbian and bisexual women have higher rates of smoking, which could account for some of the increase. It's also possible that lesbian/bisexual women live in poorer neighborhoods where there are more pollutants. As noted in the section on smoking, more lesbian and bisexual women are exposed to smoke in the workplace and at home than are heterosexual women.

What Is an Asthma Attack?

An asthma attack may include coughing, chest tightness, wheezing, and trouble breathing. The attack happens in your body's airways, which are the paths that carry air to your lungs. As the air moves through your lungs, the airways become smaller, like the branches of a tree are smaller than the tree trunk. During an asthma attack, the sides of the airways in your lungs swell and the airways shrink. Less air gets in and out of your lungs, and mucous that your body makes clogs up the airways even more. You can control your asthma by knowing the warning signs of an asthma attack, staying away from things that cause an attack, and following your doctor's advice. When you control your asthma:

- you won't have symptoms such as wheezing or coughing,
- you'll sleep better,
- you won't miss work or school,
- you can take part in all physical activities, and
- you won't have to go to the hospital.

What Causes an Asthma Attack?

An asthma attack can happen when you are exposed to "asthma triggers." Your triggers can be very different from those of someone else with asthma. Know your triggers and learn how to avoid them. Watch out for an attack when you can't avoid the triggers. Some of the most common triggers are:

- **Tobacco Smoke.** Tobacco smoke is unhealthy for everyone, but especially people with asthma. If you have asthma and you smoke, quit smoking. "Secondhand smoke" is created by being near a smoker and breathing in their smoke. Secondhand smoke can trigger an asthma attack. If you have asthma, people should never smoke near you, in your home, in your car, or wherever you may spend a lot of time.
- **Dust Mites.** Dust mites are tiny bugs that are in almost every home. If you have asthma, dust mites can trigger an asthma attack. To prevent attacks, use mattress covers and pillowcase covers to make a barrier between dust mites and yourself. Don't use down-filled pillows, quilts, or comforters. Remove stuffed animals and clutter from your bedroom. Wash sheets and blankets weekly.
- **Outdoor Air Pollution.** Outdoor air pollution can trigger an asthma attack. This pollution can come from factories, automobiles, and other sources. Pay attention to air quality forecasts on radio, television, and the Internet and check your newspaper to plan your activities for when air pollution levels will be low.
- **Cockroach Allergen.** Cockroaches and their droppings can trigger an asthma attack. Get rid of cockroaches in your home by removing as many water and food sources as you can. Cockroaches are often found where food is eaten and crumbs are left behind. At least every 2 to 3 days, vacuum or sweep areas that might attract cockroaches. Use roach traps or gels to cut down on the number of cockroaches in your home.
- **Pets.** Furry pets can trigger an asthma attack. If you think a furry pet may be causing attacks, you may want to find the pet another home. If you can't or don't want to find a new home for the pet, keep it out of the person with asthma's bedroom. Bathe pets every week and keep them outside as much as you can. People with asthma are not allergic to their pet's fur, so trimming the pet's fur will not help your asthma. If you have a furry pet, vacuum often. If your floors have a hard surface, such as wood or tile, damp mop them every week.
- **Mold.** Breathing in mold can trigger an asthma attack. Get rid of mold in your home to help control your attacks. Humidity, the amount of moisture in the air, can make mold grow. An air conditioner or dehumidifier will help you keep the humidity level low. Get a small tool called a hygrometer to check humidity levels and keep them as low as you can—no higher than 50%. Humidity levels change over the course of a day, so check the humidity levels more than once a day. Fix water leaks, which let mold grow behind walls and under floors.
- **Smoke From Burning Wood or Grass.** Smoke from burning wood or other plants is made up of a mix of harmful gases and small particles. Breathing in too much of this smoke can cause an asthma attack. If you can, avoid burning wood in your home. If a wildfire is causing poor air quality in your area pay attention to air quality forecasts on radio, television, and the Internet and check your newspaper to plan your activities for when air pollution levels will be low.
- **Other Triggers**
  - Infections linked to influenza (flu), colds, and respiratory syncytial virus (RSV) can trigger an asthma attack. Sinus infections, allergies, breathing in some chemicals, and acid reflux can also trigger attacks.
  - Burning incense or candles, of any kind, can be a source of particulate matter, which may trigger an asthma attack in some individuals.
  - Physical exercise; some medicines; bad weather, such as thunderstorms or high humidity; breathing in cold, dry air; and some foods, food additives, and fragrances can also trigger an asthma attack.
  - Strong emotions can lead to very fast breathing, called hyperventilation, that can also cause an asthma attack.

How Is Asthma Treated?

Medications and staying away from things that can trigger an attack are the main treatments. Everyone with asthma does not take the same medicine. **Some medicines can be breathed in (inhaled),** and some can be taken as a pill. Asthma medicines come in two types—quick-relief and long-term control. Quick-relief medicines control the symptoms of an asthma attack. If you need to use your quick-relief medicines more and more, visit your doctor to see if you need a different medicine. Long-term control medicines help you have fewer and milder attacks, but they don't help you while you are having an asthma attack.

Asthma medicines can have side effects, but most side effects are mild and soon go away. Ask your healthcare provider or pharmacist about the side effects of your medicines. With your healthcare provider's help, make your own asthma action plan. Decide who should have a copy of your plan and where he or she should keep it. Take your long-term control medicine even when you don't have symptoms.

In conclusion, this chapter has discussed some of the most common chronic illnesses that affect people particularly as they age. Lesbian and bisexual women may have higher rates of some of these disorders, such as asthma, and similar rates to heterosexual women on most of the others. All of these disorders are preventable to some extent through physical activity and healthy eating. In addition, the symptom severity can be reduced by making healthier choices related to activity and food, and finding healthier ways to deal with stress.

Resources

The basic information about the physical health disorders described in this chapter comes from the Centers for Disease Control and Prevention (www.cdc.gov). They provide information for consumers and healthcare providers about diagnosis, treatment, and statistics about who gets what disorder.

REFERENCES

Agrawal, R., Sharma, S., Bekin, J., Conway, G., Bailey, J., et al. (2004). Prevalence of polycystic ovaries and PCOS in lesbian women compared with heterosexual women. *Fertility and Sterility, 82*, 1352-1357.

American Cancer Society, Surveillance Research, 2013.

American Cancer Society (2013). Cancer Facts & Figures 2013. **Atlanta: American Cancer Society.** Available on the web at http://www.cancer.org/research/cancerfactsstatistics/index

American Cancer Society (2011). Colorectal Cancer Facts & Figures 2011-2013. **Atlanta: American Cancer Society.** Available on the web at http://www.cancer.org/research/cancerfactsstatistics/index

Austin SB, Pazaris MJ, Rosner B, Bowen D, Rich-Edwards J, Spiegelman D. Application of the Rosner-Colditz risk prediction model to estimate sexual orientation group disparities in breast cancer risk in a U.S. cohort of premenopausal women. *Cancer Epidemiol Biomarkers Prev. 21*(12):2201-8, 2012.

Austin SB, Pazaris MJ, Nichols LP, Bowen D, Wei EK, Spiegelman D. An examination of sexual orientation group patterns in mammographic and colorectal screening in a cohort of U.S. women. *Cancer Causes Control.* 24(3):539-47, 2013.

Boehmer, U., Miao, X., Linkletter, C., Clark, M.A. (2012). Adult health behaviors over the life course by sexual orientation. *American Journal of Public Health. 102*(2):292-300, 2012.

Brandenburg DL, Matthews AK, Johnson TP, Hughes TL. Breast cancer risk and screening: a comparison of lesbian and heterosexual women. *Womens Health.* 45(4):109-30, 2007.

Brown, JP & Tracy J.K (2008). Lesbians and cancer: An overlooked health disparity. *Cancer Causes & Control, 19*, 1009-1020.

Case P, Austin SB, Hunter DJ, et al. (2004). Sexual orientation, health risk factors, and physical functioning in the Nurses' Health Study II. *Journal of Womens Health (Larchmt). 13*(9):1033-47, 2004.

Cochran, S D., & Mays, V.M. (2007). **Physical health complaints among LGB and homosexually experienced heterosexual individuals: results from the California Quality of Life Survey.** *American Journal of Public Health, 97*, 2048-2055.

Cochran, S.D., & Mays, V.M. (2012). Risk of breast cancer mortality among women cohabiting with same sex partners: findings from the national health interview survey, 1997-2003. *Journal of Womens Health* (Larchmt). 21(5):528-33, 2012.

Cochran, S.D., & Mays, V.M. (2014). Mortality risks among persons reporting same-sex sexual partners: Evidence from the 2008 General Social Survey, National Death Index Data Set. *American Journal of Public Health,*

Conron, K.J., Mimiaga, M.J. & Landers, S.J. (2010). A population-based study of sexual orientation identity and gender differences in adult health. *American Journal of Public Health, 100*(10), 1953-1060.

DeSutter, P., Dutre, T., Vanden, Meerschant, F., Stuyver, I, Van Maele, G., & Dhont, M. (2008). PCOS in lesbian and heterosexual women treated with artificial donor insemination. *Reproductive Biomedicine Online, 17,* 398-402.

Dilley, J., Simmons, K.W., Boysun, M.J., Pizacani, B.A., & Stark, M.J. (2010). Demonstrating the importance and feasibility of including sexual orientation in public health surveys: Health disparities in the Pacific Northwest. *American Journal of Public Health, 100*(3), 460-467.

Eliason, M.J. (2014). Chronic physical health problems in sexual minority women: Review of the literature. *LGBT Health, 1* (4), 258-269.

Farmer, G.W., Jabson, J.M., Bucholz, K.K., & Bowen, D.J. (2013). A population-based study of cardiovascular disease risk in sexual minority women. *American Journal of Public Health,* published online ahead of print, doi: 10.2105/AJPH.2013.301258.

Fredriksen-Goldsen, K., Kim, H., Barkan, S.,Muraco, A., & Hoy-Ellis, C.P. (2013). Health disparities among lesbian, gay, and bisexual older adults: results from a population-based study. *American Journal of Public Health*, e1-e8; doi: 10.2105/AJPH. 2012.301110.

Frisch, M, Smith, E, Grulick, A, & Johansen, C (2003). Cancer in a population-based cohort of men and women in registered homosexual partnerships. *American Journal of Epidemiology 157*, 966-972.

Gaudet, M.M, Gapstur, S.M., Sun J, Diver WR, Hannan LM, Thun MJ. (2013). Active smoking and breast cancer risk: original cohort data and meta-analysis. *Journal of the National Cancer Institute,* 105(8):515-25. doi: 10.1093/jnci/djt023. Epub 2013 Feb 28.

Margolies, L. Lesbians and breast cancer risk. Downloaded 9/4/13 from http://www.cancer-network.org/cancer_information/lesbians_and_cancer/lesbians_and_breast_cancer.php.

Mays, V.M., Yancey, A.K., Cochran, S.D., Weber, M., & Fielding, J.E. (2002). Heterogeneity of health disparities among African American, Hispanic, and Asian American women: Unrecognized influences of sexual orientation. *American Journal of Public Health, 92*(4), 632-639.

National Cancer Institute (2006). What you need to know about cancer of the colon and rectum. National Institutes of Health, US Department of Health and Human Services. Available on the web at www.cancer.gov/cancertopics/types/colon-and-rectal

Smith, H. A., Markovic, N., Matthews, A. K., Danielson, M. E., Kalro, B. N., Youk, A. O., et al. (2011). A comparison of polycystic ovary syndrome and related factors between lesbian and heterosexual women. *Women's Health Issues, 21,* 191–198.

Zaritsky E, & Dibble S.L. (2010). Risk factors for reproductive and breast cancers among older lesbians. *Journal of Womens Health (Larchmt), 19*(1):125-31.

Chapter 7: Disability

A disability is a condition that interferes with a person's ability to function in the world, and to do activities of daily living, like dressing, bathing, preparing a meal, and getting about. Disabilities can be mainly physical mobility differences or related to mental health or intellectual/cognitive differences. Lesbian and bisexual women with disabilities are an invisible segment of an already invisible minority group, and may be stigmatized in lesbian communities in ways we rarely think about.   For example, the terminology we use, such as "sexual identities," places the emphasis on our sexual differences as lesbian and bisexual women. In other words, we are defined in society primarily by our sexuality. On the other hand, people with disabilities are often treated as children, and rendered asexual, so doubly invisible as potential lesbian/bisexual women. The language of pride and resiliency that we often use as lesbian/bisexual women, such as independent, strong, athletic, and so on, may unintentionally place greater value on able-bodiedness than on our other characteristics (O'Toole & Brown, 2003). We all want to be able to "do it for ourselves" but there are multiple ways of doing, and different ways to be "able." Some women are born with a disability and others acquire them later from accidents or illnesses. The coming out experience and sexual identity milestones might be experienced differently by these groups: women who are already out and in relationships before acquiring a disability are perceived differently than women who have the disability first, then come out.

DISABILITY IN LESBIAN/BISEXUAL WOMEN

The research shows that we are more prone to having disabilities, but there has been so little detailed study of the issues that we cannot say what kind of disabilities or how they impact our communities. In the past few years, statewide health surveys have started asking questions about sexual identity, so we have some data on the frequency of disabilities in the population. Unfortunately, these big health surveys ask only a question or two about any issue, so they provide superficial information. In regards to the question about having a disability that impairs activities of daily living, lesbian and bisexual women are more likely to say "yes" than heterosexual women. In a study of women over 50 from Washington state, 44% of lesbian/bisexual compared to 37% of heterosexual women had a physical disability (Fredriksen-Goldsen, Kim, Barkan, et al., 2013). A national study of LGBT people with an average age of 65, found that 53% of lesbians and 51% of bisexual women reported a disability (Fredriksen-Goldsen et al, 2013). Neither study asked about the types of disability or how long the woman had the disability, or how it affected her life.

Susan Cochran and Vickie Mays of UCLA (2007) looked at California women on three questions about disability, as shown below. This study suggests that there may not be a big difference in the number of women who have major physical disabilities, so the differences compared to heterosexual women might be related to mental health, substance abuse, or other types of disability. A lifetime of struggling with mental health symptoms or the long-term consequences of drug, alcohol, or tobacco use on the body and mind may account for the higher rates of disability among lesbian and bisexual women. There is no evidence that genetic disorders or disabilities acquired very early in life would be any more common among lesbian/bisexual women.

Figure 7.1. Disability among California women (from Cochran & Mays, 2007)

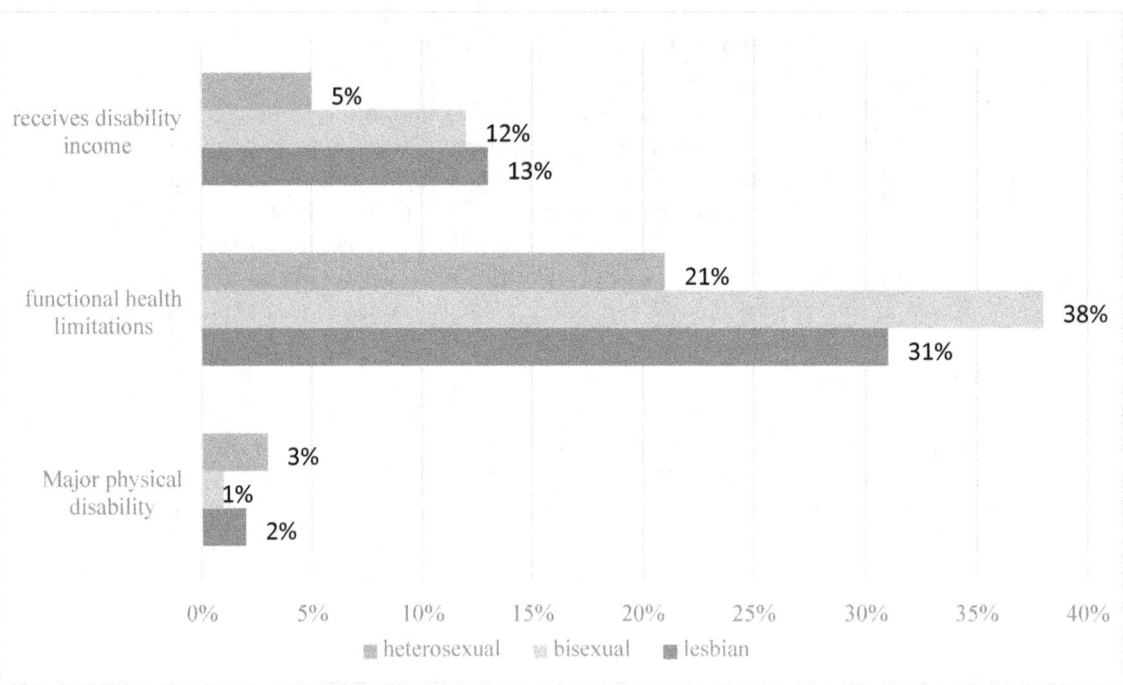

Legend: heterosexual, bisexual, lesbian

Category	heterosexual	bisexual	lesbian
receives disability income	5%	12%	13%
functional health limitations	21%	38%	31%
Major physical disability	3%	1%	2%

Inclusion in Lesbian Communities

Whether the disability is genetic and lifelong or acquired later in life, the way that lesbian and bisexual women's communities address disabilities is critical. Inclusion is a key component of a healthy community. Some women with disabilities have found our communities to be less than welcoming. One woman interviewed by Whitney (2006, p. 40), said,

> "We are seen, and see ourselves, as outsiders. Outside the mainstream, rejected by the disability community, excluded by the lesbian world. We have no community of our own."

Why have so many able-bodied lesbian and bisexual women ignored the needs of disabled women? Some think that people with disabilities remind us of our own mortality, spark fears of becoming disabled ourselves (which is always a possibility), and create discomfort because we don't know how to communicate in a sensitive way, with people who are different from us. We might not even recognize women with disabilities as being lesbian or bisexual because of the stereotypes that disability renders a person asexual. As we age, we may become more aware of the need for physically accessible spaces, and more aware of the needs of community members with visual and hearing differences. Our communities have work to do to deal with our own ableism and we have to be willing to make mistakes and learn from them.

DIFO Research on Disability

DIFO actively recruited women with disabilities to our program. The DIFO team analyzed data from the women with disabilities in our first round of groups (Eliason, Martinson, and Carabez, 2015). In our initial pool of 126 women, 52 reported having a disability, so we are able to provide at least some description of the strengths and challenges of women with disabilities compared to women without disabilities. We found some differences and many similarities between lesbian/bisexual women with and without physical disabilities. Here are ways that disabled and not disabled women were the same: both groups were an average age of 61, both groups were well-educated, with about half having graduate degrees from college, and both groups were equally likely to be out to family, friends, coworkers, and health care providers. They were equally likely to be in relationships and be satisfied with their relationships.

Some of the most significant ways that disabled women differed from nondisabled women were in terms of economic resources. Their annual household income as about $42,500 compared to $77,700 for women who were not disabled. Disabled women were more likely to be on some form of public assistance for health care rather than private insurance, and more were unable to work. In terms of sexual orientation measures, the women with disabilities were more likely to report a "butch" identity (22%) than the non-disabled women (7%), and were more likely to identify as gender queer (6%) and have a transgender partner (10%) than disabled women (none reported either a gender queer identity or a transgender partner). Disabled women were also less likely to feel a strong connection to a lesbian/bisexual women's community (19%) than nondisabled women (31%). Women with disabilities were also larger women, with a higher weight and a higher BMI. Did weight contribute to the disability, or did challenges with physical activity because of the disability cause weight gain? We could not answer this question.

Some of the largest differences between women with and without disabilities were related to experiences with discrimination. Some of these findings are shown in the figure below. Women with disabilities had more frequent experiences of being treated differently and more poorly than did women without disabilities. When asked about the source of discrimination, most disabled women said it was because of their weight (41%) or sex/gender (32%), compared to nondisabled women who reported weight discrimination (27%) and sex/gender (23%) at lower rates. Few women in either group thought that they were discriminated against because of their sexuality, which makes sense, because sexuality is not a visible difference to strangers.

Figure 7.2. Discrimination experiences of disabled and nondisabled lesbian and bisexual women (from Eliason, Martinson, & Carabez, 2015)

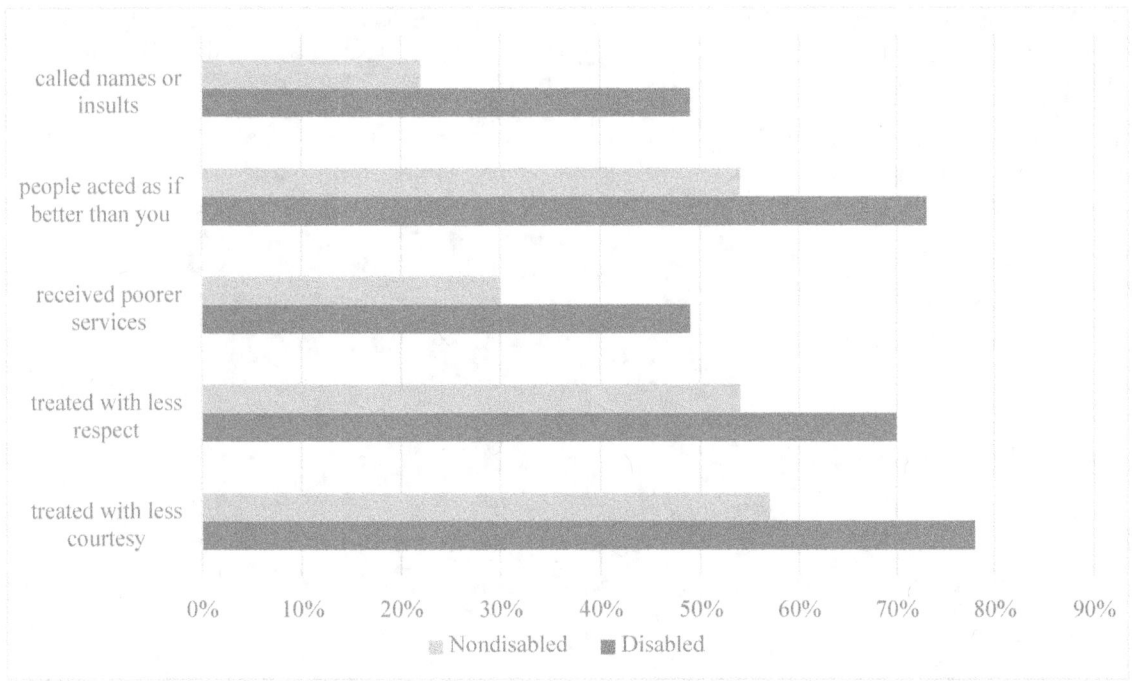

One of the women who helped us to design the DIFO program to be more sensitive to the issues of women with disabilities made a provocative statement in one of our meetings. She said, "we have been in training all of our lives to be independent elders" (Corbett O'Toole, 2014). How very true, and how sad that our lesbian and bisexual communities have not yet fully included women with disabilities who could add so much wisdom and practical advice about accommodations for changing bodies as we age.

In conclusion, we have much to learn yet about the experiences of lesbian and bisexual women with disabilities. The lack of financial resources in most lesbian/bisexual women's communities may interfere with a goal of full physical inclusion, and a combination of ableism and fears of becoming disabled oneself may interfere with full social inclusion.

Resources:
Fabled Asp (Fabulous/Activist Bay Area Lesbians with Disabilities) (www.fabledasp.com)

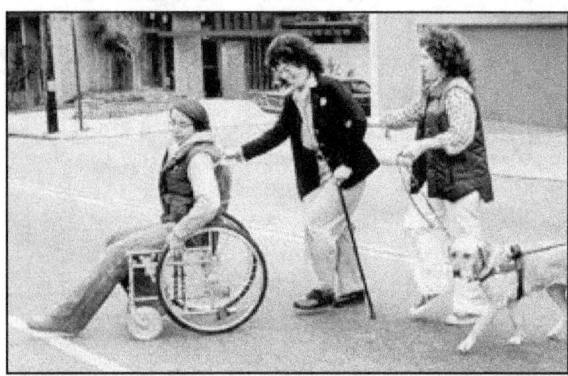

REFERENCES

Brownworth, V.A. & Raffo, S. (1999). *Restricted access: Lesbians on disability.* Boston: Seal Press.

Cochran, S D., & Mays, V.M. (2007). Physical health complaints among LGB and homosexually experienced heterosexual individuals: results from the California Quality of Life Survey. *American Journal of Public Health, 97,* 2048-2055.

Eliason, M.J., Martinson, M., & Carabez, R. (2015). Sexual minority women with disabilities. *LGBT Health,* 2(1),

Fredriksen-Goldsen, K., Kim, H., & Barkan, S. (2012). Disability among lesbian, gay, and bisexual adults: Disparities in prevalence and risk. *American Journal of Public Health, 102,* 16–21.

O'Toole, C.J., & Brown, A.A. (2003). No reflection in the mirror: Challenges for disabled lesbians accessing mental health services. *Journal of Lesbian Studies, 7(*1), 35-49.

Whitney, C. (2006). Intersections in identity—identity development among queer women with disabilities. *Sexuality and Disability, 24*(1), 39-52.

Chapter 8: Sexual Health

An active sex life is a goal for many lesbian and bisexual women as they age, but there are no guidelines about what constitutes a "normal" or healthy sex life. For some, the choice to be celibate feels right; others identify as asexual and seek out intimacy in different ways—they may prefer relationships with women, but not sex. But most lesbian/bisexual women wish to continue to be sexual as they age, because sex has so many beneficial effects on one's health and wellbeing. In fact, research has found that an active sex life:

- Keeps the immune system healthier
- Boosts libido
- Improves bladder control…and reduces incontinence which affects about 30% of women
- Lowers blood pressure
- Can be a form of exercise (burns 5 calories per minute: compared to 1 calorie per minute watching TV; sex raises the heart rate)
- Lowers heart attack risk
- Decreases pain
- Improves sleep (prolactin, a natural relaxer, is released after orgasm)
- Eases stress and improves relationship satisfaction

Common changes in the body that affect sexuality as we age include:

- We start to dry up! Skin and mucus membranes get drier, and easier to tear. This includes the vagina. Luckily, we can easily buy lubrication at the drug store along with our skin moisturizer.
- We are slower to get to orgasm. This makes sense since we tend to get slower in everything else! Some women, though, get self-conscious about taking longer and may avoid sex because of fears that our partners will get tired of trying to bring them to orgasm.
- Health problems like arthritis and joint issues may interfere and require adjustments in sexual positions.
- Medications for, or chronic health problems like heart disease or diabetes, might decrease our perceptions of sexual desire or alter our perceptions of our own attractiveness.

OVERCOMING NEGATIVE SOCIALIZATION ABOUT SEX

Sometimes we choose to self-medicate or soothe negative emotions related to our anxieties about the physical body and being sexual with our partners/girlfriends. Fears related to intimacy and sexual activity seem to underlie some substance abuse. Where do these fears and anxieties about sex/intimacy come from? The answer is in socialization about sex—the things we are taught by parents, family, religion, school, and peers about sexuality. These social norms about sex are highly gendered and women learn very different norms about sex than do most men. These norms are changing, partly as a result of greater access to information about sexuality on the internet, but lots of that information is also biased and stereotypical. Most of us were not socialized to be the initiators of sex, and some of us got virtually no sexuality education at home or school. If we did, it did not include anything about sex with women! Here are some common myths that are spread by informal socialization about sex:

- Men are supposed to initiate sex; women are the gatekeepers who say no. Where does this leave lesbian and bisexual women in relationships with other women? Do you think it is hard for women to learn to initiate sex?
- Women are taught that menstruation is "dirty," "messy," and something to hide. How do you feel about your own menstruation and that of your partner?
- Many of us were taught that women's role is as a mother. How does this affect how women view sex? menopause? Do you think lesbian/bisexual women are different?

- Male sexuality is defined as active and dominant; female sexuality as passive and submissive. Again, where does this leave women who have sex with other women? What happens when both members of a couple are passive?
- Sex is defined in so many contexts as "penetration." Heterosexual penis in the vagina sex is almost the only kind of sex that is covered in school sex education, and stands as the prototype for sexual activity. It ignores all the other sensual and sexual activities that provide pleasure and intimacy.
- Sex is defined as orgasm, leading to unrealistic expectations that orgasm is always the goal. It may prevent us from engaging in very pleasurable activities that would enhance our relationships, just because we don't have time or energy for an orgasm. Sometimes what we need is sensuality.
- Many of us were taught that "lesbian sex" is sinful or immoral. Some are taught that any pleasure in sexual activities is sinful; that sex is a duty to procreate not a means of experiencing pleasure. How have religious or moral beliefs affected your sexual relationships in the past?
- Societal stereotypes imply that older women are asexual, grandmotherly types. Is it harder to stay sexual as we age? Why? How?

All of these myths and stereotypes about sexuality can lead to feelings of shame and guilt in women who internalized them. Women who have anxieties about sex and the body may use alcohol or drugs to loosen up inhibitions, eat and gain weight to avoid being seen as a sexual being, or engage in any number of other unhealthy coping mechanisms. When we come out as lesbian or bisexual, no one gives us "sex education" about how to behave with our partners, how to express what we want or don't want in a sexual relationship, or how to even start a conversation about sex without triggering our own or her anxieties. As women get older and their bodies change, they may have to re-negotiate how they practice sexuality with a partner. To start to re-frame negative feelings about the body and sexuality, consider these questions:

- What parts of your body give you pleasure? How?
- Consider the parts of your body that give you anxiety…try stroking those parts and telling them they are ok just the way they are. How does it feel to be kind and gentle to your own body? You can be your own best lover!

SEXUALLY TRANSMITTED INFECTIONS

Most sexually transmitted infections (STIs) can be passed from one woman to another, so lesbian/bisexual women do need to consider using safer sex techniques especially when in new or open relationships. Some of the common STIs in lesbians include bacterial vaginosis (a shift in the normal bacteria in the vagina from lactobacillus to an overgrowth of bugs that can cause problems like pelvic inflammatory disease and increase susceptibility to other STIs). One study (Marrazzo et al., 2002) found 27% of lesbians compared to 24% of heterosexual women had bacterial vaginosis (they were younger women, though, and we don't know what happens over time). Chlamydia is also a very common STI with around 7% of women who only have sex with women reporting it. Genital herpes affects around 3% of women who have never had sex with men, and more who have, so it can obviously be spread between women (Marrazzo, 2010).

The typical sex education in a primary care office—use a condom—just does not work in female same-sex relationships! In general, though, just use common sense. Most infections are spread by direct contact with bodily fluids, so using barriers between you and the fluid reduces risks. This might include gloves, dental dams (or non-microwaveable Saran wrap for a less expensive and easier to find option), and putting condoms on penetrative sex toys. Carefully wash sex toys between uses because some viruses, like the ones that cause herpes and HPV, can live for a longtime on a sex toy. Sex during menstruation carries slightly more risk than sex during other times.

THE ROLE OF CHILDHOOD SEXUAL ABUSE (CSA)

Many studies now confirm that lesbian and bisexual women are more likely to report a history of childhood sexual abuse (Aaron & Hughes, 2007; Alvy, Hughes, Kristjanson, & Wilsnack, 2013; Austin et al, 2008; Balsam et al, 2005; Corliss, et al, 2002; Hughes et al, 2010; Stoddard et al, 2009). The figure below shows some very recent figures on both sexual and physical abuse in childhood.

Figure 8.1. Rates of child abuse by sexual identity (Anderson, Hughes, Zou, & Wilsnack, 2014)

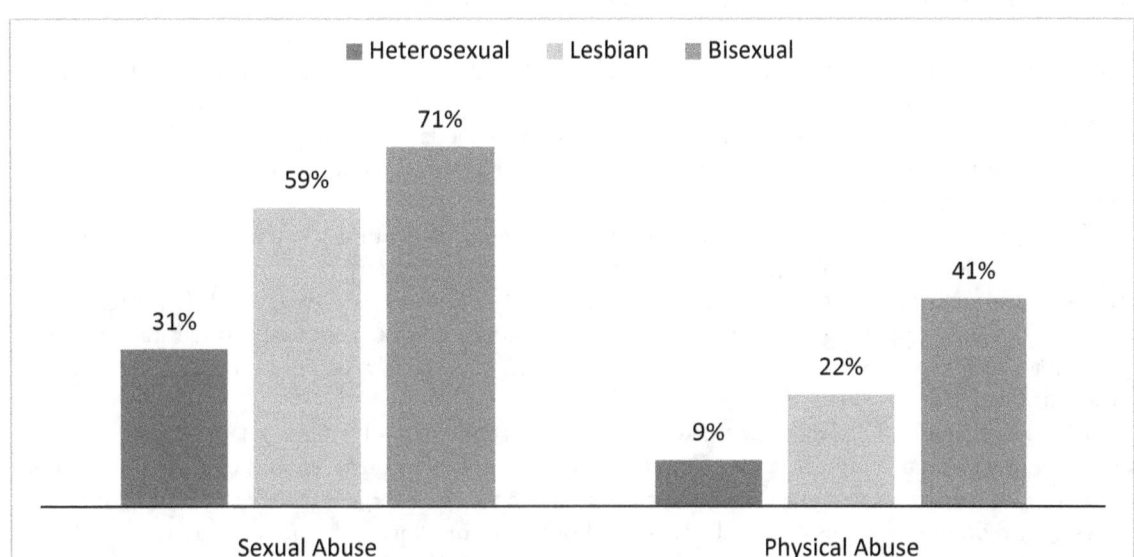

We do not yet know the reason for this. Some suggest that lesbian/bisexual women have learned how to be more open and talk about vulnerable topics, stemming from their experience of coming out. Therefore, they are more willing to share other highly personal information, such as abuse histories, than are heterosexual women. Another possibility is that there is a real difference, and lesbian/bisexual women really did experience more abuse. Perhaps it is one factor that contributes to a minority sexual identification. But why bisexual women have such an extremely high rate of abuse is a mystery.

Just knowing that the rates of abuse are higher does not tell us anything about how the abuse history affects a woman's sexual functioning in adulthood. For many heterosexual women, there are long-term consequences, with some formerly abused women becoming very sexually active, and others unable to have sex without mood-altering substances. It is likely that a sexual abuse history has widely mixed effects on lesbian/bisexual women, and may underlie the higher rates of substance abuse, mental health problems, and possibly, higher weight/BMI. Smith and colleagues (2010) found that women who were considered obese were more likely to have a history of childhood sexual abuse, regardless of sexual identity than women at other weight levels (see also Aaron & Hughes, 2007). In another study, lesbians with a BMI of 30 or more reported higher rates of lifetime sexual abuse (64%) than heterosexual women with similar BMIs (44%) (Lehavot, Molina, & Simoni, 2012), suggesting that childhood abuse experiences had even greater impact on weight of lesbians than heterosexual women.

Women who feel that sexual abuse histories are negatively affecting their current lives could benefit from seeking therapy to help them release any feelings of shame, guilt, or self-blaming that may stand in the way of their future happiness. Finding a therapist who is comfortable dealing with lesbian/bisexual women's sexuality is critical to success.

LESBIAN BED DEATH: FACT OR FICTION?

We have all heard this term---it is a common source of jokes by lesbian stand-up comics. So is it true? The term lesbian bed death is often attributed to a heterosexual sociologist, Pepper Schwartz, who did a study in the late 1970s and early 80s about the sex lives of American couples. She included heterosexual, gay male, and lesbian couples in the study, and found that long-term lesbian couples had less sex than the other two types of couples, and reported less variety in their sex lives as well. The fact that this term, lesbian bed death, entered our community vocabulary suggests there might be some truth to the concept, however, there has not been a lot of research on lesbian or bisexual women's sexuality. Some lesbian authors, however, have speculated on the causes of lesbian bed death. Joanne Loulan, a well-known lesbian sex therapist of the 1970s proposed that the lesbian tendency to fuse or merge might be the culprit. She suggested that lesbians spend so much time cuddling and petting each other, and get so emotionally enmeshed that it destroys the sex drive. That is, we like the sensual parts of touching and caressing (what some label as foreplay) but stop there. The problem might be how we define sex. If as noted above, we define sex as penetration or as orgasm, we leave out a wide range of activities that could be considered sex.

Leslie Lange, author of Dyke Drama, proposed that lesbian bed death is just a natural stage in the lesbian relationship cycle. The first phase, romance, includes sex marathons and frequent surges of sexual desire. The body eventually cannot keep up the pace, so we are forced into phase two, which Lange calls the "lesbian sexual rejuvenation phase." The tragedy is that many couples do not recognize this natural slowing down of the sexual activity and break up before they can advance to stage 3, which is a more moderate and sustainable sex life.

Another factor might be boredom. It takes work to stay actively involved in a relationship, try new things, and continue to romance our partners. Sometimes it is just easier to break up and develop a new crush with the surge of adrenalin rush that goes with it. Or we do not have the energy to break up, so just settle for a celibate lifestyle. In other cases, the so-called lesbian bed death occurs during the peak of career and family. This couple are so highly involved in child care, planning brunches and lesbian concerts, running a community non-profit, and reading for the monthly book club meetings, that they are too tired for sex.

At this point, there is no real evidence that lesbians experience a greater slowing down or higher rates of celibate relationships than heterosexual women. All relationships change over time, and if we are not comfortable talking directly about sex, our sex lives may disappear. One study of lesbians over 50 (Averet et al, 2012) found that about 1% reported having sex every day; 11% once a week; 12% once a month, 20% a few times a year, and 45% reported no sex in the past year. But part of the lack of sex was explained by changes in the perceptions of the importance of sex from 45% saying it was very important to them before the age of 55, but only 20% rating sex as very important after the age of 55. They reported that their relationships were now more mature, stable, and emotionally closer. The study found that women who were more positive about aging were also more likely to be satisfied with their sex lives. Another study (Cohen & Byers, 2014) surveyed almost 600 women who had been in committed relationships with other women for at least a year. The vast majority reported affectionate behaviors every day (82% kissing, 92% hugging or cuddling, 53% full body contact). 72% reported oral sex in the past month and most had touched their partners breasts or genitals in the past month. There was a decrease in genital activities in couples that had been together for 10 years or more, and some had lower sexual satisfaction, but the majority of couples stayed sexually active. One area where female same-sex couples differ from women in relationships with men is in the duration of sex. The women in the Cohen and Byers study reported that sex lasted about 57 minutes; this is in comparison to heterosexual women who reported a duration of 18 minutes!

There is much less information available on the sex lives of bisexual women unless you take a look at internet pornography, which would lead you to conclude that they spend 90% of their waking hours in sexual activities. We might assume that bisexual women in relationships with other women would be similar to relationships between two lesbians, but there is a need for research on whether female same-sex relationships differ based on the individual identities of the women involved.

INTIMATE PARTNER VIOLENCE

One of the taboo topics in some lesbian/bisexual women's communities is that of intimate partner violence (called domestic violence in older studies). Intimate partner violence in women in relationships with other women were invisible in the mainstream research because feminist researchers once thought violence was "gendered" so that men were the perpetrators and women the victims. Now we know that power dynamics are not restricted to gender stereotypes. In some studies up to 50% of lesbians report sexual abuse by a female partner and about the same numbers report physical abuse in a lifetime (Blasko, 2010). The motivations for abuse in same-sex relationships are similar to the dynamics of other-sex relationships: control, fears of loss, fear of abandonment, and growing up in a violent household. Butch and femme partners are equally likely to be victims of abuse, unlike other-sex relationships where the masculine partner is more likely to be a perpetrator. In same-sex couples, the abuser may hold "heterosexist" control over the victim by threatening to out the victim. Some researchers suggest that fusion in lesbian relationships (a very high degree of emotional attachment and interdependence) might be a risk factor for violence.

The following are examples of the behaviors that might occur in an abusive relationship: intimidation, isolating the partner from friends and family, minimizing the violence or the conflict, denying that abuse is happening (normalizing abusive behavior), blaming the abused person for the perpetrator's behavior (you made me do it), withholding money or goods, coercion, insults, and threats. If any of this is happening in your relationship, consider talking to a counselor, healthcare provider, or contacting a women's shelter if you fear for your safety.

In conclusion, many factors influence the sex lives of lesbian and bisexual women, including previous experiences with violence and abuse. How each member of a couple or relationship define sex, how they communicate with each other about their needs and desires, and the stress on the relationship and in general will all impact the frequency and satisfaction with sexual activities. Most female same-sex couples report high levels of satisfaction with their relationships and sexual lives, but those who are not satisfied often feel they lack options for dealing with their dissatisfaction.

REFERENCES

Aaron, D. & Hughes, T. (2007). Association of childhood sexual abuse with obesity in a community sample of lesbians. *Obesity, 15*, 1023-1028.

Alvy, L.M., Hughes, T.L., Kristjanson, A., & Wilsnack, S. (2013). Sexual identity group differences in child abuse and neglect. *Journal of Interpersonal Violence, 28*, 2088-2111,

Austin, S.B., Jun, H.J., Jackson, B., Spiegelman, D., Rick-Edwards, J., Corliss, H., et al., (2008). Disparities in child abuse victimization in lesbian, bisexual, and heterosexual women in the Nurses' Health Study II. *Journal of Women's Health, 17*, 595-606.

Averet, P., Yoon, I., & Jenkins, C.L. (2012). Older lesbian sexuality: identity, sexual behavior and the impact of aging. *Journal of Sex Research, 49*(5), 495-507.

Balsam, K., Rothblum, E., & Beauchaine, T. (2005). Victimization over the lifespan: A comparison of LGB and heterosexual siblings. *Journal of Consulting and Clinical Psychology, 73*(3), 477-487.

Blasko, K.A., (2010). "she didn't mean to hit me." Lesbian intimate partner violence. In S. Dibble & P. Robertson (Eds), Lesbian Health 101. San Francisco, CA: UCSF Nursing Press, pp. 305-322.

Cohen, J. & Byers, E.S. (2014). Beyond lesbian bed death: enhancing our understanding of the sexuality of sexual minority women in relationships. *Journal of Sex Research, 51*(8), 893-903.

Corliss, H., Cochran, S.D., & Mays, V.M. (2002). Reports of parental maltreatment during childhood in a U.S. population-based survey of homosexual, bisexual, and heterosexual adults. *Child Abuse and Neglect, 26*, 1165-1178.

Garcia, J., Lloyd, E., Wallen, K., & Fisher, H. (2014). Variation in orgasm occurrence by sexual orientation in a sample of U.S. singles. *Journal of Sex and Medicine*, doi:10/1111/jsm.12669.

Lehavot, K., Molina, Y., & Simoni, J.M. (2012). Childhood trauma, adult sexual assault, and adult gender expression among lesbian and bisexual women. *Sex Roles, 67*, 272-284.

Marrazzo, J. et al., (2002). Characteristics of vaginal flora and bacterial vaginosis in women who have sex with women. *Journal of infectious Diseases, 185*(9), 1307-1313.

Marrazzo, J. (2010). "Can I get herpes from my girlfriend?" Lesbians' sexual health. In S. Dibble & P. Robertson (Eds), Lesbian Health 101. San Francisco, CA: UCSF Nursing Press, pp.55-66.

Stoddard, J.P., Dibble, S.L., & Fineman, N. (2009). Sexual and physical abuse: A comparison between lesbians and their heterosexual sisters. *Journal of Homosexuality, 56*, 407-422.

Chapter 9: Spiritual Health and Well-Being

One critical aspect of health and wellbeing is spiritual health. One can be sound of body and mind, but if feeling a lack of meaning and connection in life, health can not be optimal. In this chapter, we explore some of the differences between religion and spirituality, and describe how either religion or spirituality can boost our sense of overall health. Some scholars of religion/spirituality have found that people with same-sex attractions or who were gendered differently than others, historically were considered people who were bridges between the material world and the spiritual world. They served as healers, shamans, or had some other special place in the organization of the group. The rise of mono-theism (one god religions), colonization, and blending of church and state led to the undermining or destruction of many of these cultural groups.

SPIRITUALITY

Some lesbian/bisexual women prefer to explore a more personal form of spirituality than engage in formal religions. These practices and beliefs are typically not based in formal places or have rigid doctrines or rules. They can take many forms. Some women feel spiritual when in nature, or when gardening, or when dancing. Others gain a sense of spirituality through meditation or yoga practices, or through creative expressions like writing or painting. Some like collective practices and rituals whereas other prefer solitary activities. But what exactly is the spirit?

Some philosophers have distinguished between the soul and the spirit in this way: the soul is the unique characteristics of the individual. We all have different experiences and different gifts and talents to bring to the world, so the soul is our uniqueness. The spirit on the other hand, is the force that connects us to other people, other living beings, and the earth. It is collective and shared by all. Most of us seem to be driven to want more connection in our lives, and do not feel healthy if we feel isolated or disconnected. Spirit may also be related to feeling purpose or meaning in life. So whether we name it as spirituality or merely as a need for connection and meaning, we share a drive as humans to feel part of a larger collective. Some of us just label this drive as "humanity." As humans, we need to feel that we have some role to play in life, and that we are connected to others. For many, religion contains the elements that the person needs to feel spiritual. Religion provides the beliefs and practices and the social order. For others, religion is too confining, or the belief systems too rigid or not aligned with their personal beliefs, and alternatives to religion are sought.

When some lesbian and bisexual women have been rejected by family or religious communities because of religious objections to their sexuality, the drive to connect may be channeled through other means than religion. Some celebrate sex or drug use as ways to expand the mind and feel that sense of connection with a larger life force. Some women felt spiritual for the first time in their lives when they discovered gay or lesbian bars and the tight-knit communities that were forged in many of them. Some found transcendence (an expanding of consciousness) through alcohol or drug use or sexual practices.

For many developmental psychologists and philosophers alike, aging is associated with greater spiritual needs as we face our own mortality. For some lesbian and bisexual women, working within the AIDS movements of the 1980s and 90s started this process of facing one's mortality. Others had experiences with loss or life-threatening illnesses earlier in life. But at some point, we all need to make peace with the fact of death and dying and prepare ourselves. Some women who were atheist or did not think much about religion or spirituality when younger turn to spirituality to try to understand death as they age. Having some type of faith or belief system around what happens after death is a comfort to many people. One of the developmental tasks of old age is to come to some level of acceptance about dying.

Practicing Spirituality in Our Communities

Spiritual teacher Angeles Arrien always declared, "Relationship is a rigorous spiritual practice" meaning that how we treat others is a barometer of our spiritual health. We are tested in relationships to act with integrity and wisdom. When we are solid with our own spiritual practice and commitments, our relationships are deeper and stronger, and our communities thrive. When we treat each other with respect and compassion, we are practicing our spirituality.

In early lesbian/bisexual women's organizing, often principles such as sitting in circle to avoid hierarchy, letting every voice be heard, and consensus building were important practices. These three practices are found in many spiritual traditions around the world. The circle is a sign of wholeness and connection, and everyone in the circle has an equal place in the group. There is no "head" of the table that indicates a leader. In addition, many early lesbian collectives shared group facilitation. In practical terms, every meeting or gathering needs someone to move the process along, but when that duty is shared, more people feel a part of the group. Hearing every voice (deep listening) is also important so that we do not allow our assumptions about individuals to go unchallenged, and so that everyone is part of the process. Finally, consensus building is a non-violent method of reaching decisions; painful and sometimes lengthy, but also necessary for all perspectives and options to be entertained before coming to a group decision. Collectives organized in this way often failed when some women grew weary of the process, or when the purpose of the collective was not clear. If some women came into a group with an agenda that was not aligned with the purpose, it could create chaos. But when the process works, members often feel a deep sense of connection and meaning in their work. Those early lesbian feminist and queer collectives happened 20, 30, or even 40 years ago. What have we learned about ourselves and our communities since then that could help us build those sacred communities again? As we age, our need is even greater for deep, spiritual communities.

RELIGION

Religion refers to organized groups that have doctrines, rituals, leadership structures, and a formal set of rules and beliefs. There are over 20 major religions in the world today, and many of those have multiple subtypes (like Christianity for example). Data from 2010 shows approximate numbers of people worldwide who affiliate with each one. Christianity is the largest religion in the world, in terms of numbers who practice the faith. Curiously, they included atheists in this list of religions! The third most common "religion" is to have no affiliation to organized religion.

1. Christianity 2.1 billion
    2. Islam 1.3 billion
    3. Secular/Irreligious/Agnostic/Atheist 1.1 billion
    4. Hinduism 900 million
    5. Chinese traditional religion 394 million
    6. Buddhism 376 million
    7. Primal indigenous 300 million
    8. African traditional and diasporic 100 million
    9. Sikhism 23 million
    10. Juche 19 million
    11. Spiritism 15 million
    12. Judaism 14 million
    13. Bahá'í Faith 7 million
    14. Jainism 4.2 million
    15. Shinto 4 million
    16. Cao Dai 4 million
    17. Zoroastrianism 2.6 million
    18. Tenrikyo 2 million
    19. Neopaganism 1 million
    20. Unitarian Universalism 800,000
    21. Rastafari movement 600,000

LGBT People and Religion
Lesbian and bisexual women have many different types and degrees of affiliations with religion: some were raised in a particular religion and continue to practice it in adulthood; some were raised in a religion, but rejected it for some reason. They may practice another religion or engage in a spiritual practice not associated

with formal religion. Others were not raised in any particular religion and they may or may not adopt a religious or spiritual practice as adults. Like the general population, lesbian and bisexual women are leaving formal religions and labeling themselves as spiritual but not religious in greater numbers in past years.

A survey done by the Pew Research Center found that LGBT people are much less likely to be affiliated with a formal religion than the broader American population, with 48%, or more than double the percentage of the general public that say they are not religious. Most LGBT Americans, 52%, do have a religion, but for only 17%, religion is "very important" in their lives. Of those who are religious, most are Protestant (27%) or Catholic (14%). The survey also reported that one-third of LGBT people felt that there was a conflict between their religious beliefs and their sexual or gender identities. This is echoed in the data from the general population, where 74% of white evangelical Protestants and a majority (55%) of all U.S. adults with a religious affiliation say homosexuality conflicts with their religious beliefs. Among adults in the general public, there is a greater tendency for frequent church attenders to believe that homosexuality is wrong. The chart below shows the percentage of LGBT people's religious affiliations compared to the general public (from the Pew Study, 2011).

Table 9.1. Religious/spiritual affiliations by sexual orientation (from Pew, 2011).

	LGBT	General Public
Christian	42%	73%
Jewish	2%	2%
Other religions	8%	4%
Atheist/Agnostic	17%	6%
No religion in particular	31%	14%
Total unaffiliated with a religion	48%	20%

Nearly all of those surveyed said at least one of the major religious institutions were "unfriendly" to LGBT people: 80%- said Islam, Mormonism and the Catholic Church were unfriendly and 75% said evangelical churches were unfriendly. A substantial number (30%) said they had been made to feel unwelcome at a place of worship. Rejection by religion/religious people is a major source of stress for lesbian/bisexual women, particularly when it underlines family rejection.

The Pew study lumped all LGBT people together. A study in Chicago looked just at lesbian and bisexual women and found the following differences between lesbian/bisexual women and the general population of women. When asked: 'How religious you would say you are?' ('religious' in this question was defined as 'how actively one currently follows the teachings of a specific religion and participates in that religion'), 44% said that they were not at all religious or only somewhat religious (45%). On the other hand, when asked about spirituality (how often one spends time thinking about the ultimate purpose of life or one's own relationship to a higher power in life) the majority of lesbian/bisexual women said that they were very spiritual (48%) or somewhat spiritual (46%); only 6% were not at all spiritual. Thinking of your own experience, were you raised in a formal religion? What does that religion have to say about LGBT people? Do you still affiliate with that religion or have you changed your beliefs and practices? What are your current beliefs?

Figure 9.1. Religious affiliations of women from Chicago by sexual orientation (Hughes et al., 20

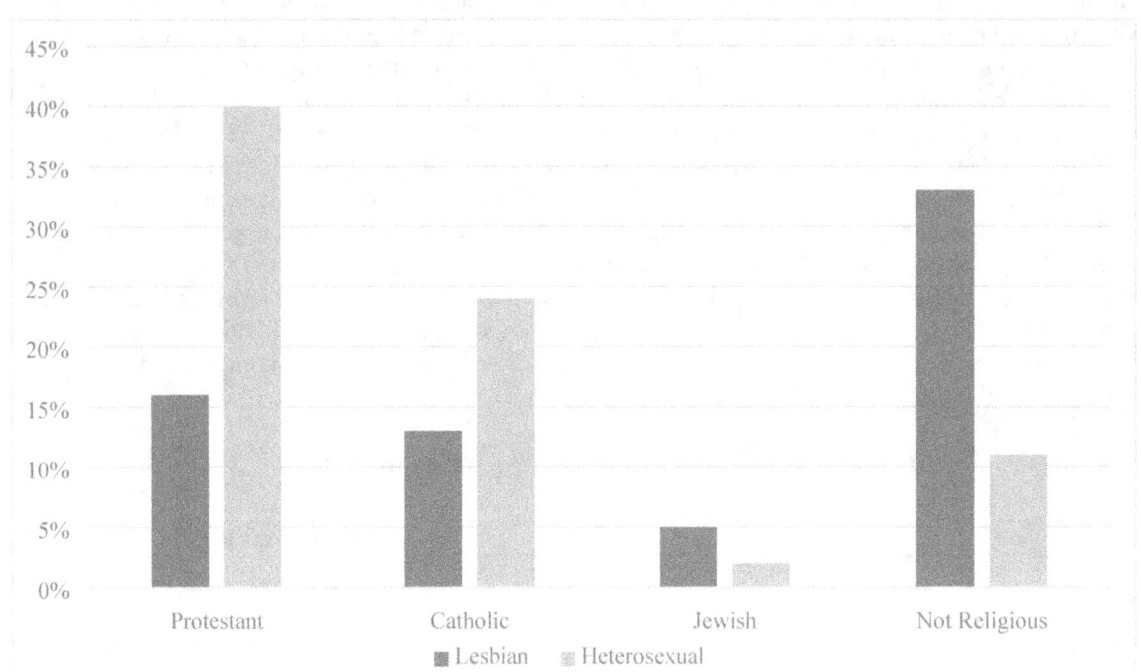

Resources for dealing with homophobia of religions

<u>Organizations or groups within organized religion</u>:
Dignity (gay Catholics)
Integrity USA (Episcopalian)
Keshet (Jewish)

<u>LGBT Churches</u>:
Metropolitan Community Church: non-denominational Christian church to serve LGBT communities

<u>LGBT-Inclusive Mainstream Churches</u>:
Unitarian Universalist
United Church of Christ
Unity Churches (see http://www.unity.org/resources/lgbt) for resources

<u>Alternative Religions</u>:
Neopagan/Wiccan/Pagan and other earth-based spiritual groups (these tend to be bridges between formal religion and more personal spiritual systems as they are loosely organized with no rigid doctrines).

REFERENCES
Hughes, T.L.
Pew Trust (2013). A survey of LGBT Americans. www.pewsocialtrends.org.

PART TWO:
CAUSES AND CONTRIBUTORS TO HEALTH PROBLEMS

As noted earlier, most chronic health problems stem from similar underlying causes. Instead of taking each problem separately, such as depression or asthma, we can look at the broader influences on health that are organized along the ecological model. Some factors will be specific to certain health problems, such as living in a highly polluted environment may put us at risk for cancers or breathing problems. Other factors, like racism and heterosexism, can influence a wide variety of health outcomes. Each chapter focuses on one level of influence, but keep in mind that they are all overlapping and one level influences each of the others. These five chapters are based on the ecological model of health that was introduced in Chapter 1. As a reminder, the ecological model looks like this. The innermost circle is the individual, the next ring represents interpersonal level, or relationships, the next ring is the community and the institutions within the community, and the outer rings are the broader societal level influences like laws, policies, and politics that impact our health and well-being. These rings of influence might change somewhat according to age and life course status.

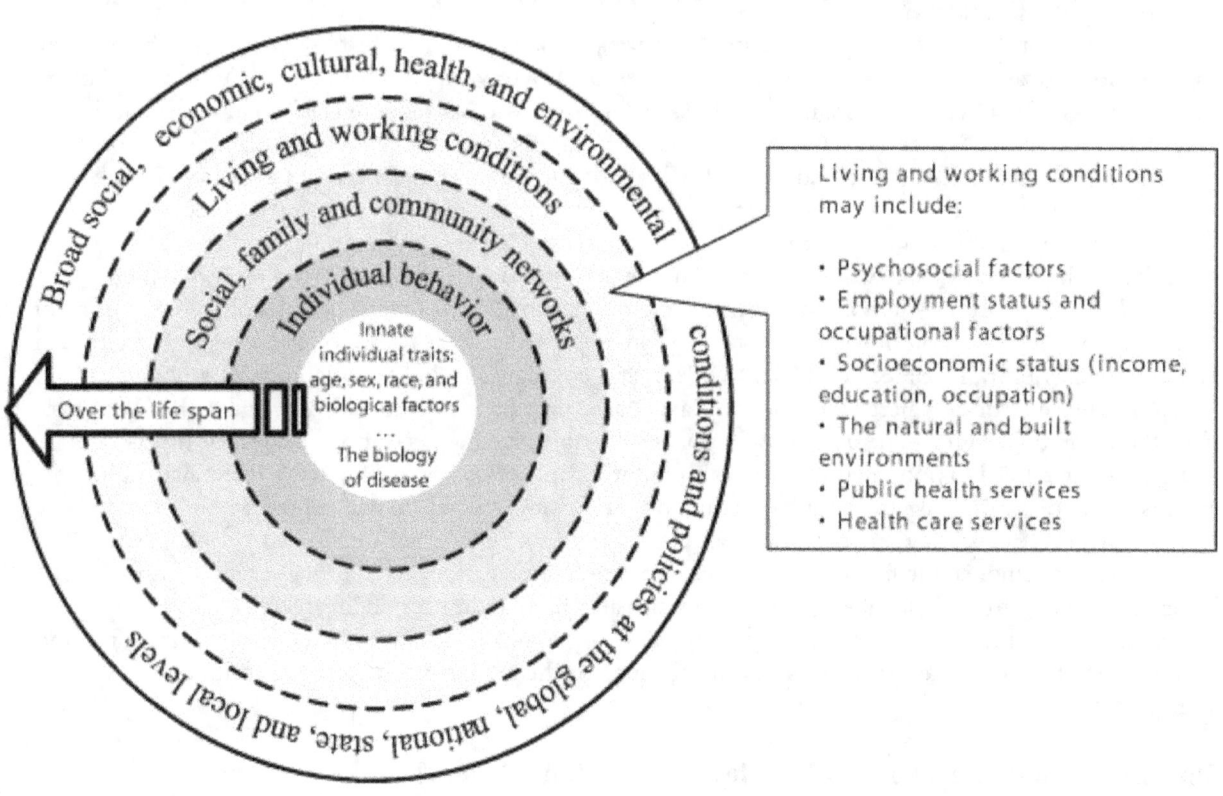

Chapter 10: Individual Level Factors

"I wish that I could find a way of eating and exercise that the weight would come off naturally and I wouldn't be so focused on it, that I could focus on my life, not my weight" (respondent in Yost & Chmielewski, 2010, p. 154).

Most research, as well as news stories and magazine articles on health, and particularly those that focus on weight, have blamed the individual person for poor nutrition, lack of physical activity, or poor choices about how to manage stress. These media reports often imply that people are overweight, or have health problems because they were just too lazy or lacked self-discipline. Yet even within the individual level, there are a host of other influences that affect weight, whether one engages in healthy behaviors, and whether a chronic illness develops. This section focuses on those variables that are mainly at the level of the individual person. Many of them were discussed in more detail in earlier chapters, so are mostly just listed here. It is important to see the multitude of factors that affect health so that we do not focus on just one or two issues and think that we will automatically be healthier. Good health means attending to physical, mental, spiritual, and political issues. As the quote that starts this chapter notes, so much media focuses on weight that many of us tend to define our health by the number on the scale when the reality is much more complicated.

Demographic Factors

In the general population, some characteristics that are associated with greater frequency of health problems include more advanced age, racial/ethnic minority identity, poverty, and lack of higher education. All of these factors are associated with more stigma and stress. These same factors seem to hold up in lesbian and bisexual communities. Yancey, Cochran, Corliss, & Mays (2003) studied over 1200 lesbians from Los Angeles County and found that those who had higher BMIs tended to be older and were less educated. Dibble and colleagues (2012) found 85% of a sample of African American lesbian/bisexual women exceeded expectations for healthy weight. Bianca Wilson and coauthors (2011) found that 37% of the African American lesbian and bisexual women in their sample had experienced weight-related discrimination. They collected data on BMI but did not report this data in this article. In the general population, women of color (with the possible exception of some subsets of Asian American women) tend to report higher weight than white women (Befort, Nazir, & Perri, 2012). Wilson and colleagues found that higher BMI among lesbian/bisexual African American women was associated with higher frequency of weight-related oppression that in turn predicted greater depression symptoms and subjective ratings of poor health. BMI was also independently related to poorer subjective health ratings. But as we saw in Chapter 5, just having a higher BMI is not necessarily a negative health outcome by itself. Some studies do not tell the whole story about health when they focus only on body size as an outcome.

These demographic factors, such as age and race/ethnicity, are linked to higher level forms of oppression, but at the individual level, one's identities also have an impact on lifestyle risk factors by increasing levels of daily stress and feelings of powerlessness. We have little or no control over most of the demographic factors as they are associated with the luck of the draw concerning what communities we were born into.

Physical Activity Levels: Aren't all lesbians softball players?

Among the population as a whole, lack of exercise is one factor in poor health. However, the few studies that have assessed physical activity among lesbian/bisexual women are quite contradictory. One study found that lesbians were <u>more </u>likely to engage in vigorous activity than heterosexual women (Aaron et al, 2001), another study found <u>similar</u> rates of physical activity (Fredriksen et al, 2010), and yet a third study reported <u>lower </u>rates of physical activity (Valanis et al, 2000). These differences may be related to age or other differences in the people studied. For example, lower rates of activity may be found in those who already have higher BMI (Yancey, et al, 2003). Fredriksen and colleagues (2010), using a random population sample from one state, reported that 17% of both lesbian and bisexual women reported a lack of regular exercise, but this was not different than heterosexual women's activity levels.

Danielle Brittain and her coauthors (2006) asked groups of lesbians aged 22 to 61 about the barriers to physical activity, and found several lesbian/bisexual specific concerns. Many women had an expectation that one had to be "out" to participate on a lesbian sports team and those who were not out had concerns about being seen exercising with a known lesbian partner. They also reported a reluctance to share locker rooms with heterosexual women for fear that the heterosexual women would feel uncomfortable or think they were looking at them. Finally, they reported a lack of social support to exercise. In the next study, they recruited lesbian/bisexual women to complete an internet survey (Brittain and colleagues, 2008). This study found that lack of time was the biggest barrier for lesbians to be active, but they also reported being worried about how their bodies looked when they exercised. Lack of exercise is certainly a factor for some lesbians, but as a group, lesbians may be more willing to engage in moderate to vigorous activity than heterosexual women if they can identify appropriate, safe, and accessible exercise options. Many communities have some recreational or sport related opportunities for lesbian and bisexual women, such as softball teams, soccer, rugby, and hiking groups. Many of these activities might be geared to younger and more healthy lesbian and bisexual women, and heavier and older women may not feel included or safe in these activities. Most communities lack facilities that can help women with disabilities to be as active as they would like.

So how does this fit with stereotypes that lesbians are more athletic than heterosexual women, and likely to be involved in vigorous activities ("sporty dykes")? As is true of all stereotypes, the reality is that some lesbian/bisexual women are very active and some are not, and no generalizations can be made. Chapter 18 addresses physical activity in more detail and offers a physical activity routine that all women, at any ability level, can do as a starter.

Gender Expression: Are butch and femme lesbians different?

Lesbian and bisexual women tend to have greater diversity of gender expression than heterosexual women and range widely on a masculinity/femininity scale (Levitt & Horne, 2002). However, only a few studies have examined potential differences in health behaviors or outcomes or risk factors related to gender expression. Singh and colleagues (1999) found that butch-identified lesbians had a greater waist-to-hip ratio than femme-identified lesbians/bisexual women or heterosexual women (in other words, they had bigger bellies!).

Lehavot and colleagues (2012) found that lesbians with butch identities were more likely to report childhood traumas than femme identified women who were more likely to experience greater victimization in adulthood. Butch-identified women tend to come out at earlier ages and experience more discrimination, minority stress, and substance use (Lehavot & Simoni, 2011; Rosario et al, 2008). Femme-identified women are more able to conceal their sexual identity in public, but as a consequence, they may suffer greater levels of internalized homophobia because they feel shame or guilt for not always revealing their sexuality (Hiestand et al, 2005; Lehavot & Simoni, 2011). Feinstein, Goldfried, & Davila (2012) found that childhood gender nonconformity (being a tomboy or not very feminine) was associated with greater levels of experiences of discrimination, which in turn was associated with greater internalized oppression, depression, sensitivity to rejection, and social anxiety. If greater masculinity in women is associated with a rejection of feminine beauty standards, then butch lesbians may feel less pressure to conform, and thus may be satisfied with carrying greater weight. In fact, some butch women deliberately choose to bulk up to appear more powerful. Maybe the greater experiences of discrimination and childhood traumas underlies body image problems. Femme-identified women may share more of the same concerns about weight and body appearance as heterosexual women, since they share at least some of the same values about femininity and appearance. This means that femme women may feel more pressure to engage in the unhealthy dieting practices that may damage health. More research is needed to test these hypotheses about the role of gender expression in lesbian/bisexual women's health. What have you noticed about differences in health and health-related behaviors in femme versus butch women? How do you identify along a butch-femme continuum? How do you think it affects your health, or your health behaviors?

Mental Health Disorders

As reported in an early chapter, several studies over the past 30 years have identified higher rates of depression and other mood disorders among lesbian and bisexual women compared to heterosexual women.

Elevated rates of mental disorders have been reported in lesbian/bisexual adult respondents in large-scale health surveys that have defined sexual orientation based on self-identity (Jorm, Korten, Rodgers, Jacomb, & Christensen, 2002; Cochran, Mays & Sullivan, 2003; Cochran et al., 2007; Conron, Mimiaga, & Landers, 2010; Bostwick et al., 2010; Hughes, Szalacha, & McNair, 2010) or on gender of sexual partners (Gilman et al., 2001). Depression and anxiety disorders were 1.5 times more common in LGB people than in comparable heterosexual individuals (King et al., 2008). People with mental health problems often have co-occurring substance abuse and physical health problems that affect their overall health status. Some think that when one is depressed, there is less motivation to take good care of one's self and more tendency to engage in emotional eating and other health-damaging behaviors.

Eating Disorders and Body Image

Chapter 5 addressed this issue, but clearly body dissatisfaction and eating disorders can profoundly affect our health. Eating disorders are associated with unhealthy nutritional patterns like weight-cycling and dangerous dieting behaviors. All women struggle to some extent with body image issues in our youth-oriented, thin-focused, ableist culture. Linda Bacon has proposed that weight-cycling and the negative effects of dieting are responsible for the health problems that healthcare professionals link to higher body weight (2010).

Alcohol, Tobacco, and Other Drug Use (ATOD)

Chapter 4 discussed ATOD use. There is a significant body of research finding higher rates of ATOD use and abuse among sexual minority women compared to heterosexual women (for a summary, see Drabble & Eliason, 2013). ATOD use, particularly alcohol use, may contribute to weight concerns via the empty calories, and the same factors that underlie ATOD use/abuse may also underlie having a higher weight (i.e., sexual abuse, mental health symptoms, minority stress, and community norms). In addition, some women who smoke hesitate to attempt to quit because of their concerns about gaining weight, and smoking cessation programs need to address this concern. Studies have found that lesbian and bisexual women are roughly twice as likely as heterosexual women to smoke (Eliason & Drabble, 2010), and smoking has been linked to many negative health consequences. A population-based study in Massachusetts found that for LGB respondents, smoking and obesity were both related to higher rates of asthma than in the general population (Landers et al, 2011), showing how these health issues intersect.

Coping Strategies

A few studies have looked at the ways that lesbian and bisexual women cope with stress and difficult life circumstances. In the general population, unhealthy coping (using substances, avoiding conflict, blaming others) is associated with poorer health and adaptive coping (communicating about conflict, relaxation and calming strategies, good self-care) with better health. Some studies of LGB people suggest that active coping strategies, such as seeking out solutions for problems, are associated with positive attitudes about one's sexuality and in turn, better psychological adjustment (Miranda & Storms, 1989) and lower levels of depression (Zea, Reisen, & Poppen, 1999). Unhealthy coping strategies were found in one study to combine with internalized homophobia to produce more challenging psychological distress symptoms (Szymanski & Owens, 2008). Lehavot (2012) found that unhealthy coping, particularly behavioral disengagement and self-blame, were related to poorer physical and mental health. In her study, bisexual women reported both a higher rate of unhealthy coping methods and worse mental and physical health than lesbians. Thus far, there has been no research examining whether lesbian/bisexual women are more or less likely to engage in overeating or eating unhealthy foods in response to stress than heterosexual women. But we know that emotional eating is a common problem for many people.

Lesbian/Bisexual Women's Tendency to Seek Health Care Services

Lesbian and bisexual women might be reluctant to seek out health care services for physical or mental health symptoms because of fear of encountering discrimination or poor quality of care (summarized in Eliason, Dibble, DeJoseph & Chinn, 2009). However, recent data suggest that this may not true of all subsets of lesbians, or may be changing as the climate in society has improved. One study of California women (Grella and colleagues, 2011) found that lesbian and bisexual women were more likely to seek out substance abuse and mental health services than heterosexual women, even when they had no diagnosed disorder. This seemed to confirm what some researchers said earlier: because lesbian/bisexual women go through the self-analysis process of coming out, they may put more value on that process and use therapy to improve quality of life.

Studies of women with substance use disorders also found that lesbian/bisexual women were more likely to attend 12 step meetings than heterosexual women (Jessup & Dibble, 2012; McCabe et al, 2012) and surveys of lesbian/bisexual women found that they are more likely to seek out and receive individual counseling (Jones & Gabriel, 1999; Jorm et al, 2002). Finally, lesbian and bisexual women use alternative and complementary health options such as acupuncture, meditation, and homeopathy, more often than heterosexual women (Smith, Matthews, Markovic et al, 2010; Matthews, Hughes, Osterman, & Kodl, 2005). This willingness to deal with one's emotional and adjustment problems and seek solutions outside of mainstream bio-medicine suggest that lesbian/bisexual might be more open to group educational, therapy, and support groups than heterosexual women, especially if these treatment options are tailored to their needs. It may be that there is still reluctance to seek out medical services, but not mental health, substance abuse, or alternative complementary medicine services because the later are perceived as more safe and inclusive environments than settings for physical health.

Definitions of Health

Sarah Fogel and colleagues (2012) asked an open-ended question on an online survey to 198 lesbian and bisexual women: "What does healthy mean to you?" The women noted that health has an emotional component (being happy, peaceful, energetic, free from stress, comfortable with one's own body), and includes sleeping well, having an average weight, being pain-free, disease-free, and not out of breath. The respondents suggested that there were three benefits of a healthy body: energy, strength, and the ability to do what she wants to do. Other studies have found similar findings: lesbians often do not associate health with losing weight (Roberts, et al., 2010) like heterosexual women often do.

Disabilities

Lesbian and bisexual women with disabilities are mostly invisible in the research literature on health outcomes. This is of concern, since most of us will experience disability in our lifetimes. Chapter 7 dealt with disability. In some stereotypical thinking, disability is equated with poor health but of course, one can have a disability and be very healthy. We need more research to study how women adapt and reach their ultimate health within the limitations (and potentials) of a disability. For many women with disabilities, finding adaptive equipment and assistance to engage in physical activity is a challenge. Gyms and swimming pools often are not set up for people with disabilities.

Resilience

This concept refers to our capacity to bounce back from stressful or traumatic experiences, and people vary widely on this quality. Those who are resilient may experience discrimination, but not have negative consequences. One way to increase one's resilience is to build a supportive social network or community. Other ways to build resilience might be to meditate and strengthen one's inner resources or objectively view our lives in ways that help us stay more positive and grounded. We have focused on the subsets of lesbian and bisexual women who have some negative health outcome in much of this book, but in reality, most are healthy and well-adjusted. We need to study the protective factors that allow many lesbian/bisexual women to be resilient.

Genetic and Familial Factors

There is no evidence that lesbian and bisexual women are any different than heterosexual women in terms of genetic factors. The research on the genetics of sexual orientation is still not clear, especially for women, and even if there were a "gay gene" it would not necessarily be associated with any health outcomes. It would probably be more like eye color—a trait that is not associated with any health outcomes. So lesbian/bisexual women have the same genetic challenges as heterosexual women: some forms of breast cancer and Alzheimer's disease appear to be genetic, and some family patterns are related more to food behaviors (eating preferences in families, such as believing dessert should be served after every meal), or occupations like coal-mining where many family members have lung diseases. It is important to assess your own personal risks and when possible, reduce the risk factors that you have control over. Angelina Jolie re-ignited discussion in the media about having a double mastectomy to prevent a genetic form of breast cancer. There is no easy answer as to whether that route is the right one for any individual, and if you have the breast cancer gene, you need to do a lot of research and talk to several health care providers about your options.

Conclusions About Individual Level Factors

In summary, there are a host of individual level factors that impact our health. We have control over some of them, but many of them are experiences that happened to us when we were children, are genetic factors, or related to life circumstances that are not easy to change. If we focus only on these individual factors, we suffer from the delusion that we are mostly at fault for any problems we have. In reality, every problem in the result of many factors, over which we have control of only a few things.   The next few chapters outline the social determinants of health.

REFERENCES

Aaron, D., Markovic, N., Danielson, M., Honnold, J., Janosky, J., & Schmidt, N. (2001). Behavioral risk factors for disease and preventive health practices among lesbians. *American Journal of Public Health, 91*, 972-975.

Alanko, K., Santtila, P., Witting, K., Varjonen, M., Jern, P., Johansson, A., van der Pahlen, B., & Sandnabba, K. (2009). Psychiatric symptoms and same-sex attraction and behavior in light of childhood gender atypical behavior and parental relationships. *Journal of Sex Research, 46*, 494-504..

Befort, C., Nazir, N., & Perri, M. (2012). Prevalence of obesity among adults from rural and urban areas of the U.S. *Journal of Rural Health, 28*(4), 392-397.

Bostwick, W.B., Boyd, C.J., Hughes, T.L., & McCabe, S.E. (2010). Dimensions of sexual orientation and the prevalence of mood and anxiety disorders in the United States. *American Journal of Public Health, 100*(3), 468-475.

Brittain, D., Gyurscik, N., & McElroy, M. (2008). Perceived barriers to physical activity among adult lesbians. *Women in Sport and Physical Activity Journal, 17*, 68-79

Brittain, D., Baillergeon, T., McElroy, M., Aaron, D., & Gyuraski, N. (2006). Barriers to moderate physical activity in adult lesbians. *Women and Health, 43*, 75-92.

Cochran, S D., & Mays, V.M. (2007). Physical health complaints among LGB and homosexually experienced heterosexual individuals: results from the California Quality of Life Survey. *American Journal of Public Health, 97*, 2048-2055.

Cochran, S.D., Sullivan, J.G., & Mays, V.M. (2003). Prevalence of mental disorders, psychological distress, and mental health services use among lesbian, gay, and bisexual adults in the United States. *Journal of Consulting and Clinical Psychology, 71 (1)*, 53-61

Conron, K. J., Mimiaga, M. J. & Landers, S. J. (2010). A population-based study of sexual orientation identity and gender differences in adult health. *American Journal of Public Health, 100*, 1953–1960.

Dibble, S.D., Eliason, M.J., & Crawford, B. (2012).). Correlates of wellbeing among African American lesbians. *Journal of Homosexuality, 59*, 820-838.

Dillworth, T. M., Kaysen, D., Montoya, H. D., & Larimer, M. E. (2009). Identification with mainstream culture and preference for alternative alcohol treatment approaches in a community sample. *Behavior Therapy, 40*(1), 72-81.

Feinstein, B.A., Goldfried, M.R., & Davila, J. (2012). The relationship between experiences of discrimination and mental health among lesbians and gay men. *Journal of Consulting and Clinical Psychology, 80*(5), 917-927.

Fogel, S., Calman, L., & Magrini, D. (2012). Lesbians' and bisexual women's definition of health. *Journal of Homosexuality, 59(9)*,

Fredriksen-Goldsen, K., Kim, H., Barkan, S. Balsam, K., & Mincer S. (2010). Disparities in health-related quality of life: A comparison of lesbian and bisexual women. American *Journal of Public Health, 100*(11), 2255-2261.

Gilman, S.E., Cochran, S.D., Mays, V.M., Hughes, M., Ostrow, D., & Kessler, R.C. (2001). Risk of psychiatric disorders among individuals reporting same-sex partners in the National Comorbidity Survey. *American Journal of Public Health, 91*, 933-939.

Grella, C.E., Cochran, S.D., Greenwell, L., & Mays, V.M. (2011). Effects of sexual orientation and gender on perceived need for treatment by persons with and without mental disorders. *Psychiatric Services*, 404-412.

Hiestand, K.R., & Levitt, H.M. (2005). Butch identity development: The formation of an authentic gender. *Feminism and Psychology, 15*, 61-85.

Hughes, T., Szalacha, L.A.,& McNair, R. (2010). Substance abuse and mental health disparities: comparisons across sexual identity groups in a national sample of young Australian women, *Social Science and Medicine;71*(4):824-31

Jorm, A., Korten, A., Rodgers, B., Jacob, P., & Christensen, H. (2002). Sexual orientation and mental health; results from a community survey of young and middle-aged adults. *British Journal of Psychiatry, 180,*

King, M., Semlyen, J., Tai, S.S., Killaspy, H., Osborn, D., Popelyuk, D., et al. (2008). A systematic review of mental disorder, suicide, and deliberate self harm in lesbian, gay, and bisexual people. *BMC Psychiatry, 8*:70. Retrieved June 8, 2009 from http://www.ncbi.nlm.nih.gov/pmc/articles/PMC2533652/.

Lehavot, K. (2012). Coping strategies and health in a national sample of sexual minority women. *American Journal of Orthopsychiatry, 82*(4), 494-504.

Lehavot, K., & Simoni, J. M. (2011a). The impact of minority stress on mental health and substance use among sexual minority women. *Journal of Consulting and Clinical Psychology, 79*(2), 159-170.

Levitt, H.M., & Horne, S.G., (2002). Explorations of lesbian-queer genders: Butch, femme, androgynous, or "other." *Journal of Lesbian Studies, 6*, 25-39.

Levitt, H.M., Puckett, J.A., Ippolito, M.P. & Horne, S.G. (2012). Sexual minority women's gender identity and expression: Challenges and supports. *Journal of Lesbian Studies, 16*, 153-176.

Matthews, A. K., Hughes, T. L., Osterman, G. P., & Kodl, M. M. (2005). Complementary medicine practices in a community-based sample of lesbian and heterosexual women. *Health Care for Women International, 26*(5): 430-47.

Roberts, S.J., Stuart-Shor, E.M., & Oppenheimer, R.A. (2010). Lesbians' attitudes and beliefs regarding overweight and weight reduction. *Journal of Clinical Nursing, 19*, 1986-1994.

Rosario M., Schrimshaw, E.W., Hunter, J., & Levy-Warren, A. (2007). The coming out process of young lesbian and bisexual women: Are there butch/femme differences in sexual identity development? *Archives of Sexual Behavior, 38*, 34-49.

Singh, D., Vidaurri, M., Sambarano, R.J., & Dabbs, Jr, J.M. (1999). Lesbian erotic role identification: behavioral, morphological, and hormonal correlates. *Journal of Personality and Social Psychology, 76*, 1035-1049.

Valanis, B.G., Bowen, D., Bassford, T., Whitlock, E., Charney, P., & Carter, R. (2000). Sexual orientation and health. *Archives of Family Medicine, 9*, 843-853.

Wells, B.E., Bimbi, D.S., Tider, D., Van Ora, J., & Parsons, J.T. (2006). Preventive health behaviors among lesbian and bisexually identified women. *Women's Health, 44*(2), 1-13.

Wilson, B.D., Okwu, C., & Mills, S.A. (2011). The relationship between multiple forms of oppression and subjective health among Black lesbian and bisexual women. *Journal of Lesbian Studies, 15*, 15-24.

Yancey, A.K., Cochran, S.D., Corliss, H.L., & Mays, V.M. (2003). Correlates of overweight and obesity among lesbian and bisexual women. *Preventive Medicine, 26*(6), 676-68.

Yean, C., Benau, E.M., Dakanalis, A., Hormes, J.M., Perone, J., & Timko, C.A. (2013). The relationship of sex and sexual orientation to self-esteem, body shape satisfaction, and eating disorder symptomatology. *Frontiers in Psychology,4*, doi: 10.3389/fpsyg.2013.00887.

Yost, M.R. & Chmielewski, J.F. (2011). Narrating rural lesbian's lives: body image and lesbian community in central Pennsylvania. *Journal of Lesbian Studies, 15*, 148-165.

Chapter 11: Interpersonal Level Factors

"She is not a junk food eater and I am a junk food eater…She wasn't a big dessert [eater] before I met her. And now she eats desserts at night time" (lesbian respondent in Reczek, 2012, p. 1117).

Humans are social animals and have interdependent relationships with many other people. The direct interactions and complex relationships we have with important people in our close social networks have a profound impact on us as individuals. Our health is influenced by significant others, our close friends, ex-lovers, coworkers, family of origin, and other people we interact with on a regular basis. Some of these experiences that are rooted in our childhood continue to impact us for the rest of our lives, such as experiences of child and adolescent abuse. When we come out as lesbian or bisexual, often the greatest challenges in our lives are related to changes in the social relationships with the people closest to us. Rejection by family members or close friends can also impact our health dramatically. This chapter gives just a few examples of how interpersonal dynamics affect our health.

Child and Adult Experiences of Abuse and Trauma

Several studies have now reported that lesbian and bisexual women are more likely to report that they were exposed to trauma and abuse as children (Austin et al., 2008; Balsam et al, 2005; Corliss et al, 2002; Hughes et al, 2010; Stoddard et al, 2009). This includes sexual abuse as well as physical and emotional abuse. Some experts have suggested lesbian and bisexual women, because they have already gone through the emotionally challenging process of coming out, may be more likely to share other personal information, such as childhood trauma experiences. So the difference may be a difference in reporting rather than in actual rates of abuse.

We know that the experience of childhood trauma can affect a person well into their adulthood. Women who report child abuse are more likely to have larger bodies (and be in the category of "obese" according to biomedical standards: Aaron & Hughes, 2007; Lehavot, Molina, & Simoni, 2012; Smith and colleagues, 2010) and may be more likely to have eating disorders (Midei & Matthew, 2011). Many women cope with stress and trauma with emotional eating; some deliberately try to hide their sexuality behind a larger body to seem less sexually desirable.

One study found that bisexual women reported higher rates of sexual traumas than lesbian or heterosexual women (Long et al., 2007), but there is not enough research on this to draw any conclusions. Some researchers have found child and adolescent abuse experiences to be linked to anti-gay beliefs of the perpetrators, particularly in women who are gender non-conforming (Alanko et al, 2009; D'Augelli et al, 2006). There is little research to suggest whether lesbian/bisexual women who were abused because of their perceived sexuality manifest different symptoms later on, or if female partners react to and deal with long-term symptoms of abuse in their partners differently than do male partners. Old stereotypes suggested that sexual abuse by a man in childhood would influence a woman's sexual identity later on, turning her off to sexual relationships with men. Obviously this cannot be the only explanation for a lesbian identity, because heterosexual and bisexual women also report high rates of childhood sexual abuse, but it may be one of many factors that influence some women to be lesbians. We need more research to understand how a sexual abuse history affects female same-sex relationships.

Significant Other Relationships

Intimate relationships profoundly affect our mental and physical health and wellbeing, and even our health behaviors. Fogel and colleagues (2012) found that over half of overweight lesbians reported also having an overweight partner, and our own DIFO program found the same result—almost 60% of participants who were heavier also had larger bodied partners. Markey and Markey (2013) found that 42% of the female same-sex couples they studied were in the same weight category and only 34% consisted of one with a "normal" weight and a heavier partner. General population studies also find that having an overweight spouse or partner is a predictor of higher weight. Similar findings are true for alcohol, drug, and tobacco use; we are more likely to use if our partners or close friends use. Sometimes we take on health-damaging behaviors to please partners or feel more connected, or because our social norms are altered into accepting unhealthy behaviors as "normal," because everyone in our close social network engage in those behaviors. Another alternative explanation is that there is nothing wrong with having a larger body and since lesbian and bisexual women are more satisfied with a larger body, more lesbian/bisexual women in relationships are heavier women.

Some lesbian therapists described a concept called "lesbian fusion" or "merger" that described a pattern of relating in female same-sex partners. Fusion indicates an even greater sense of closeness and influence on each other because of lack of validation of their relationships in their families of origin and society as a whole (Kurdek, 2004). This greater influence on each other may include health-related behaviors, such as how and what we eat, how much physical activity we get, and how we deal with stress in our lives. Significant other relationships may be more stressful for lesbian and bisexual women because of the lack of validation of relationships in society at large and the stress of maintaining family of origin relationships along with same-sex relationships (Frost & Eliason, 2013). Whether our relationships are fused/merged or not, partners influence our health.

Reczek and Umberson (2012) examined gendered patterns of health behavior. They noted that traditional gender stereotypes expect women to be the health educators and enforcers of health behaviors in relationships whereas men are expected to engage in bad health behavior or be inattentive to their health. How does this play out in same-sex relationships? They found that same-sex couples reported more cooperative health work dynamics whereby both partners promoted health in the other. In another study, Reczek (2012) looked at the specific patterns by which partners might influence health behaviors, and identified three mechanisms by which lesbian, gay, and heterosexual married couples affected each other's health:

- The first pattern "unilateral diffusion" is where one partner consistently influences the other in a negative or positive way. In half of the heterosexual couples, the husband was identified as the "bad influence" but only 1/3 of same-sex couples reported one was a bad influence.
- The second type was "bilateral diffusion" whereby couples more or less equally influenced each other. Over half of the same-sex couples and only 10% of the heterosexual couples reported this.
- Finally, some individuals focused on personal responsibility for health and did not try to influence their partner's health behaviors. This was far more common in heterosexual couples and only 1 lesbian respondent endorsed this pattern.

Thus it appears that same-sex couples are more equal in sharing of health education, influence, and beliefs than are heterosexual couples. This fits with other research showing more equality in same-sex relationships than in other-sex relationships.

Relationship satisfaction is another factor that might be a major influence on health. In studies of the general population, and a few studies of same-sex relationships, those who are legally married have greater health benefits—they are more satisfied with their relationships and those relationships seem to lead to better physical health and mental health (Wright, LeBlanc, & Badgett, 2013). Legal marriage is still relatively new for same-sex couples, so more information will available in the years to come. It is important to note, though, that not all lesbian/bisexual women would choose marriage if it were available to them, and they might still be very satisfied with their relationships. Some lesbian/bisexual women express feminist concerns with the institution of marriage and prefer other types of relationships.

Intimate Partner Violence

Many lesbian and bisexual women have experienced abuse from both male and female partners in their lifetimes. One study found that 39% had been sexually or physically abused by a male partner and 11% by a female partner, and that psychological abuse was even more common, and cut across race, ethnicity, and social class boundaries. When significant others become abusive, there are few resources for the battered partner to turn to in the community (Balsam, Rothblum, & Beauchaine, 2005; Murray & Mobley, 2009). Sometimes women encounter abuse in their first lesbian relationship, before they have developed support systems in sexual minority communities, and when they face or fear rejection from family of origin for coming out (McDonald, 2012). If the significant other is not a U.S. citizen, immigration laws have often not treated that relationship as legitimate and partners risk separation by deportation (Lewis, 2010). For all of these reasons, lesbian/bisexual victims of abuse are less likely to call the police for help.

Lesbian/Bisexual Women and Their Exes

Lesbian and bisexual women seem to maintain longer and more intense relationships with ex-lovers than do heterosexual women, and in many cases, these relationships may take on features of family. There is not much research on the influence (positive or negative) of ex-lovers on health behaviors, but they are often integrated in close social networks or families of choice and it is possible that they may have more influence on the individual than other friends. This added close relationship can be a source of stress or support, depending on the nature of the relationship.

Family of Choice/Social Networks

Older lesbians tend to form informal networks with other lesbians for support (Cohn & Hastings, 2011; D'Augelli, 1987), or with LGBT communities, and many form family-like networks with close friends and ex-lovers (Weinstock & Rothblum, 2004; Weston, 1991). In general population studies, spouses and close friends are highly influential on individual lifestyle choices such as eating patterns and physical activity (Cunningham, Vaquera, Maturo, & Narayan, 2012). Lehavot (2012) suggested that social support is a protective factor for health and may both strengthen a person's individual level coping strategies and provide group-level support that acknowledges the higher level societal factors that affect one's health. For example, in many lesbian/bisexual women's communities, feminist activities and philosophies support the community at the group level by pointing out that common problems that women face are because of societal level structural barriers, not any individual short-coming (Szymanski & Owens, 2009). As attitudes in society have been changing for the better, more lesbian and bisexual women are reporting that their close social networks include a mix of heterosexual friends and co-workers, along with LGBT people. Everyone needs a supportive network of family and friends to get through normal life challenges and the aging process.

Family of Origin Issues

Rejection or invalidation by family of origin may be a significant source of minority stress for many lesbian/bisexual women. Some women cope with the stresses of family of origin with unhealthy strategies, and many experience depression, anxiety, and other psychological distress that is directly related to being rejected by the people who are supposed to love and support you unconditionally. In addition, whether we have currently have close, distant or non-existent relationships with family of origin, they were our original source of information about health practices. We learned how to define health, we learned about comfort foods and eating to please others, we learned attitudes about physical activity, responses to stress, and much more from our families of origin. Sometimes before any change toward health promotion can be successful, we have to re-examine the messages we got from family.

Conclusions about Interpersonal Factors

We need other people, but often the ways that we learned to communicate as children/youth, and the traumas we have suffered at the hands of others, affect our ability to connect and feel support from other people. Building our intimate relationships and close social networks is critical to our health, so it behooves us to pay close attention to how we treat others in our networks and who we let in or keep out of our lives.

REFERENCES

Alanko, K., Santtila, P., Witting, K., Varjonen, M., Jern, P., Johansson, A., van der Pahlen, B., & Sandnabba, K. (2009). Psychiatric symptoms and same-sex attraction and behavior in light of childhood gender atypical behavior and parental relationships. *Journal of Sex Research, 46,* 494-504.

Alvy, L.M., Hughes, T.L., Kristjanson, A., & Wilsnack, S. (2013). Sexual identity group differences in child abuse and neglect. *Journal of Interpersonal Violence, 28,* 2088-2111,

Austin, S.B., Jun, H.J., Jackson, B., Spiegelman, D., Rick-Edwards, J., Corliss, H., et al., (2008). Disparities in child abuse victimization in lesbian, bisexual, and heterosexual women in the Nurses' Health Study II. *Journal of Women's Health, 17*, 595-606.

Balsam, K.F., Lehavot, K., Beadnell, B., & Circo, E. (2010). Childhood abuse and mental health indicators among ethnically diverse lesbian, gay, and bisexual adults. *Journal of Consulting and Clinical Psychology, 78*(4), 459-468.

Balsam, K., Molina, Y., Beadnell, B., Simoni, J., & Walters, K. (2011). Measuring minority stress: The LGBT People of Color B Scale. *Cultural Diversity and Ethnic Minority Psychology, 17*(2), 163-174.

Balsam, K., Rothblum, E., & Beauchaine, T. (2005). Victimization over the lifespan: A comparison of LGB and heterosexual siblings. *Journal of Consulting and Clinical Psychology, 73*(3), 477-487.

Brown-Saracino, J. (2011). From the lesbian ghetto to ambient community: The perceived costs and benefits of integration for community. *Social Problems, 58* (3), 361-388.

Cohn, T. & Hastings, S. (2011). Rural lesbian life: narratives of community, commitment, and coping. *Journal of Lesbian Studies, 15*, 141-147.

Corliss, H., Cochran, S.D., & Mays, V.M. (2002). Reports of parental maltreatment during childhood in a U.S. population-based survey of homosexual, bisexual, and heterosexual adults. *Child Abuse and Neglect, 26*, 1165-1178.

Cunningham,S., Vaquera, E., Maturo, C.C., & Venkat Narayan, K.M. (2012). Is there evidence that friends influence body weight? A systematic review of empirical research. *Social Science and Medicine, 75*, 1175-1183.

D'Augelli, A., Collins, C., & Hart, M. (1987). Social support patterns of lesbian women in a rural helping network. *Journal of Rural Community Psychology, 8*(1), 12-22.

D'Augelli, A., Grossman, A.H., & Starks, M.T. (2006). Childhood gender atypicality, victimization, and PTSD among LGB youth. *Journal of Interpersonal Violence, 21*, 1462-1482.

Fogel, S., Young, L., Dietrich, M., & Blakemore, D. (2012). Weight loss and related behavior changes among lesbians, *Journal of Homosexuality, 59*, 689-702.

Frost, D. & Eliason, M.J. (2013). Challenging fusion in female same-sex relationships: An Inclusion of Other in Self (IOS) approach. Psychology of Women Quarterly, *doi:10.1177/0361684313475877*

Kurdek, L. A. (2004). Are gay and lesbian cohabiting couples really different from heterosexual married couples? *Journal of Marriage and Family, 66*, 880-900.

Lehavot, K., Balsam, K.F., & Ibrahim-Wells, G.D. (2009). Redefining the American quilt: Definitions and experiences of community among ethnically diverse lesbian and bisexual women. *Journal of Community Psychology, 37*(4), 439-458.

Logan, L.S. (2013). Status homophily, sexual identity, and lesbian social ties. *Journal of Homosexuality, 60*, 1494-1519.

Lyle, J. Jones, J. & Drakes, G. (1999). Beauty on the borderland: On being black lesbian and beautiful. *Journal of Lesbian Studies, 3*(4), 45-53.

Ludwig, M.R., & Brownell, K.D. (1999). Lesbians, bisexual women, and body image: An exploration of gender roles and social group affiliation. *International Journal of Eating Disorders, 25*, 89-97.

Maor, M. (2012). The body that does not diminish itself: Fat acceptance in Israel's lesbian queer communities. *Journal of Lesbian Studies, 16*(2), 177-198.

Reczek, C. (2012). The promotion of unhealthy habits in gay, lesbian, and straight intimate partnerships. *Social Science and Medicine, 75*, 1114-1121.

Reczek, C., & Unberson, D. (2012). Gender, health behavior, and intimate relationships: Lesbian, gay, and straight contexts. *Social Science and Medicine, 74*, 1783-1790.

Smith, H.A., Markovic, N., Danielson, M.E., Matthews, A., Youk, A., Talbott, E.O., Larkby, C., & Hughes, T. (2010). Sexual abuse, sexual orientation, and obesity in women. *Journal of Women's Health, 19*(8), 1525-1532.

Stoddard, J.P., Dibble, S.L., & Fineman, N. (2009). Sexual and physical abuse: A comparison between lesbians and their heterosexual sisters. *Journal of Homosexuality, 56*, 407-420.

Swami, V. & Tovee, M. (2006). The influence of BMI on the physical attractiveness preferences of feminist and nonfeminist heterosexual women and lesbians. *Psychology of Women Quarterly, 30*, 252-257.

Szymanski, D.M. & Owens, G.P. (2008). Do coping strategies moderate or mediate the relationship between internalized heterosexism and sexual minority women's psychological distress? *Psychology of Women Quarterly, 32*, 95-104.

Szymanski, D.M. & Owens, G.P. (2009). Group-level coping as a moderator between heterosexism and sexism and psychological distress in sexual minority women. *Psychology of Women Quarterly, 33*, 197-205.

Taub, J. (1999). Bisexual women and beauty norms: A qualitative examination. *Journal of Lesbian Studies, 3*, 27-36.

Thayer, A. N. (2010). *Community Matters: The exploration of overweight and obesity within the lesbian population.* PhD Dissertation, Virginia Polytechnic Institute and State University.

Thompson, B.Y. (2012). The price of community from bisexual/biracial women's perspectives. *Journal of Bisexuality, 12,* 417-428.

Walters, M..C. (2011). Straighten up and act like a lady: a qualitative study of lesbian survivors of intimate partner violence. *Journal of Gay and Lesbian Social Services, 23,* 250-270.

Wen, M., & Kowaleski-Jones, L. (2012). The built environment and risk of obesity in the U.S.: Racial-ethnic disparities. *Health and Place, 18,* 1314-1322.

Wichstrom, L. (2006). Sexual orientation as a risk factor for bulimic symptoms. *International Journal of Eating Disorders, 39,* 448-453.

Wilson, B.D., Okwu, C., & Mills, S.A. (2011). The relationship between multiple forms of oppression and subjective health among Black lesbian and bisexual women. *Journal of Lesbian Studies, 15,* 15-24.

Wright, R.G., LeBlanc, A.J., & Badgett, L. (2013). Same-sex legal marriage and psychological wellbeing: findings from the California Health Interview Survey. *American Journal of Public Health, 103(*2), 339-346.

Chapter 12: Community Level Factors

"I do feel very comfortable in the community and I feel it's very accepting of very different body images that aren't portrayed by the media or the heterosexual world," but also "lesbian community is just as fat-phobic as the heterosexual community" (respondents in Yost & Chmielewski, 2011, p. 160).

Communities are complex social networks and can be defined in many ways. Community might be the neighborhood or town or region where we physically live. Community might be a group of people we identify with, such as lesbian and bisexual women or LGBT or women's communities that exist in many places. Community might be a social network of friends, acquaintances, even people we never met but associate with online, such as a Facebook network. Most of us belong to many communities, some based on our identities, some on our interests or beliefs, and some on physical spaces.

At the community level, individuals experience "cross-cutting social circles" or intersections among the webs of social groups based on the different identifications and interests of the individual, and some of these have different social norms. Belonging to a wide number of sometimes competing social networks and communities can be stressful, but can also offer opportunities for forging more fluid and creative responses to oppression (Pastrana, 2010). One study that reviewed the effects of different factors on one's health and well-being found that having a strong sense of belonging to at least one community was as powerful an effect on one's health as quitting smoking (Holt-Lunstad et al, 2013). Other recent research suggests that feeling alone and alienated may be a better predictor of addiction than any biological factors, also pointing to the power of community connection.

For lesbian and bisexual women who might be rejected by some communities, the need for a safe and inclusive community where one can feel a strong sense of belonging, is critical to good health. In this chapter, community is simplified into two main divisions: lesbian community and mainstream community, but with recognition that there are many sub-communities under each grouping. In this chapter, the term "lesbian community" is used because that is what most of the literature focuses on. Lesbian community has always included bisexual women whether they were open and accepted as bisexual or not.

LESBIAN COMMUNITY

Research on LGBT communities in general shows that a strong sense of community has many potential health enhancing effects. Community:

- Decreases depression and anxiety (Lehavot & Simoni, 2011)
- Decreases stress (Doty et al, 2010)
- Increases life satisfaction and decreases loneliness (Keleher et al, 2010)
- Increases self-esteem (Beals et al, 2009)
- Increases relationship satisfaction (Jordan & Deluty, 2000)
- Increases chances of being out (to healthcare providers among others) (Kwon, 2013)

The concept of community is sometimes more of an illusion than a reality. Sometimes we have a warped sense of what a community should look like. If we idealized *The L Word*, we may lament that we don't hang out with our friends everyday at the coffee shop or have enough elaborate dinner parties. The reality of community is more complicated than what we see in the media. Most women acknowledge that there is an LGBT or lesbian community, but they differ on their opinions about how it is constituted and what effects it has on individual members. Lugones (2008) said that "lesbian community is the context in which lesbians create new value" and Hostetler (2012) defined LGBT community as having a shared history of discrimination, stigma, and political movements. So we may seek LGBT community for a sense of sharing a history with gay and bisexual men and transgender individuals, or we may seek out specifically lesbian/bisexual women's communities for a more intimate and close sharing of both history and values as women.

Some research has shown that lesbian community is not so much a place or real people as an "ambient community" or a sense of belonging that comes from informal voluntary and emotional ties with others of shared interests or philosophies with whom one feels safe and accepted (Brown-Sracino, 2011). In reality, there is no one "lesbian community" or "lesbian/bisexual women's community" but instead, clusters of loosely connected smaller social or political sub-groups based on geography, interests, age, race, ethnicity, social class and income level, political issues, sexual styles, and many other factors. Physical communities also vary in the degree to which they offer lesbian/bisexual women specific activities and resources, such as health clinics, educational programs, social and recreational activities, political organizations, and so on.

Gay and bisexual men's organizing has been centered around HIV/AIDS activism since the 1980s, and has always had a strong bar and party culture. Women's communities historically have had less access to the economic resources and public spaces that gay male communities have had, and existed more in private spaces. Lesbian communities have been more influenced by feminist movements for gender equality than have gay/bisexual men's communities, although of course, many gay/bisexual men are much more knowledgeable about feminism than most heterosexual men. Because of the lack of financial resources, women have created informal support networks and loose collections of non-hierarchical organizations, often affiliated with a feminist orientation in many locations across the country, both urban and rural (Hostetler, 2012). Men gather at the bar or sports arenas; women in private homes and coffee shops. Men party; women organize. Of course, these are generalizations that are not always true, but lesbian and women tend to be involved in a wider variety of political organizing than gay/bisexual men.

Tensions in Lesbian Communities

Much has been written about lesbian communities, but there is less research about the ways that bisexual women have created communities. Many bisexual women feel that lesbian communities are rejecting of bisexual women, depending on whether they are oriented to lesbian feminist or separatist ideas versus more inclusive LGBT worldviews. If bisexual women are in relationships with women, they often have access to lesbian community events and organizations, but if in relationships with men, may feel unwelcomed in those spaces. Similarly, there have been pockets of transphobia in lesbian communities as well, particularly related to transgender women seeking involvement in lesbian activities and organizations. But there is also a sense of betrayal expressed about transgender men, many of whom identified as lesbian before transitioning. Feeling alienated and not belonging is a risk factor for health problems. Many lesbian communities have struggled with issues related to bisexuality and to transgender issues, and the conflicts have often created rifts in the community around inclusion versus exclusion. For example, where do you stand on the issue of the Michigan Women's Music Festival? They have been the source of controversy for many years for publicly stating that the festival is for womyn-born women. Although they do not actively police the grounds, they create an atmosphere that feels unwelcoming to many who call themselves women or lesbians.

Lesbian and bisexual women of color may also feel less involved in lesbian communities particularly those based on lesbian separatist principles, which emerged mostly out of white, middle class women's value systems and experiences (Alimahomed, 2010). White lesbians sometimes assume that they are enlightened about all forms of oppression just because of living with the oppression of sex and sexual orientation. Unfortunately other oppressions must be unlearned through an active process of engagement and commitment to social justice—we do not automatically shed all prejudices when we come out. For both white bisexual women and queer women of color regardless of sexual identifications, invisibility in lesbian or LGBT communities can lead to feeling like an outsider or on the margins of all their communities. Other women who may not feel fully integrated into lesbian community might be women with disabilities, poor lesbian and bisexual women, old lesbian and bisexual women, women in butch-femme relationships, and those with different religious/spiritual beliefs than are common in their local communities. The struggles about the boundaries of communities—who is on the outside and who is in, cause stress and emotional pain for many women on both sides of the borders.

Lesbian Community Norms about Weight/Body Image

Chapter 5 focused on lesbian community norms about the body. To sum this up, the research suggests:

- Lesbian and bisexual women are more accepting of a wider diversity of body shapes, sizes, and functioning in their friends, partners, and for themselves, than are heterosexual women, but some lesbian and bisexual women are fat-phobic, ableist, and have body shame and dissatisfaction. Yost and Chmielewski (2011) put it this way,

  "although women believe the lesbian community in the abstract to be accepting of larger women, women who are in fact heavier do not feel this support and acceptance in any concrete way" (p. 161).

- Coming out often leads to feeling better about one's own body and feeling less pressured by societal feminine beauty standards, but again, the media, other women, and other dominant expectations for women's appearance affect lesbian and bisexual women. It's hard to totally escape the focus on looks in our society.
- More lesbian and bisexual women are involved in fat positive, Health At Every Size, and other body and sex positive movements than are heterosexual women. However, some start to feel greater dissatisfaction with their bodies or their weight as they age and feel that they cannot carry the same weight as they did when younger. They may fear expressing this concern about weight and aging for fear of being rejected by fat-positive communities that were so helpful and supportive at an early stage of life.
- Some lesbian communities have appearance norms that feel too restrictive for some women, such as an emphasis on an androgynous look or an "earth mother" look. The community norms vary widely depending on many factors such as the age of the group, race/ethnicity, education, geographic region, and so on. Los Angeles "A-list" lesbians have a very different look than Wisconsin working class dykes. Whatever the norms, some women may feel pressure to try to fit in.

Geographic Differences in Lesbian Communities

Geography, or where you live, may play a significant role in how lesbian communities are organized, and what community norms they adopt. Rural areas have historically been more racially homogeneous and politically and religiously conservative. Kazyak (2012) proposed that female masculinity is normative in many rural settings and differs from the ways that female masculinity is expressed in urban settings. Masculinity is more highly valued in rural areas so that butch lesbians may be accepted in ways that more feminine gay men rarely are. Masculinity is equated with "country style," and particularly early in the coming out process, some women are inclined, or pressured, to reject traditional femininity and become more androgynous or masculine in their appearance. Along with the rejection of femininity is a rejection of the thinness imperative (Yost & Chmielewski, 2011). In urban areas, there may be much more diversity of gender and sexual expressions, thus, less pressure to be androgynous or butch. There are more diverse subsets of the lesbian and bisexual population so that any individual may be able to find a group that is compatible with one's own interests and appearance norms. Lots of research finds that rural lesbians are less likely to be out in all aspects of their lives, and face more blatant discrimination, particularly from conservative religions, than do urban lesbian/bisexual women. On the other hand, as the expense of living in LGBT-friendly cities has increased, older lesbian and bisexual women may be displaced to suburbs and rural areas for financial reasons, and may be creating strong social networks and communities where none existed previously.

The Role of Gay Bars

Bars are an example of the paradox of many lesbian communities, with both positive, life-affirming qualities, and health-damaging qualities. In many locations across the country, gay bars have played a role as LGBT community centers for lesbian/bisexual women. At one time, many communities had a number of lesbian bars, but over time and with the growing health-consciousness of many lesbian/bisexual women (and the economic struggle to sustain any business that caters to a very small and economically deprived segment fo the community), few lesbian bars exist today. However, even today, gay bars thrive and are among the very few places where some women can feel free to be themselves. Particularly in rural areas, gay bars are the center of support, acceptance, and education about one's own community. But women who frequent gay bars are exposed to high levels of drinking, drug use, smoking, and "bar food" or unhealthy fried or processed foods. Women who spend their leisure time in bars are likely to meet their partners and close friends in those venues, increasing the risk for a heavier drinking, using, smoking social network (Rosario, 2008) and a generally unhealthier lifestyle. Some lesbian/bisexual women's community norms may be more permissive about the acceptability of drug and heavy alcohol use than are heterosexual women's communities. When gay bars are prevalent and widely accepted as "community centers," there may be more permissive attitudes about alcohol and drugs, and less support for sobriety. Cochran, Grella, and Mays (2012) found that LGBT respondents were more likely to report that it was "ok" for people to use marijuana, cocaine, hallucinogens, and drink 4-5 alcoholic beverages per day, than were heterosexual respondents. This more libertarian attitude about drugs and alcohol may extend to other potentially health damaging behaviors as well. The attitude is that everyone should have the right to do whatever they want with their own bodies. Sometimes, though, community norms need to be altered to support health (but not to demonize those who choose otherwise or who have little choice in their behaviors). A visit to a lesbian or LGBT Alcoholic Anonymous meeting will show just how damaging those permissive attitudes about drugs and alcohol have been on some individual's lives.

Informal Support Networks and Community Activities

Lesbian/bisexual women's communities have always created a wide range of informal support networks such as community potlucks, book clubs, sports and recreational activities, music festivals, political groups, collectives to publish books or start new organizations, and performances. Many lesbian and bisexual women distrust mainstream services such as those offered by hospitals or community health agencies, and prefer to be in lesbian/bisexual-specific groups or settings in "lesbian community." This "do it for ourselves" mentality has created many opportunities for community connection for lesbian and bisexual women.

MAINSTREAM COMMUNITY

Lesbian and bisexual women do not exist in isolation, but are imbedded in mainstream communities of place, identity, and interest. These mainstream communities have a wide diversity of inclusiveness of lesbian/bisexual women, and can be a source of stress or a source of comfort and resiliency. Just a few aspects of mainstream communities are explored here.

Built and Physical Environment

Lower income is associated with living in neighborhoods with fewer resources for healthy living. Low income neighborhoods are often lacking in healthy food options, over-represented by fast food, have higher crime and pollution rates, less walkable areas, and higher stress over all (Wen & Kowaleski-Jones, 2012). Because of the combination of sexism and heterosexism, lesbian and bisexual women in relationships have lower household incomes than heterosexual couples or male same-sex couples (Sears & Badgett, 2012), forcing them into lower income neighborhoods. Lower income and lower education neighborhoods may be associated with higher rates of anti-gay discrimination and violence. These neighborhoods' gyms, rec centers, and parks may be perceived as unsafe for some lesbian and bisexual women.

Home ownership typically gives a person more financial stability as they age. Because of the lower income levels, fewer lesbian/bisexual women may own their own homes, creating greater risk as they age. In states without legal marriage, it is more challenging to protect one's interest in a home that might be in a lover's name. If one tries to put the house in the other's name, she may be subject to a transfer tax or estate tax (not applicable if the couple are legally married). Surveys of homeless individuals rarely have asked questions about sexual orientation. San Francisco does a homeless count every two years, and in 2013 added a question about sexual orientation. The city officials were surprised to find that almost 30% of the homeless population were LGBT, compared to 15% in the general population of the city—so the rate was double of what would be expected (SF Examiner, Oct 7, 2013). Of the older homeless individuals, many were because of evictions, but data were not divided by gender so it's impossible to know how many were older lesbian and bisexual women.

Workplace Communities

Most lesbian and bisexual women work, or worked prior to retirement, and fewer were home-makers than older heterosexual women. The workplace can be a stressful place for lesbian and bisexual women if they do not feel fully included and valued, and many have experienced the gamut of negative responses from being ignored or left out to being fired for being lesbian or bisexual.

Religious/Spiritual Communities

What would it be like to live in the neighborhood with a fundamentalist church like the Westboro Baptist Church, that targets LGBT people? Many lesbian and bisexual women must live near people who hate us. This is even more challenging when one's own religious or spiritual family preaches intolerance and labels us as sinners. With the rise of fundamentalism in recent years, lesbian and bisexual women are faced with hatred in their neighborhoods, by business owners in their towns, by editorials in the local newspaper, by political campaigns, and by billboards on the way to work. These constant assaults from the religious right are one form of micro-aggression that affect us almost every day.

Political Communities

Lesbian and bisexual women are much more likely than heterosexual women to have liberal or radical political views, but often must live in communities where right-wing and fundamentalist religious groups have tainted the politics of the community. Living through hateful campaigns against same-sex marriage, adding gender identity to human rights codes, or just hearing local politicians engage in gay-bashing speeches can take a toll on one's health and wellbeing. Many lesbian and bisexual women are affiliated with progressive politics, but have to endure family dinners, workplace conversations, or community events that are homophobic.

Conclusion: Community Level Influences

As so many experts say, "It takes a village…" to do whatever needs to be done. We cannot do it all on our own, and we need supportive communities. Consider what you can do to build a stronger community for yourself. What kind of community do you want? How do you find that community? What can you do to make the mainstream community in which you live and/or work safer for lesbian/bisexual women? How can you help to make the lesbian/bisexual women's community more inclusive and capable of providing the social and emotional support we need to thrive as we age?

REFERENCES

Alimahomed, S. (2010), Thinking outside the rainbow: women of color redefining queer politics and identity. *Social Identities, 16*, 151-168.

Beals, K, Peplau, L., & Gable, S. (2009). Stigma management and well-being: the role of perceived social support, emotional processing, and suppression. *Personality and Social Psychology Bulletin, 25*, 867-879.

Brown-Saracino, J. (2011). From the lesbian ghetto to ambient community: The perceived costs and benefits of integration for community. *Social Problems, 58* (3), 361-388.

Cochran, S.D., Grella, C., & Mays, V.M. (2012). Do substance use norms and perceived drug availability mediate sexual orientation differences in patterns of substance use? Results from the California Quality of Life Study II. *Journal of Studies of Alcohol and Drugs,*

Hostetler, A.J. (2012). Community involvement, perceived control, and attitudes toward aging among lesbians and gay men. *International Journal of Aging and Human Development, 75*(2), 141-167.

Jordan, K., & Deluty, R. (2000). Social support, coming out, and relationship satisfaction in lesbian couples. *Journal of Lesbian Studies, 4*(1), 145-164.

Kazyak, E. (2012). Midwest or lesbian? Gender, rurality, and sexuality. *Gender and Society, 26*(6), 825-848.

Keleher, J., Wei, M., & Liao, K. (2010). Attachment, positive feelings about being a lesbian, perceived general support, and well-being. *Journal of Social and Clinical Psychology, 29*, 847-873.

Kelly, L. (2007). Lesbian body image perception. The context of body silence. *Qualitative Health Research, 17*, 873-883

Keridwen, L (2012). Karma eaters: the politics of food and fat in women's land communities in the United States. *Journal of Lesbian Studies, 16(*1), 108-134.

Kwon, P. (2013). Resilience in lesbian, gay, and bisexual individuals. *Personality and Social Psychology Review*, doi: 10.1177/1088868312490248.

Lehavot, K., & Simoni, J. M. (2011). The impact of minority stress on mental health and substance use among sexual minority women. *Journal of Consulting and Clinical Psychology, 79*(2), 159-170.

Lugones, M. (2003). *Theorizing coalition against multiple oppressions*, Latham, MD: Rowman & Littlefield, p. 189.

Rosario, M. (2008). Elevated substance use among lesbian and bisexual women: Possible explanations and intervention implications for an urgent public health concern. *Substance Use and Misuse, 43*(8/9), 1268-1270.

Sears, B., & Badgett, L. (2012). Poverty in LGBT community. *Tides*, Issue 4.

Wen, M., & Kowaleski-Jones, L. (2012). The built environment and risk of obesity in the U.S.: Racial-ethnic disparities. *Health and Place, 18*, 1314-1322.

Yost, M.R. & Chmielewski, J.F. (2011). Narrating rural lesbians lives: body image and lesbian community in central Pennsylvania. *Journal of Lesbian Studies, 15*, 148-165.

Chapter 13: Institutional Level Factors

There is so much bias, even today, against lesbian and bisexual women in the major institutions of society. Institutions are the large organizational forces that impact our daily lives, including healthcare systems, the media, education, the legal system, law enforcement, political systems, and corporations. They are sometimes somewhat hidden influences, other times, we directly confront the bias. In this chapter, we focus on healthcare systems, as lesbian/bisexual women must access healthcare systems more often as we age, but the other systems are also important to our health. When politicians run campaigns based on anti-LGBT sentiment, our quality of life and sense of being safe in the world is threatened. When corporations are granted the right to discriminate against us based on religious beliefs of its owners (e.g. the Hobby Lobby Supreme Court decision), we are threatened.

When we must use health care institutions, we often encounter fat bias and overwhelming pressure from healthcare providers to diet and lose weight. We often encounter lack of knowledge about lesbian/bisexual women's health issues. We face a few healthcare providers who are hostile or uncomfortable taking care of us. Some research has examined the role of stigma of sexual identity in creating/maintaining health problems, accessing care, and disclosure of sexual identity, or has examined the experience of fat people in healthcare, but so far few studies have examined the intersection of fat and sexual identity. Likewise, we don't have much research on other intersections, such as race/ethnicity and sexuality or disability and sexuality. Healthcare settings are places where stigma gets enacted, so this section starts with a brief discussion of stigma.

STIGMA

Stigma results from visible or invisible human characteristics that have been designated as "deviant" by societal institutions—those deviant groups include lesbian, bisexual, queer, woman, fat, not white, poor, disabled, and many others. Some authors argue that individuals with a concealable stigma can easily hide and avoid the prejudice and resultant discrimination that accompanies visible differences (e.g. Goffman, 1963). Others suggest that the energy it takes to hide a stigmatized identity takes an enormous toll on one's health and wellbeing (Pachankis, 2007). People with visible differences (such as skin color or greater body mass or gender non-conformity) are constantly "out," but people with hidden forms of difference such as sexual identity must continually make decisions about disclosure, sometimes multiple times per day (Pachankis, 2007). Some authors refer to this as "stigma management" (Meyer, 2007) and it adds a level of stress to daily life. In the U.S., stigma regarding lesbian and bisexual women primarily comes from two sources: medicine (sickness) and religion (sin). There is a link between sin and illness stories in many religious objections to same-sex desire. Medical discourses are based on ideas of disease or biological abnormality, and some of the most potent sources of stigma come from psychiatric notions of sickness, abnormality, or mental illness. In 1973 the American Psychiatric Association removed sexual orientation from the Diagnostic and Statistical Manual of Mental Disorders (DSM), but a minority of mental health providers still advocate "reparative" therapies. The sin and sickness messages continue to impact health care institutions, limiting access to health care services and affecting the quality of care received once in the system. We just don't know what kind of treatment we will get when we enter any new place; clinic, hospital, social service agency, or senior center.

HEALTH CARE ENCOUNTERS

This section addresses a number of issues that arise when lesbian/bisexual women have to seek health care services, including decisions whether to disclose to providers, encountering fat stigma and shaming, and access and quality of care issues.

Disclosure

Do lesbian and bisexual women reveal their hidden sexual identities to healthcare providers? This is not a simple yes or no question. There are at least four aspects of disclosure (Eliason & Schope, 2001):

115

- Active disclosure = directly telling your healthcare provider that you are lesbian or bisexual
- Passive disclosure = assuming that the healthcare provider will figure out that you are lesbian or bisexual because you brought a female partner to the visit, wore an LGBT-affirmative t-shirt, or said, "that's my partner," or something else that implies you are lesbian or bisexual, but without actually telling the provider that you are lesbian/bisexual.
- Passive nondisclosure = the typical healthcare provider doesn't ask so you don't tell.
- Active nondisclosure = you actively lie about your sexuality to avoid negative outcomes.

Which of these strategies have you used and how did they work for you?

Eliason, Dibble, DeJoseph, and Chinn (2009) proposed that there are at least three levels of influence on disclosure decisions: the individual patient, the health care provider, and the institution. On the individual patient level, factors that may predict disclosure include age, gender, racial/ethnic identity, religion, comfort with own sexuality, comfort with one's own gender, degree of internalized homophobia, past experience with health care, type of presenting problem (one might be less likely to disclose for an acute problem and more likely for a problem that involves on-going care), and whether the individual has a partner (someone who needs to be involved in health care decision-making). At the provider level, LGBTQ people may be more likely to choose female health care professionals because of a belief that women are more accepting of diverse sexual identities; some perceive that younger health care professionals are more accepting than older ones. Other provider considerations are body language, verbal language, reputation in the community, and whether the health care professional provides an opportunity for patients/clients to disclose. At the institutional level are the policies and procedures such as nondiscrimination policies, staff training, whether benefits are extended to domestic partners of same-sex couples, the written language on the forms, the atmosphere of the waiting room/reception areas, and whether the agency/institution has a reputation in the LGBT community.

Durso and Meyer (2012) reported on the factors that predicted whether 400 LGB people would disclose to health care providers. Nondisclosure was higher among bisexual men (39%) and women (33%) than lesbians (14%) or gay men (10%), and age, immigration status, medical history, education, level of internalized homophobia and connectedness to LGBT community predicted disclosure. Austin (2013) found similar predictors among southern lesbians (n=934), and also reported that non-urban lesbians were less likely to disclose than urban lesbians. Eliason & Schope (2001) reported that most LGBT respondents (over 50%) had a positive or neutral response from their disclosure, however, many others reported anger, hostility, discomfort, disgust, embarrassment, fear, and/or shock on the part of the provider. Another stressor related to health care is how and when the partner or family will be involved in care, and how they will be treated. In states with no recognition of same-sex relationships, partners without power of attorney may be denied access to their loved ones and have difficulty receiving information about their progress (Boehmer & Case, 2004; Rondahl et al, 2006).

Weight stigma

Qualitative studies have noted that larger women feel stigmatized by their weight, and often find that health care providers are judgmental or interpret any health problem in relation to their weight (Buxton & Snethen, 2013; O'Hara & Gregg, 2012). Even healthcare providers who specialize in treatment of larger people exhibit weight bias (Schwartz, Chambliss, Brownell, Blair, & Billington, 2003). The quote below sums up the experience of many larger women in seeking healthcare:

> *"You should eat less and exercise more and lose weight. If it was that easy everyone would do it, it's shaming. It's the same thing with the gowns, I'm not going to say, 'This gown is too small.' Those things are hard, I just don't sit around my house eating Snickers, there is a host of other things going on." (Lesbian respondent in Seaver, Freund, Wright, Tjia, & Frayne, 2008, p. 221).*

There are challenges to fat stigma now from many venues. Some scholars in biomedicine are challenging the notion that weight predicts health problems and are examining other factors that may create both weight gain and health problems (Bacon & Aphramor, 2011; Flegal & Graubard, 2009). It is quite

116

challenging to figure out whether heavier weight causes health problems, or whether it is the stigma related to being fat that causes health problems. It could be some combination of both. Esther Rothblum (2015) has published a plea to lesbian and bisexual women to take the lead in challenging fat stigma, as we would benefit greatly from a more body-positive climate, and we already have experience in challenging stigma.

Accessing Health Care Services

The research is really mixed on this issue. Do lesbian and bisexual women avoid care because of fears of discrimination or poor quality care? Some recent research shows that lesbian and bisexual women use health care services at the same or even higher rate than the general population of women. For example, one study (Bakker, Sandfort, Wanwesenbeek, van Lindert, & Westert, 2006) found that lesbians were 2.06 times more likely to see a mental health provider, and were equivalent to heterosexual women in seeing medical specialists (see also Mosack, Brouwer, & Petroll, 2013; Tjepkema, 2008). Grella and colleagues (2011) found that lesbian and bisexual women were more likely to seek mental health and substance abuse treatment than heterosexual women, even in the absence of a diagnosed problem, suggesting that they may be more willing to address quality of life issues in therapy. Some research finds that lesbian and bisexual women might be more likely to use alternative and complementary therapies because of discrimination experiences or mistrust of mainstream health care. Matthews and colleagues (2005) found that 42% of lesbians had experienced discrimination in health care compared to 35% of heterosexual women, and lesbians were more likely to use meditation/visualization, chiropractic services, massage, and mental health support groups than heterosexual women (see also, Dillworth, Kaysen, Montoya, & Larimer, 2009; Smith, Matthews, Markovic, et al., 2010; Tjepkema, 2008).

On the other hand, Lewis, Derlega, & Clarke (2006) noted that lesbian/bisexual individuals often expect to encounter discrimination and prejudice when they access services and as a result, may delay, not access services, not disclose, and/or feel reluctant to talk about their experiences as LGBTQ to health care professionals. Rounds, McGrath, & Walsh (2013) reported that LGBT people raised the potential for poor quality of care as a concern for accessing care. Some studies report that lesbian and bisexual women are less likely than heterosexual women to get pap tests and mammograms (Powers, Bowen, & White, 2001; Cochran et al, 2001), or conduct self-breast exams (Wells, Bimbi, Tider, et al., 2007), but other studies found no differences (e.g. Mosack et al., 2013). More research is needed to address whether women who accessed services disclosed their sexual or gender identities to the health care professional, and whether there are differences in accessing routine screening versus care for specific physical or mental health symptoms. We know very little about the health care seeking behaviors of older lesbian and bisexual women since the earlier studies did not consider whether there might be age differences in health care seeking.

HEALTH CARE PROVIDERS

When lesbian and bisexual women access healthcare services, they too often encounter providers who have had little or no education about their needs (Abdessamad et al, 2013; Eliason, Dibble, & Robertson, 2012; Obedin-Maliver et al., 2011; Sanchez, Rabatin, Sanchez, Hubbard, & Kalet, 2006). If not overtly discriminatory, patients encounter ignorance and heterosexism in healthcare settings (Rondahl, Innala, & Carlsson, 2006: Rounds, et al., 2013). In some recent studies of medical and nursing school curriculum, many schools had no content at all about LGBT health issues, and of those that did have some content, it was typically less than one hour per year of the program. Health care providers lack knowledge about the terminology related to sexuality and gender, confuse gender identity and sexual identity, do not ask the right questions to identify lesbian and bisexual patients, and many are uncomfortable when a patient does come out. So what happens is that the patient must educate the provider on how to address her and her partner(s), and what health issues might be different for her compared to heterosexual women. When we are in a vulnerable patient role, particularly with serious illnesses, this is an unfair burden to put on us.

In addition, lesbian and bisexual women often encounter providers who have been trained in biomedical ideas that obesity is the root cause of much chronic illness, and who encourage patients to diet and exercise more without consideration of all the other factors in their lives (O'Reilly & Sixsmith, 2012). If lesbian/bisexual patients experience a combination of homophobia and fat phobia in a healthcare provider, they may be even more inclined to delay or avoid healthcare.

Conclusion: Institutional Level

In conclusion, sexual minority women often experience differential treatment, lack of knowledge, and sometimes discriminatory or poor quality care when they access healthcare services, stemming from biases about sexual orientation and fat people, as well as other stigmatizing social identities. Disclosure to health care providers can be frightening when you have no idea how the provider might respond. If there is one time when you don't want to have to be an activist and fight for your own rights, it's when you are sick or injured.

REFERENCES

Abdessamad, H., Yudin, M.H., Tarasoff, L.A., Radford, K.D., & Ross, L.E. (2013). Attitudes and knowledge among obstetrician-gynecologists regarding lesbian patients and their health, *Journal of Women's Health, 22,* 85-93.

Austin, E. (2013). Sexual orientation disclosure to health care providers among urban and non-urban southern lesbians. *Women's Health, 53,* 41-55.

Bacon, L., & Aphramor, L. (2011). Weight science: evaluating the evidence for a paradigm shift. *Nutrition Journal,* 10:9 http://www.nutritionj.com/content/10/1/9.

Bakker, F.C., Sandfort, T.G.M., Wanwesenbeeck, I., van Lindert, H., & Westert, G.P. (2006). Do homosexual persons use health care services more frequently than heterosexual persons: Findings from a Dutch population study. *Social Science and Medicine, 63,* 2022-2030.

Boehmer, U. & Case, P. (2004). Physicians don't ask, sometimes patients tell: disclosure of sexual orientation among women with breast carcinoma. *Cancer, 101,* 1882-1889.

Buxton, B.K., & Snethen, J. (2013). Obese women's perceptions and experiences of healthcare and primary care providers. *Nursing Research, 62,* 252-259.

Cochran, S.D., Mays, V.M., Bowen, K., Gage, S., Bybee, D., Roberts, S., Goldstein, R., Robison, A., Rankow, E., & White, J (2001). Cancer-related risk indicators and preventive screening behaviors among lesbians and bisexual women. *American Journal of Public Health, 91,* 591-597.

Dillworth, T. M., Kaysen, D., Montoya, H. D., & Larimer, M. E. (2009). Identification with mainstream culture and preference for alternative alcohol treatment approaches in a community sample. *Behavior Therapy, 40*(1), 72-81.

Durso, L.E., & Meyer, I. (2012). Patterns and predictors of disclosure of sexual orientation to healthcare providers among lesbians, gay men, and bisexuals. *Sexuality Research and Social Policy,* doi.10.1007/x13178-012-0105-2.

Eliason, M.J., Dibble, S., De Joseph, J., & Chinn, P. (2009). *LGBTQ Cultures: What healthcare professionals need to know about sexual and gender diversity.* Philadelphia: Lippincott.

Eliason, M.J., Dibble, S.L., & Robertson, P. (2011). Lesbian, gay, bisexual and transgender physician's experiences in the workplace. *Journal of Homosexuality,* 58, 1355-1371

Eliason, M. J., & Schope, R. (2001). Does "Don't Ask, Don't Tell" apply to health care? Lesbian, gay, and bisexual people's disclosure to health care providers. *Journal of the Gay and Lesbian Medical Association, 5*(4), 125-134.

Flegal, K. M., & Graubard, B.I. (2009). Estimate of excess deaths associated with body mass index and other anthropometric variables. *American Journal of Clinical Nutrition, 89*(4), 1213-1219.

Grella, C.E., Cochran, S.D., Greenwell, L., & Mays, V.M. (2011). Effects of sexual orientation and gender on perceived need for treatment by persons with and without mental disorders. *Psychiatric Services,* 404-412.

Lehavot, K., Balsam, K.F., & Ibrahim-Wells, G.D. (2009). Redefining the American quilt: Definitions and experiences of community among ethnically diverse lesbian and bisexual women. *Journal of Community Psychology, 37*(4), 439-458.

Lewis, R., Kholodkov, T., & Kerlaga, V. (2012). Still stressful after all these years: A review of lesbian and bisexual women's minority stress. *Journal of Lesbian Studies, 16(1),* 30-44.

Matthews, A. K., Hughes, T. L., Osterman, G. P., & Kodl, M. M. (2005). Complementary medicine practices in a community-based sample of lesbian and heterosexual women. *Health Care for Women International, 26*(5): 430-47.

Meyer, I.H. (2007). Prejudice and discrimination as social stressors. In Meyer, I.H. & Northridge, M. (Eds). *The health of sexual minorities: Public health perspectives on lesbian, gay, bisexual, and transgender populations.* NY: Springer, pp 242-267.

Mosack, K.E., Brouwer, A.M., & Petroll, A.E. (2013). Sexual identity, identity disclosure, and health care experiences: Is there evidence for differential homophobia in primary care practice? *Women's Health Issues, 23,* e341-e346.

Obedin-Maliver, J., Goldsmith, E., Stewart, L., White, W., Tran, E., Brenman, S.. et al. (2011). LGBT-related content in undergraduate medical education. *JAMA*, 306:971-977.

O'Hara, L., & Gregg, J. (2012). Human rights casualties from the 'war on obesity': why focusing on body weight is inconsistent with a human rights approach to health, *Fat Studies, 1(1)*, 32-46.

O'Reilly, C. & Sixsmith, J. (2012). From theory to policy: Reducing harms associated the weight-centered health paradigm. *Fat Studies, 1*(1), 97-113.

Pachankis, J. (2007). The psychological implications of concealing a stigma: A cognitive-affective-behavioral model. *Psychological Bulletin, 133(2)*, 328-345.

Powers, D., Bowen, D.,& White, J. (2001). The influence of sexual orientation on health behaviors in women. *Journal of Prevention and Intervention in the Community, 22(2)*, 43-60.

Röndahl, G., Innala, S., & Carlsson, M. (2006). Heterosexual assumptions in verbal and non-verbal communication in nursing. *Journal of Advanced Nursing, 56(40*, 373-381.

Rothblum, E (2015). Commentary: Lesbians should take the lead in removing the stigma that has long been associated with body weight. *Psychology of Sexual Orientation and Gender Diversity*, doi:.org/10.1037/sgd0000065.

Rounds, L.E. McGrath, B.B., & Walsh, E. (2013). Perspectives on provider behaviors: A qualitative study of sexual and gender minorities regarding quality of care. *Contemporary Nurse, 44*, 99-110.

Sanchez, N.F., Rabatin, J., Sanchez, J.P., Hubbard, S., & Kalet, A. (2006). Medical students' ability to care for LGBT patients. *Family Medicine, 38(1)*, 21-27.

Schwartz, M. B., Chambliss, H. O., Brownell, K. D., Blair, S.N., & Billington, C. (2003). Weight bias among health professionals specializing in obesity, *Obesity Research, 11*, 1033-1039.

Seaver, M.R., Freund, K.M., Wright, L.M., Tjia, J., & Frayne, S.M. (2008). Healthcare preferences among lesbians: A focus group analysis. *Journal of Women's Health, 17*, 215-225.

Smith, H., Matthews, A., Markovic, N., Youk, A., Danielson, M., & Talbott, E., (2010). A comparative study of complementary and alternative medicine use among heterosexually and lesbian-identified women: data from the ESTHER project. *Journal of Alternative and Complementary Medicine, 16(*11), 1161-1170.

Tjepkema, M. (2008). Health care use among gay, lesbian, and bisexual Canadians. *Health Reports, 19(1)*, 53-62.

Wells, B.E., Bimbi, D.S., Tider, D., Van Ora, J., & Parsons, J.T. (2006). Preventive health behaviors among lesbian and bisexually identified women. *Women's Health, 44*(2), 1-13.

Chapter 14: Societal Level Factors

"If you're a woman you already know that you're making 59 cents to a male dollar. If you're a queer woman who is non-white, how much of that 59 cents are you making? There are tolls that get paid all the way along that don't get looked at" (respondent in Lehavot, Balsam, & Ibrahim-Wells, 2009, p. 451)

The societal level is where all the forms of oppression get maintained because the laws, policies, and power to control others are institutionalized at this level—in law enforcement, education, welfare, government, health care policies, healthcare education and training programs, religion, and the media. This chapter deals with race, class, gender and sexuality in the most detail, but also notes some of the other forms of oppression experienced by lesbian and bisexual women.

INSTITUTIONALIZED SEXISM

Forces of oppression that affect all women, such as differential pay for equal work, sexual violence, sexual harassment, and stereotypes about women that limit our potential, deeply affect lesbian and bisexual women. Figure 14.1 below shows the wage gap by gender.

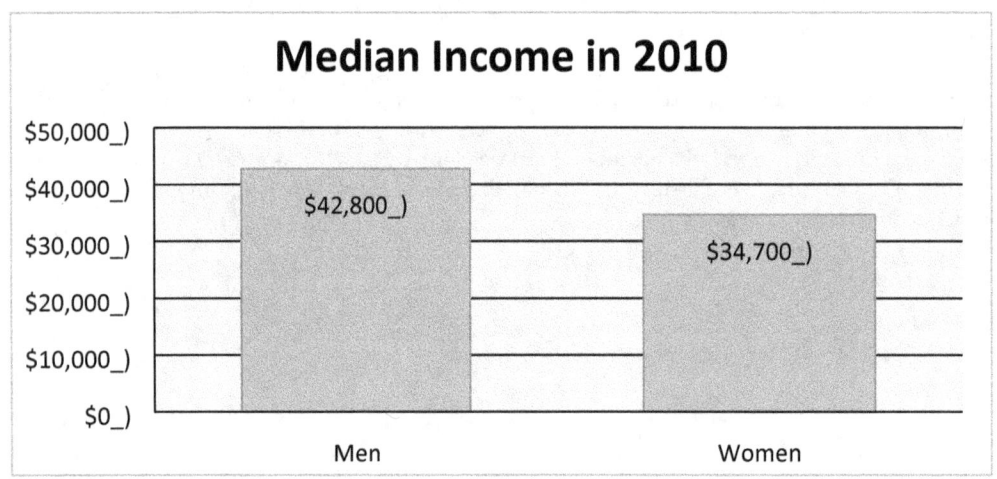

The media ruthlessly promotes youth and painfully thin bodies, and even lesbian-themed movies often fall into Hollywood beauty standards. Older and/or larger women are shown as pathetic or the butt of the joke. Lesbian and bisexual women often encounter sexism in the broader LGBT community from men and also from women without exposure to feminism. In fact, in many communities the term "feminism" is used to mean "lesbian." In addition, women who do not conform to societal gender norms in their appearance or behavior are more likely to experience discrimination and violence than gender-conforming women (Feinstein, Goldfried, & Davila, 2012), and some may also experience exclusion and negativity from lesbian feminist communities that emphasize androgyny (Sullivan, 2003).

As noted above, sexism impacts income level and job advancement, and creates financial stress that affects access to health resources and to healthy food, gym memberships, and time to engage in healthful activities. In addition, lesbian/bisexual women who are parents may face additional stigma associated with same-sex parenting and stereotypes about the role of single-sex role models for children. There is a sexist belief that all children need a male role model in their lives to be well-adjusted. How many female same-sex couples have been made to feel inadequate because of this?

One of the pernicious effects of sexism on women's health is the objectification of women's bodies in the media. Many authors note that ongoing experience with objectification in the media and by parents, teachers, peers, and others in communities, leads to internalization and self-objectification. Most women begin an ongoing process of "body surveillance" at an early age and experience body shame and often disordered eating behaviors (Bacon & Aphramor, 2014). In recent years, media messages about fat bodies have changed from a focus on "beauty" to a focus on "health." Thus, the fat woman now is scrutinized as a unhealthy object or vector of disease that puts a burden on the health care sector and in turn, society as a whole. This is quite similar to the ways that being lesbian or bisexual has been pathologized as a disorder, and one that puts burden on society. For example, all the political messages about same-sex marriage as a "threat" to heterosexual marriage is based on a notion of special rights and added burden to society.

Internalized Sexism

When women believe the negative stereotypes about women that circulate in the culture, the internalization produces self-hatred and shame. Many women deep down feel there is something wrong with them; that any problems they encounter in relationships or in the workplace and in many other settings, is the result of not being smart enough, or being too emotional, or having an inferior body. If one is taught from the time of birth to hate women or consider women as less than men, than what kind of relationship can we have with other women? This internalizing of sexism sets up competition among women and petty jealousies and rivalries.

INSTITUTIONALIZED HETEROSEXISM

Heterosexism and sexism are inter-related concepts, and much of the opposition to LGBT people stems from deeply ingrained societal stereotypes based on sex/gender. Heterosexism is the belief that the only "normal" or "natural" options for relationships are for one man and one woman in a legal marriage. Heterosexism is displayed in the lack of legal recognition of relationships, such as lack of marriage or civil unions in many states, the use of anti-gay rhetoric in political campaigns and religious discourses, the lack of sexuality education in schools, and the inability to address employment, housing, or educational discrimination based on sexuality. All of these forces of oppression impact the lesbian or bisexual woman's daily existence and add to the total levels of stress. Heterosexism and sexism can be internalized and result in shame, guilt, fear, low self-esteem, and self-harm at the individual level.

Religion has played a large role in creating the stigma that increases risk for health problems in lesbian and bisexual women, and the educational system in the U.S. perpetuates the stereotypes about lesbian and bisexual women by remaining silent about sexual orientation and allowing school bullying based on sexuality, sex/gender, and gender expression to continue. Chapter 9 dealt with religion, which is a major factor in both experiences of discrimination and in internalized oppression.

Internalized heterosexism

As has been noted many times in this book, internalized heterosexism, or feelings of disgust, shame, guilt, self-hatred, inferiority about one's sexual desires, is at the root of most of the health problems that lesbian and bisexual women experience. Internalized heterosexism is related to a wish to not be lesbian or bisexual, a fear of associating with people who look visibly LGBT or queer, a sense of inferiority, and most of all, guilt and shame. These distressing feelings of low self-worth can underlie substance abuse, depression, anxiety, suicide behaviors, and emotional eating. It's hard to completely resist internalizing some of the negative messages, because we are exposed to them constantly from early childhood on. Even well-adjusted, out and proud lesbian and bisexual women may sometimes have doubts.

RACISM AND CLASSISM

These two forms of oppression related to race and socioeconomic status, are combined here. Some authors think that they cannot be separated—that racism affects one socioeconomic status profoundly, and the negative effects on health are the product of the class difference. Others argue that there are some critical differences in racism and classism. Women of color have experienced some unique issues with white lesbian/bisexual women that differ somewhat from experiences of poor women, regardless of race, and women of color with good financial means and middle class or higher status, still experience racism in some aspects of lesbian community. Figure 14.2 shows how income is doubly impacted by the combinations of race and sex. Income level is the greatest predictor of health outcomes, and this shows that African American and Latina women are most affected by the income gap in the U.S. A relationship consisting of two lesbian/bisexual women of color is likely to be economically disadvantaged.

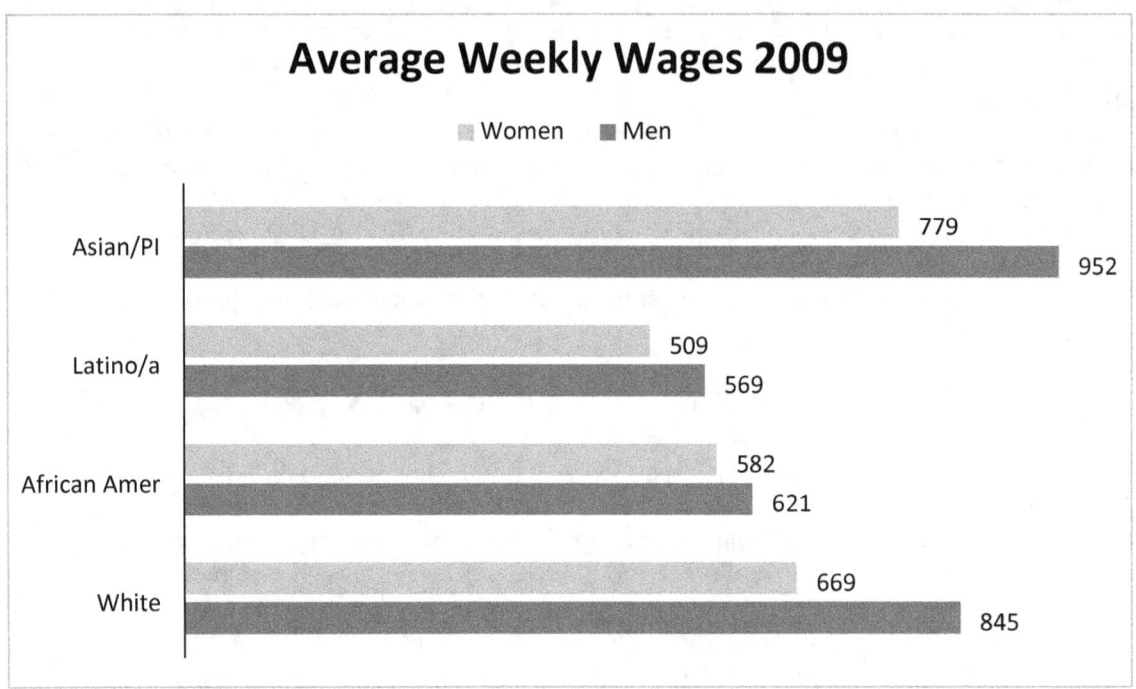

Lesbian communities have often been criticized for their lack of attention to issues of race and class. When the community focuses on Olivia cruises and Dinah Shore weekend trips, they may exclude many women who could never afford these outings. The challenge becomes to create communities that allow all women to participate in whatever way they can, and feel a sense of belonging.

Other Forms of Oppression

As noted at the beginning of this book, oppression gets written on the bodies of those who live under the stressful conditions of unfair treatment, threat of violence, and unequal access to health information and services (Krieger, 2005). Lesbian and bisexual women may also experience ageism, ableism, oppression related to their religious or spiritual beliefs and practices, and other intersecting forces that impact their daily lives. Finally, there is a growing body of research on fat stigma and the negativity of societal discourses toward larger bodies. Large women face ridicule and harassment from physicians, family members, and even strangers. There appears to be growing institutionalized policies that oppress larger people, such as employment discrimination, having to pay for two airline tickets because seats have been made smaller, and poor treatment by health care providers. People with disabilities also face many challenges because of institutionalized ableism that values only a certain type of productivity and functionality.

INTERSECTIONALITY

Minority stress has impact on lesbian and bisexual women at all levels of the ecological model. Several studies now have identified that minority stress consists of two components: 1) internalized oppressions that impact individual and interpersonal well-being, and 2) external sources of discrimination, harassment, and violence that cause psychological distress in sexual minority individuals (Meyer, 2003). Internalized oppression comes from constant exposure to sexist and heterosexist (and racist, ageist, classist) messages through-out one's life. It is difficult for anyone to totally resist the negative messages, and all people internalize them to some extent, but some have more negative exposures than others and may develop self-doubt, guilt, depression, and anxiety about their sexual desires. Likewise, nearly all lesbian/bisexual women have experienced or witnessed some degree of external discrimination related to being women or to having a sexual minority identity. But minority falls short as a theory when we consider lesbian and bisexual women who have multiple oppressed minority identities, such as the Native American bisexual disabled woman of 70 years of age.

To truly understand the impact of minority stress, feminist theories of intersectionality are needed that identify the potential interactive and complex relationships among social identities and community identifications (Bowleg, 2012). Lesbian and bisexual women have to deal with both heterosexism and sexism at a minimum, and many also deal with ageism, racism, classism, ableism, and other forms of oppression, all of which contribute to minority stress. The different combinations of stigmatized identities may result in very different community subgroups. For example, some older lesbians identify with LGBT or at least gay communities and engage in mixed social and recreational activities, whereas others were influenced by feminism and separatist politics and have mostly or entirely lesbian social networks (Averett & Jenkins, 2012). Some older lesbians are bi-phobic and trans-phobic as well as preferring women-born only social spaces (McLean, 2008; Weiss, 2011). Some women of color may affiliate primarily in social networks based on race, not sexual orientation, and sometimes have to downplay their sexuality in those settings.

Conclusion: Societal Level

The societal levels of discrimination have profound effects on individual wellbeing. Internalized oppressions, however, are complex and messy phenomena, stemming from the messages that come from parents, family, religious leaders, teachers, the media, formal education, medical-psychiatric discourses, political campaigns and many more. Minority stress is not simply additive, but is intersectional, making it difficult to assess. The multiple forces of oppression, the many social identities that are adopted to varying degrees among lesbian and bisexual women, and the constantly changing public discourses about sex, gender, sexuality, health, weight, and aging all combine to create minority stress that expresses in unpredictable ways.

REFERENCES

Averett, P., Yoon, I., & Jenkins, C.L. (2013). Older lesbian experiences of homophobia and ageism. *Journal of Social Service Research, 39*, 3-15.

Bowleg, L. (2012). The problem with the phrase women and minorities: Intersectionality an important theoretical framework for public health. *American Journal of Public Health, 102*(7), 1267-1273.

Feinstein, B.A., Goldfried, M.R., & Davila, J. (2012). The relationship between experiences of discrimination and mental health among lesbians and gay men. *Journal of Consulting and Clinical Psychology, 80*(5), 917-927.

Krieger, N. (2005). Embodiment: a conceptual glossary for epidemiology. *Journal of Epidemiology and Community Health, 59*, 350-355.

Lehavot, K., Balsam, K.F., & Ibrahim-Wells, G.D. (2009). Redefining the American quilt: Definitions and experiences of community among ethnically diverse lesbian and bisexual women. *Journal of Community Psychology, 37*(4), 439-458.

McLean, K. (2008). Inside, outside, nowhere: Bisexual men and women in the gay and lesbian community. *Journal of Bisexuality, 8*, 63-80.

Sullivan, N. (2003). A critical introduction to queer theory. Edinburgh, Scotland: Edinburgh Univ Press.

Weiss, J. (2011). GL versus BT: the archeology of biphobia and transphobia within U.S. gay and lesbian communities. *Journal of Bisexuality, 11*(4), 498-502.

PART THREE: IMPROVING YOUR HEALTH

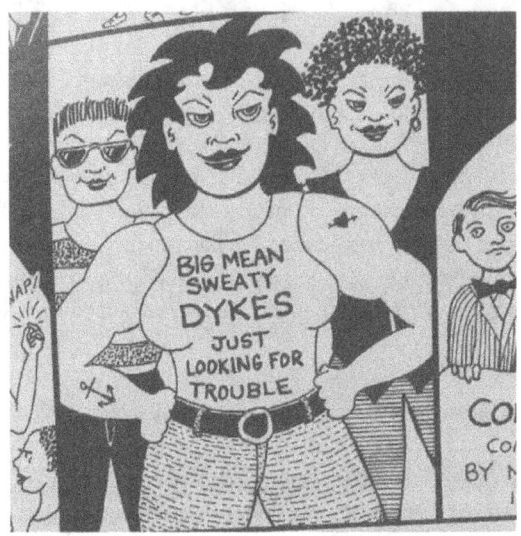

For any program designed to improve the health and wellbeing of lesbian and bisexual women to be effective, it must address all levels of the ecological model and draw from both the research on health in the general population and considerations of the unique qualities of lesbian/bisexual women's communities. So far, very few programs have been developed specifically for lesbian and bisexual women, so the chapters in this section pull from mainstream literature on physical activity, nutrition, and stress reduction and place that information within a lesbian/bisexual women's context. But getting healthier begins with making changes in behavior, so the first chapter in this section is on the nature of change. The five chapters in this section provide concrete suggestions on improving one's individual health. These chapters offer discussion or reflection questions to foster application to your own life. These chapters require some action on your part, even if that action is just noticing what is true for you, or where you are in terms of health behavior change. The final chapter summarizes the findings of the book.

.

Chapter 15. Making Changes

In a famous study of patients with heart disease, doctors told them that if they did not make some major change in their lives (change their dietary patterns, get more physical activity, stop smoking), that they would probably die in the very near future. In spite of this life and death scenario, only one out of seven followed through with making a change. Why is change so difficult that even those facing possible death cannot change these behaviors? We have probably all had the experience of resolving to change, but discovering that change is hard to sustain for more than a short period of time. We will begin this chapter with a discussion of two models of change that come from decades of research on deeply ingrained habits and change. The first is the transtheoretical model of change and the second is called Immunity to Change.

Before we go into these two models, it may be useful to look at some of the literature on how and why people make big changes in their lives. Sometimes these are called "transformative" changes, because they lead to major improvements in health and wellbeing. Marilyn Schlitz, Cassandra Vieten, and Tina Amorok, authors *of Living Deeply: The Art and Science of Transformation* (2007), suggested that there are four components to transformative change:

1. Intention: a conscious desire and commitment to change
2. Attention: a willingness to look closely at one's own patterns; to see the world through different eyes, and to wake up and stay awake
3. Repetition: practicing new patterns and skills daily to replace old habits
4. Guidance: a teacher, mentor, group, book, a program.

You probably already have intention, or you would not be reading this chapter. Most people have the intention to change some aspect of their behavior, but many never follow through and actually change. Attention is the second component. This is best understood as mindfulness. Every spiritual and religious tradition in the world has some type of contemplative practices that are meant to focus our attention inward to better understand our own motivations and expectations. These mindfulness practices can include prayer, meditation, reading sacred texts, spending time in nature to think deeply, journaling or writing memoir, working with wise elders, and so on. Mindfulness helps us to stay awake to our present—the place where life is actually lived. It helps us thrive in the present.

In regards to repetition, some experts think that it takes at least three months of practicing a new behavior before it becomes a habit. This is why substance abuse treatment in the past was usually 90 days in length. Practice is critical to change, but is so hard to maintain over time. Many of us commit to a change and practice it for a week or two, and then lapse back into the old patterns out of habit or lapse in attention.

Finally, the last component is guidance. In this case, we recommend that you attempt to make changes in your behavior with the support of a group and accurate information, such as provided in this book and elsewhere. The guidance might come from sacred texts of our lesbian/bisexual women's history, or from ancient or contemporary thinkers about the nature of good health. But this guidance must always be tempered by contemplation—does the practice meet the needs of your own unique self and body? Consider whether all four components are in place for you as you embark on any path to change.

TRANSTHEORETICAL THEORY OF CHANGE

The Stages of Change or Transtheoretical Model was initially published in the late 1970s by James Prochaska. In the 1980's, Prochaska and DiClemente (1983) worked further on this model to outline the stages of an individual's readiness to change, or the steps in their attempts to change unhealthy behaviors. The Stages of Change Model evolved from research on smoking cessation and the treatment of drug and alcohol addiction, but has also been applied to other health behaviors, such as dietary changes. Behavior change is viewed as a process, not an event, with individuals at various levels of motivation or "readiness" to change. Since people are at different points in this process, the programs or interventions should match their stage. There are six stages in the model:

1) **Pre-contemplation** - the person is unaware of the problem or has not thought seriously about change;

2) **Contemplation** - the person is seriously thinking about a change in the near future;

3) **Preparation** - the person is planning to take action and is making final adjustments before changing behavior;

4) **Action** - the person implements some specific action plan to change behavior and/or the surroundings;

5) **Maintenance** - the person continues with desirable actions, repeating the steps that have worked, while being mindful of triggers to prevent lapses and relapse; and

6) **Relapse -** the person reverts to the previous unhealthy behavior. Not everyone relapses but the majority will experience small slips or full relapses.

This is a circular or spiral model, rather than a linear model. That means people do not go through the stages one at a time and in order just once and then are done. In fact, the person may go through several cycles of contemplation, action, relapse (or recycle), or have several steps backwards before becoming free of the addictive or problematic behavior or making a relatively permanent change. This model is useful in figuring out where you are in terms of motivation, but not so helpful in increasing the motivation to change or figuring out how to move to the next stage. For that, we will consult the Immunity to Change model, which was developed for action, not just description. But let's start with your level of motivation, because it is helpful to know where you are before you decide where to go next! Think about one thing you would like to change about your current behavior, and note which of the six stages above best describes where you are right now. Write about this in your journal or discuss it with someone who will support you in making changes.

Creating Change in Old Patterns

The stages of change model outlines different places in the process of making changes, from not even thinking about change (pre-contemplation) to getting back on track after a slip-up. But the stages of change do not outline how to move from one stage to another. The concept of mindfulness is one tool for moving forward. Mindfulness comes from ancient wisdom/spiritual/religious practices, but can also be thought of as a cognitive skill or mind set for those who do not relate to the more spiritual aspects of mindfulness. Mindfulness is on a continuum from not being present at all to one's current life and living a life full of distraction, regrets of the past, fears of the future, to being fully present to one's life and making conscious decisions. The tools of mindfulness that foster making change are noticing and tracking. When we are not mindful, we are usually not paying attention to our behaviors and the consequences of our behaviors, so we do not learn from experience. We are destined to repeat mistakes and missteps if we don't pay attention to what causes them. Change requires not just paying attention (noticing), but also conscious and consistent tracking of our behaviors…what is working? What is challenging? How are different behaviors related to each other? How is my behavior linked to past experiences and old belief patterns? What is holding me back from changing? If I have a plan and know how to change, why aren't I changing? There must still be something holding us back, perhaps fears that stem from our past, such as fear of abandonment, fear of entrapment, fear of loss or pain. Formal tracking on a daily basis helps identify the patterns and see what differences the changes we are making have on our lives. The table below links the stages of change to different degrees of awareness or mindfulness. Think about where you are in terms of mindfulness, noticing, and tracking in regards to some health behavior you want to change.

Table 15.1. The relationship between stages of change and mindfulness

Stages of Change	Mindfulness	Noticing/Tracking
Pre-contemplation: Not even thinking about change	"asleep at the wheel"	Not paying attention, automatic pilot
Contemplation: First steps in thinking/considering a change	Starting to wake up	Noticing on occasion
Preparation: making plans	Seeing connections, being more present	Noticing regularly
Action: taking steps toward change	Staying present more often than lapsing into past or future	Formal tracking (journaling, reflecting on experiences, talking about it, charting behavior, recording progress)
Slip: temporary setbacks	Dozed off or stressed out	Back on automatic temporarily
Maintenance: keeping motivated to keep up healthy changes	Fully awake and present	Tracking happens automatically, daily

As you can see from this chart, moving from noticing to tracking is often associated with taking action. It may be beneficial to just track your behavior for a few weeks before taking action, and then track closely the results of your behavior change goals and actions. But if this is not enough to get the changes you want in your life, next we will consider a more complex process of making changes.

IMMUNITY TO CHANGE

Harvard professors Robert Kegan and Lisa Lahey (2009) have spent the last 20 years studying how internal resistance to change keeps us stuck in older patterns. In this manual, we focus on physical activity, nutrition, and stress reduction, but this process is helpful for making any kind of change in lifestyle or behavior. Kegan and Lahey reported that there are two kinds of preparations that people need to make to be successful at change. The first they call **technical change** that includes a need to learn new skills to accomplish one's goals. There are many programs available that teach skills; exercise classes, DVD's, personal coaches, nutritional counseling, internet information, but yet people resist getting or applying this information. That is why the second kind of change is probably the most important. **Adaptive change** involves changing one's mindset, or the internal habits and resistances to change. So change is not really about willpower or discipline, but understanding how habits form, create pathways in our brains, and how our own internal voices create mindsets that keep us from changing. Kegan and Lahey tested their system in many different settings with different types of people and found it to work better than programs that focus just on behavior or technical change alone.

Kegan and Lahey's model is a bit complicated, but if you will devote some time to working through the steps outlined below, you may find the process of change and creating new, healthier habits will be easier. The examples are framed around physical activity, but nutritional patterns and activity are very much related. For example, if we go on a calorie restriction diet, the body goes into survival mode and tries to conserve energy (Bacon, 2010). We don't have the energy to do much and just want to lounge on the sofa. If we eat foods that are high on the inflammation scale, we may feel pain or swelling in our joints that will slow us down. So in reality, changes in nutrition and physical activity need to happen together. But to simplify this immunity to change process, we will use a single example of behavior change.

The Immunity To Change Map

Kegan and Lahey proposed several steps in the process to identifying the mindsets that keep us from changing, even when there is overwhelming evidence that the change will be good for us. Use the next several pages as fodder for journaling about one of the changes that you would like to make in your life. It's important to write down the information so that you can look for the hidden assumptions and gain some insight into your own thoughts, behaviors, and hidden agendas. This process is a little hard to do alone, so consider getting a buddy or small group to work together and challenge each other to go deeper. To be most effective, make yourself a chart or "map" that looks like the one at the end of this chapter. You will fill it out over the course of several steps. It's important not to jump ahead and make yourself a "plan" for achieving your goal until you have worked through all the steps. Make several copies of the complete chart so that you can refine it as you move through the steps.

Step One: Set your goal

Set a goal for yourself that addresses something you have wanted to change for a long time now. Maybe you have tried to make this change before with limited success. It's important that this goal be SMART, that it is:

S   specific and concrete

M   measurable (you will be able to know if you meet the goal)

A   awesome (something you will enjoy and be able to stick to)

R   realistic (don't say you are going to climb Mt Everest unless you really are able to do it!)

T   time-related (establish a time frame for when you will accomplish it)

Examples:

I will use physical activity as an example through-out this section. Here are some common ways that women define their goals:

- "Get more exercise." This is obviously a poorly written goal, because it is too abstract and has no measureable or time-related components. It may not be awesome either, if you hate exercise. In fact, for most of us, the word "exercise" is dreaded. Let's just call it movement or physical activity. A better goal would be something like: "Increase walking by 5 minutes each day for 2 weeks." At the end of 2 weeks, you evaluate whether you have reached the level you want to maintain, or want to keep increasing (or maybe decrease a bit). If you enjoy walking, this is an awesome goal. You might even want to specify when and where you will walk (after work, first thing in the morning, in the local park, around the lake, in the mall in winter, and so on).

- "Try a yoga class." This is better than the first example, but still lacks information. A better goal might be "Go to the gentle yoga class at the Y once a week for three weeks." Three sessions is probably enough to determine if you like the class, the teacher, the actual yoga. You can then re-evaluate and keep going, or find another activity if this doesn't suit you.

- "Watch the DIFO physical activity video every day for a month." Well, this goal is concrete, measureable, and has a time-frame, but may not be realistic. It's 20 minutes long and most people will tire of watching it that often. A better goal might be "Watch the DIFO physical activity video once a week for 3 weeks, and try 2-3 different activities from the video every day during that time period." We will talk more about the video later.

Setting Your Personal Goal:

Write out the first draft of your physical activity goal in your journal. Next, evaluate it. Is it smart? In other words, is it:

☐ Concrete and specific

☐ Measureable

☐ Awesome

☐ Realistic

☐ Time-related?

Revise the goal if you need to and write it on your immunity to change map. Do not do anything to work on your goal yet, not until you have worked through the next several steps.

Step Two: Identifying Barriers

Next, you will identify all the things that you do, or do not do, that keep you from succeeding at your improvement goal. Make sure that these are concrete behaviors--not just feelings or thoughts. We will get to those later. Use this first step in the Immunity to Change Map to explore these issues.

Table 15.2. Immunity to Change Map. First Steps.

Barriers	Worries	Big Assumptions
What I do:	Feelings I have when I do the opposite of the barriers:	
What I don't do:	Competing Commitments:	

- Start your list in your journal. What do I do that gets in the way of my goal?

- What is it that I <u>do not do</u> that keeps me from achieving my goal?

These lists identify some of the technical changes that you might need to make to be successful. Give this some thought and when you think your list is complete, put the list on your immunity to change map. These are the technical skills you will need to address, but these behaviors and knowledge deficits alone are not enough. Technical changes are easy. If that was all there was to it, you would be successful at changing. You need to work through two more steps to get at the emotional mindset that keeps you stuck.

Step Three: Searching for the Motivations

This step is the most complicated and has two parts to it. First is the "worry box." Look at each behavior in column two (what I do and don't do that get in the way of my goal) and ask yourself this question in relation to each one: "What is the worst thing that could happen if I did the opposite of that behavior?" Let's say one of the things you do that keeps you from physical activity after work, is changing into your pajamas and settling in front of the TV. You might say: "If I did not put on my pjs the minute I got home, I might be more inclined to go for a walk after work." Do this for each item on your list of barriers to achieving your goal.

The second part of finding your motivations includes the competing commitments, or the motivations or mindsets that interfere with making changes. Are you protecting yourself from being perceived negatively by others? Are you trying to avoid dealing with your own body changes related to aging or illness? Do you think you need the approval of important others? Are you afraid of looking foolish? Are you afraid that if you increase your physical activity and meet your goals, you will still not feel healthy? You may need to consider what you learned from your family, racial/ethnic community, religion, or school about physical activity that you have carried into your adult life. So look at your list of barriers and see if you can find any common patterns or underlying beliefs that are holding you back.

Once you have the competing commitments listed in column 3, you can start to see that the improvement goal in Column 1 is the gas pedal and the competing commitments in Column 3 are the brakes. Reflect on what you have in columns 2 and 3 now and see if you can identify the hidden assumption. That is, why lies underneath the worries and the competing commitments? This step requires digging a little deeper into your unconscious mind. Notice that each step is a method of peeling the onion, finding the stuff hidden deeper and deeper.

Step 4: Finding the Hidden Assumption(s)

If no big assumption is apparent when you look at the two lists, it may be useful to repeat the "If-then" exercise on the competing commitments. Each time you do it, you may go a little deeper. Maybe you are harboring a fear of abandonment, a lack of body acceptance, a fear of being shown up as incompetent; a fear of failure; a fear of not being loved. If you have a bit of an emotional reaction when you do this, you have hit paydirt…that is, you might have found the emotional foundation where you might be stuck. This is a mindset--a belief system that may have no basis in reality. Now you can look at it more objectively and test it out.

Conclusions: The processes of change

Change is hard; otherwise we would all be healthier and happier! It's not easy to face your own motivations and assumptions, but if you really want to be successful in meeting your goals, it will take some work and deeper reflections. Unlike some of the other chapters that focused on the influences of the outside world on us as lesbian and bisexual women, when it comes to changing our lifestyle behaviors in regards to eating, moving, and reducing stress, it's an inside job!

REFERENCES

Kegan, R., & Lahey, L. (2009). *Immunity to change*. Boston: Harvard Business Park.

Prochanska, J. & DiClemente, C. (1983). Stages and processes of self change and smoking. *Journal of Consulting and Clinical Psychology, 51*, 47-51.

Schlitz, M., Vietan, C., & Amorak, T. (2007). *Living deeply: The art and science of transformation in everyday life*. Oakland, CA: Harbinger Press.

IMMUNITY TO CHANGE MAP

My improvement goal	
Barriers: What I do that gets in the way What I don't do that gets in the way	
Worries (Feelings I have when I do the opposite of the barriers). What puts on the brakes?	
Commitments (what are those worries masking?)	
The Big Assumption	

Chapter 16: Reducing Stress

This chapter addresses the many sources of stress that may directly and indirectly affect our health. Some types of stress are good, and motivate us, but many forms of stress lead us to develop unhealthy ways of coping that may damage our health. Some stress is beyond our control but we do have some control over how we react to the stress. Stress is both an event (like an illness) and our response to the event. This chapter explores where stress comes from and then talks about how to manage it in a healthier way.

Does Inequality Make Us Sick?

Several research studies have shown that chronic exposure to minority stress, whether related to sexual orientation, race, sex/gender, age, or other factors, increases the risk for health problems (Meyer, 2013). The figure below shows how this works.

Figure 16.1. The relationship between stigma and poor health outcomes.

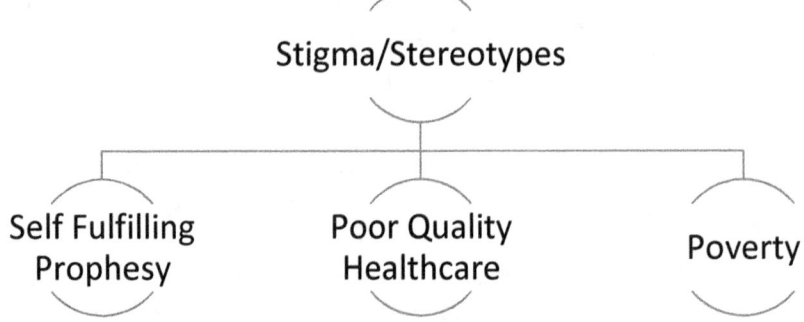

Stereotypes create the attitude that one group is less deserving or inferior to others. This results in less opportunity for people within the group to get higher education and good jobs, which increases the chance of poverty and poor or no access to health benefits. Educational institutions ignore us and do not train healthcare providers in our issues or to be respectful of us. We may respond by using unhealthy coping strategies for the stress or avoiding or delaying health care because of fears of mistreatment.

In a recent study of over 800 lesbian and bisexual women (Fredriksen-Goldsen et al, 2013), 28% of lesbians and 48% of bisexual women were living under the federal poverty level. Transgender women are even more likely to be struggling financially. A recent study (Gates, 2014) showed that lesbian and bisexual women were more likely to report not having enough money for food and using food stamps than heterosexual women, as shown in the chart below.

Figure 16.2. Food insecurity markers in women in California (from Gates, 2014)

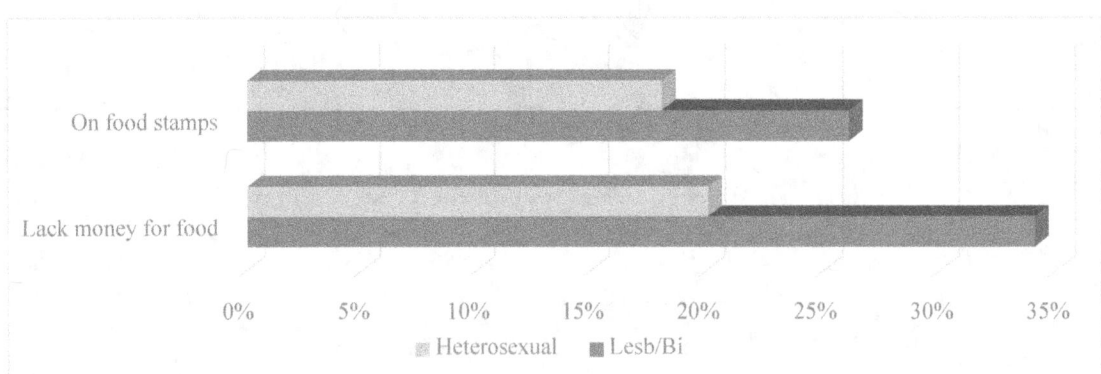

The shocking fact is that about one in three lesbian/bisexual women are "food insecure" and this affects how we eat. If we have to worry about where our next meal is coming from, we go on a survival mode that makes mindful eating more difficult. Survival mode means eating as much as we can when food is available, because unconsciously we are afraid we may not get another meal soon enough. We are on a psychological starvation mindset. Even women with adequate incomes may have to navigate healthcare systems and providers who are ignorant or even hostile, so oppression related to sexual orientation affects us all.

DIVERSITY

We share a common bond of identifying as lesbian, bisexual, queer, or a similar identity, and aging, but we are all also different in many ways. Those differences can create stress when we attempt to find inclusive communities and social networks to nurture us. Consider the following questions, and journal about any of these topics that cause you stress.

- What other identities make up your unique self in addition to your sexual orientation? (these could include race, ethnicity, language, country of origin and immigration status, socioeconomic status, religion, disability status, butch/femme identities, S&M or BDSM identities, etc.). List any identities that sometimes make you feel on the outside of a social group:

- How are these other identities related to your overall health?

- How can LGBT or lesbian/bisexual communities be more mindful of the differences among us? How can we be healthier and more inclusive as a community?

The Role of Gender Expression

One form of diversity within lesbian/bisexual women's communities is based on the gender expression continuum. Some women identify as femme, some as butch, and others as androgynous or in the middle of gender. Others do not think these terms apply to them. But when strangers see us, they notice the visible markers of identity on us: our gender, race, and physical appearance (including size and physical (dis)ability status) are the most immediately noticeable. Sexual orientation is one of the invisible or hidden identities; our gender expression is highly visible. Much of the violence against LGBT people by strangers is based on our appearance, and women who do not conform to gender expectations are the most likely to experience discrimination and violence. Butch and androgynous lesbians are more identifiable than femme lesbians. Visible lesbians—the ones who do not fit feminine stereotypes--experience more discrimination and harassment from an early age, but less visible lesbians may experience more internalized homophobia and may feel bad about not being identifiable as lesbian/bisexual (Levitt & Horne, 2002; Rosario et al, 2009).

Some transgender people are more visible while in transition. Transgender individuals may have considerable stress around "passing" as the gender with which they identify. The term "passing" in lesbian communities is often negative, meaning that the person deliberately hides their sexuality. This difference in the definition of the term "passing" may create misunderstandings between lesbian/bisexual women and transgender women.

- Where do you fall on the gender spectrum and how do others treat you on the basis of your gender expression? Is this a source of stress in your life?

The Role of Religion

Religion is another major source of anti-gay attitudes and stress that affect families' and communities' attitudes about us. If we grew up in a religion that is negative about us as women or as lesbian/bisexual women, we have to make decisions about trying to find the good in our religious life to balance that negativity, finding another less homophobic religion, opting for a spiritual practice rather than a formal religion, or rejecting both religion and spirituality. As a community, we need to find ways to support all of our members, whatever they choose about religious or spiritual beliefs and practices. But we also need to stand up against religion-sponsored ex-gay therapies that do so much harm to members of our community (Jones & Yarhouse, 2011). Research has shown that ex-gay ministries and pseudo-psychological therapies do not result in change in sexual orientation or gender identity for most people, but do increase shame, guilt, fear, depression, and suicide thoughts and attempts, and cuts off the person from LGBT support networks.

- What part does religion or spirituality play in your life now? How did you come to this place? What effect, if any, does religion play in your sense of well-being as a lesbian or bisexual woman?

Fat Stigma

Sometimes the media, and even medical professionals, talk about "the war against obesity." Some think that this language pathologizes larger people and permits others to shame those who are heavier. It may even lead to discrimination, harassment, and violence based on a person's weight, as bigger size has been labeled as "the enemy" in this war. Linda Bacon called the Intuitive Eating approach a "new peace movement" that ends the war on obesity. It allows us to make peace with our own bodies and to stop shaming others for their appearance. The war on obesity is a social justice issue related to basic human rights (O'Hara & Gregg, 2012). Some research indicates that negative attitudes about fat people may be the "last acceptable form of prejudice" (Buxton & Snethen, 2013). The majority of primary care providers have negative attitudes about their larger patients, and consider them more likely than thin or normal weight patients to be lazy, unmotivated, unintelligent, and less worthy of health care (Schwartz et al., 2003). In one study of college students, fat people were rated even more negatively than gay people or Muslims (Lautner et al, 2008). And larger patients report that their healthcare providers tend to blame every symptom they have on their weight (Cossrow et al., 2001). Check out the Health At Every Size ™ website for a downloadable handout that you can give to your healthcare providers if you have experienced fat discrimination in healthcare.

Lesbian and bisexual women have been at the forefront of fat positive movements and are well-represented in some of the most powerful writings on the topic. For example, *Shadow of a Tightrope: Writings by Women on Fat Oppression; The Fat Studies Reader; Looking Queer: Body Image and Identity in LGBT Communities* (see references for full citation of these books).

- Where do you stand in relationship to the fat positive movement? Do you accept your own body? Do you have negative attitudes about people who are larger?

Justice and Health Worksheet

This section helps you to delve into the influence of your identities on your health. Some identities will be protective factors that do not negatively affect your health and/or positively affect health, and others may be associated with health risks. List your identities in a table like the one below. Put the ones that people see first at the top (visible identities) and then list the others and note how they affect your health in a positive or negative way. Make as many rows as you need to address all of your identities.

Visible Identities	How it affects my health
Invisible Identities	How it affects my health

Now think about how you present your gender when you go out in public and show you think of yourself in your own internal self image. Use a 0 to 10 scale where 0-1 equals extremely masculine (FTM, MTF, transmasculine), 2-3 is pretty butch, 4-6 is around the middle, or androgynous, 7-8 is pretty femme, and 9-10 is extremely feminine.

How I rate myself: ____
How strangers might perceive me: ____

- If there is a difference in these numbers, why?

- Do people treat me differently because of my gender presentation? How have healthcare providers reacted?

- What responses do I usually have when I think I am being treated unfairly? How do I feel? How do I behave?

Developing Resilience

Resilience is the ability to bounce back after a stressful event, and can apply to both individuals and communities. Paul Kwon (2013) proposed that resilience has at least three components that work together to reduce reactivity to stress, and therefore, leading to better psychological health. These components are shown below:

Figure 16.2. Factors associated with resilience (from Kwon, 2013)

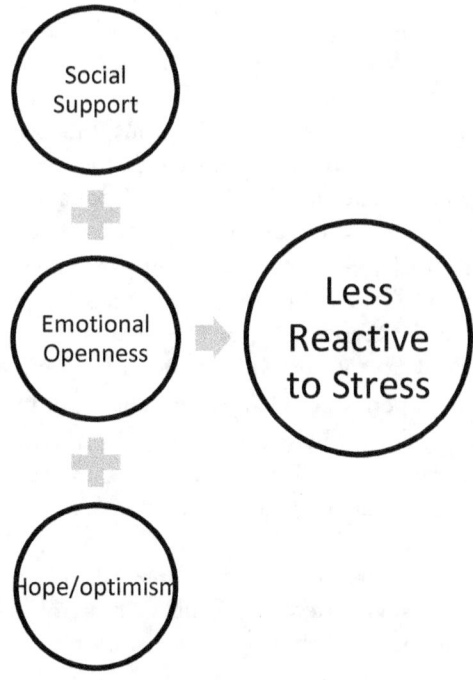

Use the chart below to think about strategies for increasing your resilience by boosting each factor.

	My current status	What I can do to strengthen this
Social Support		
Emotional Openness		
Hope/optimism		

REDUCING THE PHYSICAL EFFECTS OF STRESS

There are many ways to reduce the effects of stress on your physical and mental health. Some of these involve eliminating the stressors from your life, but often, they are life circumstances that we cannot change, so we can only change how we react to them. This section focuses on some key components of taking care of ourselves: sleep quality and napping, engaging in activism, letting go (detachment) and increasing your health literacy.

Stress and Sleep

In the past, sleep was thought of as a time when the brain shut down almost completely, but now we know it is a period of considerable mental activity organized into five distinct stages that involve differences in brain wave patterns, body temperature, release of hormones, and muscle and sensory activity. These five stages cycle about every 90 minutes so we experience 4-5 sleep cycles each night. Even in the deepest sleep, the brain is about 80% activated. Some scientists think that sleep may be more critical to health than diet, exercise, or even our genes. Sleep is also time that we consolidate new learning and memories, and gain insights about our learning.

The switch that puts us to sleep is in the hypothalamus, the center of most of our primal drives, like hunger, thirst, and sexual desire. The cells in the hypothalamus that trigger sleep are on a timer to some extent. For most of us, they keep us awake and alert between 6 am and 9 pm, so the best time to go to bed is an hour or so after 9 pm. Here is a brief description of the five stages of sleep:

- In the first stage of sleep, melatonin production increases, the muscles relax (although we may often have a big jerk, called a mycolonic twitch that startles back to awake. This is more frequent in people who are stressed, nervous, or overly tired), and the senses start to shut down a bit. Thoughts and images jump from one topic to another with no logical connection.
- Stages 2 and 3 involve brief periods of changes in brain wave patterns.
- Stage 4 is when breathing rate becomes slow and regular, the muscle are limp, and the pituitary gland is releasing chemicals that help the cells to grow, divide, and repair. This stage lasts about 30-45 minutes, and if we dream, they are dull and short dreams.
- Stage 5 is REM (rapid eye movement) sleep. The breathing rate is more rapid and the eyes may twitch. The brain is very active, but the logical centers of the brain are not activated, so the dreams are vivid, emotional, and strange, often irrational. We remember dreams from this stage in the final sleep cycle before waking up, although most of us dream for 90 minutes to 2 hours each night.

Nightmares might be produced by premature dreams that come in earlier stages. Women have more nightmares than men, although it is not known whether this is because of hormone differences or more stress in women's lives. Many older adults experience "micro-arousals" or brief moments of wakefulness during the night. They may last only a few seconds, but may occur hundreds of time during one night. These micro-arousals might be a result of being more sensitive to caffeine and alcohol, and maybe some foods, as we age.

Things that improve sleep quality:
- Exercise. Some research finds exercise during the day (but not too close to the time of going to bed) to be better than any sleeping pill.
- Natural light exposure in the day time. The body needs at least 20 minutes of natural light each day.
- Darkness at night. Those little blue LED lights from all of our electronics can disturb sleep. Any light interferes with melatonin production. The light that comes from computer screens may be a big factor. Turn off all electronics at least an hour before bedtime. In fact, start dimming the lights in your house in the hour or two before going to bed. Melatonin is released with the onset of darkness, so our bodies may not know it is bedtime if the lights are too bright.
- Winding down period. Turn off all electronics and stop stimulating activities at least one hour before bed. An active mind has trouble letting the body relax for sleep. If you read, choose something calming and peaceful, not the lesbian romance novel full of arousing and drama-laden scenes! If you watch TV, avoid action-packed or highly dramatic thrillers.

Things that mess up sleep quality:
- Alcohol. A drink may help us fall asleep initially, but as it gets metabolized, it has a stimulant effect that kicks in a few hours after falling asleep that disrupts the sleep cycle. Even one drink in the evening is enough to create a lighter sleep in the middle of the night.
- Caffeine (most older people have to restrict caffeine after noon).
- Diet. Spicy foods, high fat or high sugar foods are also arousing (and may cause GIRD that also disrupts sleep). The best bedtime snacks are complex carbs (like whole wheat crackers) with a little protein (cheese, peanut butter).
- Noise. If sleep is light, any noise can wake us. Try turning on a fan or a white noise machine.
- Electronics.

Sleep Deprivation Effects

Most people need between 7 and 8 hours of sleep each night. If deprived, even slightly, we may have "micro-sleeps" or periods of falling asleep for 3-10 seconds during the day. These are a major cause of accidents and injuries. Sleep deprivation also affects other health outcomes:
- Vaccines don't work as well
- Blood sugar and other hormone regulation is impaired
- Cortisol levels increase and so does risk for hypertension
- Leptin decreases, disrupting hunger cues, so we eat more and crave foods more often.

Poor sleep is associated with weight gain. In one study of over 68,000 women over a 16 year period, those who slept less (5 hours per night or so) gained more weight than those who slept more, even though they did not consume more calories or get less exercise. The experts think the difference is that sleep deprivation changed their metabolic rate.

The best natural sleep aids (besides exercise) are valerian and melatonin. Melatonin can increase dreaming or even nightmares in people prone to them, but can also enhance immune functioning. The best dose of melatonin is about 20 milligrams an hour before bed, according to Andrew Weil, but you should experiment for yourself to find the right dosage.

Napping

To nap or not to nap? Many of us have periods of sleepiness during the day and wonder if we should nap or whether that nap will interfere with sleep that night. Most mammals (more than 85%) are polyphasic sleepers, meaning that they sleep for short periods throughout the day. Most humans are part of the minority of monophasic sleepers, because our days are divided into two distinct periods, one for sleep and one for wakefulness. It is not clear that this is the natural sleep pattern of humans, and some evidence shows that most people in the past napped during the day. Even today, young children and elderly persons nap, and napping is a very important aspect of many cultures. As a nation, the United States appears to be becoming more and more sleep deprived. It turns out that a short nap of 20-30 minutes can help to improve mood, alertness and performance.

Naps can be described as:

- **Planned napping** (also called preparatory napping) involves taking a nap before you actually get sleepy. You may use this technique when you know that you will be up later than your normal bed time or as a way to ward off getting tired earlier.

- **Emergency napping** occurs when you are suddenly very tired and cannot continue with the activity you were originally engaged in. This type of nap can be used to combat drowsy driving or fatigue while using heavy and dangerous machinery.

- **Habitual napping** is practiced when a person takes a nap at the same time each day. Young children may fall asleep at about the same time each afternoon or an adult might take a short nap after lunch each day.

TIPS:
- A short nap is usually recommended (20-30 minutes) for short-term alertness. This type of nap provides significant benefit for improved alertness and performance without leaving you feeling groggy or interfering with nighttime sleep.
- Your sleep environment can greatly impact your ability to fall asleep. Make sure that you have a restful place to lie down and that the temperature in the room is comfortable. Try to limit the amount of noise and light. While some studies have shown that just spending time in bed can be beneficial, it is better to try to actually sleep.
- If you take a nap too late in the day, it might affect your nighttime sleep patterns and make it difficult to fall asleep at your regular bedtime. If you try to take it too early in the day, your body may not be ready for more sleep. Listen to your body cues to find the best time for you.

BENEFITS:
- Naps can restore alertness, enhance performance, and reduce mistakes and accidents. A study at NASA on sleepy military pilots and astronauts found that a 40-minute nap improved performance by 34% and alertness by 100%.
- Naps can increase alertness in the period directly following the nap and may extend alertness a few hours later in the day.
- Scheduled napping has also been prescribed for those who are affected by narcolepsy.
- Napping has psychological benefits. A nap can be a pleasant luxury, like a mini-vacation. It can provide an easy way to get some relaxation and rejuvenation.

Driving while sleepy is extremely dangerous. Getting a full night's sleep before driving is the best, but taking a short nap before driving can reduce your risk of having an accident. Sleep experts recommend that if you feel drowsy when driving, you should immediately pull over to a rest area, drink a caffeinated beverage and take a 20-minute nap. "Caffeine naps" are quite productive—if you sleep just after drinking a caffeinated beverage, you will feel doubly refreshed when you wake up in 15 minutes, when the caffeine and the nap both combine to increase your alertness.

Shift work, or working an evening or night job, may cause fatigue and performance impairments, especially for night shift workers. In one study, researchers looked at the effectiveness of taking naps and consuming caffeine to cope with sleepiness during the night shift. They found that both naps and caffeine improved alertness and performance among night shift workers and that the combination of naps and caffeine had the most beneficial effect.

In spite of the benefits, napping is not always the best option. For example, some people have trouble sleeping any place other than their own bed, making a nap at the office, in the car, or anywhere else unlikely. Other people have trouble sleeping in the daytime; it could be that certain individuals are more sensitive to the midday dip than others – those who are may feel sleepier and have an easier time napping. Here are some other negative effects:

- Naps can leave people with sleep inertia, especially when they last more than 10-20 minutes. Sleep inertia is defined as the feeling of grogginess and disorientation that can come with awakening from a deep sleep. This disorientating state usually only lasts for a few minutes to a half-hour, but it can be detrimental to those who must perform immediately after waking from a nap.
- Napping can also have a negative effect on other sleeping periods. A long nap or a nap taken too late in the day may adversely affect the length and quality of nighttime sleep. If you have trouble sleeping at night, a nap will only amplify problems.
- One study indicated that napping is associated with increased risk of heart failure in people already at risk.

Napping still has stigmas associated with it. Some people think that napping indicates laziness, a lack of ambition, and low standards, or that it is only for children, the sick and the elderly. Though these statements are false, many segments of the public may still need to be educated on the benefits of napping. A study in the research journal *Sleep* looked at the benefits of naps of various lengths compared to no naps. The results showed that a 10-minute nap produced the most benefit in terms of reduced sleepiness and improved cognitive performance. A nap lasting 30 minutes or longer is more likely to be accompanied by sleep inertia, which is the period of grogginess that sometimes follows sleep.

Stress Reduction Through Activism

Working to change the injustices in the world is a stress-reliever. Whenever we take an action to make the world a better place, we feel better about ourselves and the world. Lesbian and bisexual women are involved in all kinds of causes. Activism has many benefits—we get out and work with other people. We get to do something we are passionate about. We get to do something that has the potential to make the work a better place for future generations, thus helps us with generativity needs. Here are some examples.

Women's Organizations and Politics. Getting involved with the National Organization of Women (NOW), Planned Parenthood, women's political action committees, and other groups are ways to build solidarity and community with heterosexual women. Lesbian/bisexual women within these organizations have historically helped heterosexual women see how our struggles against sexism are connected.

Working For Justice for Lesbian/Bisexual Women. Organizations such as the National Center for Lesbian Rights, lesbian/bisexual women's health clinics, Old Lesbians Organizing Change, and local groups for and by lesbian/bisexual women.

Working for LGBT Justice. Examples are The National Gay and Lesbian Task Force, The Human Rights Campaign, Lambda Legal, The Stonewall Democrats, Legal Service Members Network, GLAAD (Gay and Lesbian Alliance Against Defamation), PFLAG (Parents and Friends of Lesbians and Gays), GSAs (gay-straight alliances in schools). This could also involve volunteering at a local LGBT community center.

Working to Reduce Ageism. Gray Panthers, Old Lesbians Organizing for Change, volunteering at local senior centers or LGBT aging groups/agencies.

Working to Reduce Racism. Belonging to the NAACP, immigration rights organizations, civil rights groups like Amnesty International.

Working for Animal Rights. These might include PETA or the Humane Society, or volunteer at a local animal shelter or be part of an animal rescue group.

Working for Environmental Justice. There are many local organizations that work on issues of pesticides and farm workers, industrial pollution in particular neighborhoods, educating about climate change, developing urban gardens, and so on.

Working for Food Justice. Lesbian and bisexual women often have more awareness of political issues in society because of our experiences with oppression. Lesbian/bisexual women are more likely to have progressive or liberal political views than heterosexual women. This may include greater consciousness around food justice and food politics. Many lesbian and bisexual women have adopted vegetarian or vegan nutritional lifestyles, are involved in organic food production or support organic farming, and are involved in food justice organizations and activities. This is highly compatible with a mindful approach to nutrition and eating.

Food justice means respecting others, helping everyone to have access to information about and actual availability of healthy foods, and teaches about how the food industries are making money off making us sick. And when the food industry makes us sick, there is a need for a "health" industry to make us well again. The weight control industry has grown to a multi-billion dollar operation that takes far too much of our hard-earned money, time and energy. There are no weight loss approaches that research has shown to be effective for more than 5% of participants in the long run. Instead, these weight loss or exercise programs often make us sicker by lowering self-esteem, contributing to weight cycling and dieting, and draining our already slim wallets. With tools like intuitive eating and mindful physical activity, we can get healthier without dieting, purchasing expensive gym memberships (and having to buy appropriate clothing so no one at the gym looks down on us), or subjecting ourselves to dangerous medications or surgeries. If we have access to accurate information about food, knowledge of the food industry, and community support, we can get healthier in a more natural and less expensive way. If we all had safe and walkable neighborhoods, and gyms and rec centers that were safe and respectful for all women, but particularly older and diverse women, we would be more inclined to be physically active.

Letting Go: Detachment

One of the components of mindfulness is learning about when to let go of stress reactions. Stress is mostly a problem created by our minds, because we latch onto to some problem and make it bigger and worse than it actually is. Meditation practices can help us to recognize when we are stressed, and help us to let the feelings wash over us and pass through. Most emotions are short-lived and only less a few seconds unless we latch onto them. A Native American story tells of two wolves that live inside each person; one is good and kind and beautiful, the other is cruel and evil. When asked which wolf will win over the person, the wise elder replies, "the one we feed." So meditation or stress-relieving breathing exercises teach us to not feed the stress and let it go. Chapter 19 includes some stress breathing activities that can be done as forms of meditation as well as part of the physical activity core strengthening activities. Taking a walk in nature, or other forms of physical activity can also reduce stress dramatically.

IMPROVING HEALTH LITERACY

Health literacy is having confidence in your ability to find, interpret, and communicate about your own health to a healthcare provider and engage in dialogues and processes to make informed decisions about your own healthcare needs. Areas that many lesbian/bisexual women find challenging and stressful are locating information about health on the internet and evaluating whether that information is valid and accurate. How do we know what to believe? In addition, many lesbian and bisexual women are uncomfortable with disclosing information about their sexuality or their relationships to healthcare providers. These topics are addressed below.

Evaluating Health Information on the Internet

As we look to improve our health, we can get bombarded with conflicting information. Some of the information we find has a few kernels of truth to it but many companies grasp on to one true fact and build an entire marketing campaign to sell a product on it. If you look hard enough you can find "experts" validating anything, including how a junk food diet is good for you. Common sense is usually a good tool to start with when evaluating health claims from the Internet.

Many web sites are promoting or selling something and even if they cite research, their interpretation of it may not take into account the group of people the information may be relevant to. For example an optimal food plan for a young athlete is and should be different than a food plan for a woman over fifty. Results of an exercise program for a one hundred lab rats is interesting but may not be practical information you can use for yourself. Companies often don't explain the limitations of "research" and as a consumer it can be very confusing what to believe.

Types of Websites

Consider the source of the information. Is the website run by a commercial interests? That is not always bad, just important to know if they are trying to sell you something. Sites that are selling products are .com. What about .org? Some of these sites are legitimate professional or consumer organizations that provide accurate information, but anyone can obtain a .org designation, so be cautious if you are not familiar with the organization, or the website seems to be selling a lot of products.

Websites run by .gov or .edu usually have more reliable information. They are government or educational sites. Several professionals have reviewed this information before it is posted, and the information is updated frequently. The information on these sites is backed by research. Keep in mind that all research is biased, though, and even scientific knowledge can be influenced by lobbyists from the food and pharmaceutical industries. No research is without flaws or some kind of bias.

- One good source to start with is Medline. Their information comes from academic/biomedical research. You can search by health topic and questions related to your age and gender. NIH: National Library of Medicine: http://www.nlm.nih.gov/medlineplus/

- Another good source of information is the Centers for Disease Control and Prevention (CDC). There is information on almost all chronic and infectious diseases, written for consumers, on this website.

- If you want to know the current research on some health program or treatment, like the effects of herbal products on sleep, or the role of Vitamins in preventing cancer, visit the Cochrane Library. They seek independent reviews of treatment alternatives from many different scholars who are qualified to judge the quality of a research study. They are definitely more academic in tone, though.

If you find a health claim on the internet, here are some guidelines for evaluating whether it might be based on research findings.
- Does the piece list the author, and does that author have some credentials that indicate they are "legitimate?"
- Is there a date on the piece so you can determine if the information is up-to-date?
- Are there references to scientific studies in research journals?
- Does the article provide evidence from research studies, or only present a few case studies?
- Is the piece slanted to one perspective, or does it present pros and cons of a health intervention?

Reliable Sources of Information on LGBT Health:

- Lavender Health (www.lavenderhealth.org)
- Centers for Disease Control (http://www.cdc.gov/lgbthealth/)
- Health Resources and Services Administration (http://www.hrsa.gov/lgbt/)
- GLMA: Health Professionals Advancing LGBT Health (www.glma.org)

Working With Your Healthcare Provider

There are many good reasons to come out to a primary care provider, or to specialists if you are going to receive ongoing treatment or care for a chronic health problem. If you want a partner or close social network to be involved in your healthcare decision-making, want them to have access to information about your condition, and want your relationships honored, you need to let health care providers know who should be involved in your care. Most healthcare providers are "heterosexist"—meaning that they assume every patient is heterosexual unless they are told directly. At the end of this chapter you will find a sample handout that you can bring along with you to your healthcare provider with personal information that you can fill in. There is a copy of this on the website if you want to download it rather than copy it from this book.

Legal Issues and Documents that Lesbian/Bisexual Women Should Know About

Legal marriage gives couples most of the rights that are covered by these documents, but not every same-sex couple wants to, or is able to marry. Here are some of the pros and cons of marriage to consider:

Why I should consider marriage	Why I should consider not marrying
Financial reasons, like tax breaks	For some couples, the tax breaks are small and if you break up, it can be costly to un-do the financial issues.
Legal reasons, like inheritance. One of the main reasons is to protect families with children.	Legal benefits can be obtained through other legal documents.
Makes the relationship "legitimate" in the eyes of the state	Does not guarantee success of a relationship: we don't have a lot of data on whether marriage makes the relationship better or last longer
It might be good for one's mental health	Not enough research to tell: any good relationship is good for one's mental health
Same-sex marriage is good for the economy and spawns a new career option: the gay wedding planner!	Same-sex marriage also means same-sex divorce; it's harder to end a relationship if married
Some argue that marriage leads to deepening of "family values" thus is good for society. It also decreases likelihood of sexually transmitted infections by encouraging faithfulness.	There are philosophical/political reasons to oppose marriage. Should government be involved in intimate relationships? Is the institution of marriage flawed? Should we work to change the system so that benefits are not tied to legal marriage or employment, but to human status? Why only two? What about relationships of 3 or more?

Legal Documents

Lesbian and bisexual women have some unique legal challenges if they are unable or choose not to legally formalize their relationships in the state, national, or international arenas. Many of the forms listed here can be downloaded and completed without the assistance of a lawyer, but an estate-planning specialist concentrating on LGBT issues is an excellent source of information and help. The following information has been adapted from National Center for Lesbian Rights and Rainbow Laws' websites: (http://www.nclrights.org/site/DocServer/NCLR_LIFELINES.pdf?docID=521 and http://www.rainbowlaw.com/free.htm). If you choose legal marriage, you will automatically get some of these rights, but you will still want to consider having many of these documents.

Living will/medical directive. In every state, people can sign documents describing their wishes concerning life-prolonging medical care. This document may be called a living will, medical directive, health care directive, directive to physicians, or declaration regarding health care, and it directs health care professionals about what you want done when you are no longer capable of making or communicating choices regarding life-prolonging and other medical care.

Durable power of attorney for health care/health care proxy. A durable power of attorney for health care (also called a "health care proxy") allows the designated person to make medical decisions for you in case you are unable to make decisions for yourself. This is a very important document for lesbian and bisexual women, since you may not want your biological family making health care decisions on your behalf. Many couples choose someone other than their partner or spouse for this duty, because it may put considerable emotional burden on the significant other.

Hospital visitation authorization. A hospital visitation authorization allows you to name all the specific individuals you will allow to visit you in case you are not able to communicate your wishes.

Authorization for consent to medical treatment of minor. The medical treatment of a minor requires authorization by the legal parents. This form allows the legal parents to permit someone other than a child's legal parents to authorize a doctor or other health care professional to provide medical services to a minor child. In states that do not recognize both parents in a same-sex couple as legal parents, this form is critical so that all parents and others involved in the care of the child are able to consent to emergency medical treatment. For couples who are considering having children, it is important to complete this document before the birth mother goes into the hospital. This form may not be legally binding, but hospitals will usually honor the authorization.

Durable power of attorney for finances. A durable power of attorney for finances allows a designated person, the "agent," to take care of your finances when you are not able to do so. A general power of attorney for finances authorizes this designated agent to take care of financial matters, including paying medical bills, cashing checks, or receiving benefits.

Wills. A will is a legal document that allows you to designate who will receive your property when you die. When someone dies without a will, their property goes to their legal heirs—parents, children, or the next closest blood relative. With the exception of the states with legal same-sex marriage, a same-sex partner is NOT considered to be a legal heir and therefore is not legally entitled to inherit property when an individual dies without a will. This is true regardless of how long people have been with their partners and regardless of the quality of their relationship with their relatives.

Trusts. You can also designate who will receive property upon your death through a revocable living trust. A living trust is similar to a will in that it allows you to say who should get what. Property left by a will goes through the court probate process - which means that the will must be proven valid, and your debts must be paid before the property is distributed. The probate process often takes about a year. With a living trust, this process is avoided and the property goes directly to the people named in the trust. In some circumstances, transferring the property through a living trust rather than a will helps to reduce or avoid some estate taxes.

Nomination of conservator or guardian for a minor. This document transfers the responsibility of the care and custody of a child to another responsible adult in the event that the child's legal parent dies or becomes physically or psychologically unable to care for the child. When the birth mother dies without providing for her children's future, biological family members are automatically given custody, even if there is a long-term same-sex partner. Usually, a person who is appointed to be the child's guardian is given physical custody of the child and authority to manage the child's financial matters.

Elder guardian/conservator. If the time comes when you are unable to manage your affairs, who will handle these matters? If someone has not been named in a durable power-of-attorney, advanced medical directive, and/or a trust, then someone will have to seek to qualify as a guardian and/or conservator. A petition will be filed in the Circuit Court of the city or county of residence asking the Judge to appoint an individual to serve as a guardian and/or conservator. A guardian is appointed to be responsible for the person, such as taking care of physical needs, medical treatment, medication and living arrangements. A conservator is appointed to attend to financial affairs, protect assets, pay bills, invest funds, and preserve resources of the incapacitated elder. The best option is to carefully plan for this eventuality and put your wishes in writing, yet hope that you can maintain control over your own environment and care.

Autopsy and disposition of remains. In the absence of written instructions, nearly every state gives relatives the right to control the disposition of a body, including funeral arrangements, upon death. As is true for wills and power of attorney for health care, in states without same-sex marriage, this right to control disposition of remains is not provided automatically to a same-sex partner.

REFERENCES

Ackerman, J. (2007). *Sex, Sleep, Eat, Drink, Dream: A day in the life of your body.* Boston: Houghton Miflin.

Buxton, B.K., & Snethen, J. (2013). Obese women's perceptions and experiences of healthcare and primary care providers. *Nursing Research, 62,* 252-259.

Levitt, H.M., & Horne, S.G., (2002). Explorations of lesbian-queer genders: Butch, femme, androgynous, or "other." *Journal of Lesbian Studies, 6,* 25-39.

O'Hara, L., & Gregg, J. (2012). Human rights casualties from the 'war on obesity': why focusing on body weight is inconsistent with a human rights approach to health, *Fat Studies, 1(*1), 32-46.

Rosario M., Schrimshaw, E.W., Hunter, J., & Levy-Warren, A. (2007). The coming out process of young lesbian and bisexual women: Are there butch/femme differences in sexual identity development? *Archives of Sexual Behavior, 38,* 34-49.

Schwartz, M. B., Chambliss, H. O., Brownell, K. D., Blair, S.N., & Billington, C. (2003). Weight bias among health professionals specializing in obesity, *Obesity Research, 11,* 1033-

Weil, A. (2005*). Healthy aging.* NY: Knoph.

What Healthcare Providers Need to Know about Lesbian and Bisexual Women

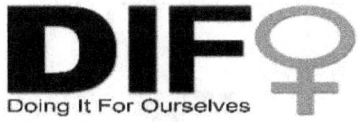

Most healthcare providers get very little or no information about the health needs of lesbian and bisexual women in their professional training or in continuing education, but times are changing and healthcare systems are now required to provide quality care to all patients. Several recent policy changes impact healthcare systems. The Department of Health and Human Services website lists some of the changes that healthcare providers should know about, from patient visitation policies to same-sex marriage to nondiscrimination of employees. See http://www.hhs.gov/lgbt/resources/reports/health-objectives-2011.html. This brochure focuses on health care issues of lesbian and bisexual women, which tend to be quite different than the needs of gay or bisexual men or transgender people.

Why is it important to know a patient's sexual orientation?

Most of the time, there are no differences in how diseases or disorders manifest, the physical symptoms, or the type of treatments by sexual orientation. The biggest differences are in how our families and relationships are structured, and who we want to have involved in our care. In the past, same-sex partners and different types of families were ignored or even discriminated against. Most healthcare providers do not ask about sexual orientation or gender identity, so do not recognize their LGBT (lesbian, gay, bisexual, and transgender) patients. If every patient is assumed to be heterosexual, it is easy to overlook the important relationships in your patients' lives that will help with dealing with illness and healing.

Health disparities of lesbian and bisexual women.

Lesbian and bisexual women have higher rates of smoking, alcohol, drug use and asthma than heterosexual women and are more likely to experience current or lifetime mood disorders (depression, anxiety, and PTSD are the most common). Because health surveys have just begun asking about sexual orientation, we do not know as much about physical health disparities. Some studies find lesbian and bisexual women are more likely to report being disabled, to live in poverty, not have a regular healthcare provider, and delay or avoid care for fear of discrimination. All of these health disparities are caused by the societal stigma association with sexual orientation that creates a more hostile or uncaring environment for many women.

What is sexual orientation?

Sexual orientation refers to a constellation of at least three factors:

1) Sexual identities are the labels that people use to refer to themselves. The most common are heterosexual, lesbian, gay, and bisexual, but some patients may use terms like queer, same gender loving (common in some African American communities), two spirit (common in some Native American communities), or other terms. Most lesbian and bisexual women would prefer if you ask about sexual identities either on your written forms or in your history-taking, because it takes the pressure off of them to find a way to tell you. Many of your patients might fear what will happen if they disclose this information to you, if you have not given off any clues of how you feel about LGBT people.

2) Sexual behaviors are what people actually do. Identities and behaviors are not always consistent over time. If you want to know if I am at risk for some problem that is related to specific sexual behaviors, such as number of male partners as a risk factor for cervical cancer, you will need to ask for this information. If you just ask for total number of sexual partners, this will be misleading since having female partners is not a risk for pregnancy or cervical cancer or some sexually transmitted infections. Remember that sexual identity does not tell you anything about a person's sexual behaviors. Women who identify as lesbian may have had past relationships with men, or even currently have sex/relationships with men. Women who identify as bisexual might currently be in a relationship with a

man, but that does not make her heterosexual. Most bisexual women are in relationships with one person at a time, despite stereotypes, but a small number of both lesbians and bisexual women are in open or poly relationships.

3) Sexual attractions are internal feelings that a person may act on or not. It might be important to ask about this because some people experience a lot of distress over having same-sex feelings, and that distress might cause mental or physical health problems. In addition, some youth may be at risk for depression and suicide attempts if they fear rejection for telling someone about same-sex attractions.

What is the difference between sexual orientation and gender identity?
Gender identity refers to whether a person identifies as male, female, transgender, or some other gender term. Gender identity and sexual orientation are different things. Some lesbian and bisexual women were born with male bodies, but their gender identity is female. They may or may not have changed their bodies through hormones and surgeries. Similarly, some people born female now identify as male (transgender men). They still have internal female reproductive organs, so need pap tests and other screenings. To be gender-inclusive, your forms or history taking need to ask about the sex a patient was assigned at birth (recognizing that some people are born with intersex differences), and their current gender identity (man, woman, transgender, other). Most lesbian and bisexual women were born with female bodies and identify as women. But they may vary in how they present themselves, with some adopting attire, hairstyles, and mannerisms that are not as feminine as typical women in this culture. Women who do not look feminine are more likely to be targeted for discrimination, harassment, and violence in public places.

Lesbian and bisexual women tend to have larger bodies than heterosexual women.
Some actively reject the body standards that society expects from women, including rejecting dieting as a dangerous behavior. They may be satisfied with larger bodies. Many lesbian and bisexual women are involved in body positive or health at every size (HAES) movements that challenge whether weight is the culprit in health problems. They are committed to being healthier, but may not be interested in talking about diets. Please do not assume that the cause of every health problem of a larger woman is because of her weight or her sexuality. We ask that you listen to us, and consider all possibilities for the cause of health problems without automatically defaulting to a talk about losing weight. Far too many of us have been the victims of fat prejudice in society and do not care to experience it in the healthcare provider's office as well.

What do we want from our healthcare providers?
- Listen to us as individuals. Do not make assumptions about us based on our sexual identity, gender presentation, weight, race/ethnicity, or any other visible characteristic.
- Accept and acknowledge our sexual identities, genders, and partners/families. When we come out to you, please acknowledge it. Say something like "Thank you for sharing that information." We don't know how to interpret silences and assume that means you are uncomfortable.
- Educate yourself and your staff. There are many resources available now.
- Make your office/unit welcoming and inclusive. The simplest things you can do are to include the words sexual orientation and gender identity in patient rights or non-discrimination policies and prominently display them. The other big thing you can do is to change your written forms to include questions about sexual and gender identities and same-sex partners.
- Participate in the Healthcare Equality Index project. The Human Rights Campaign sponsors a survey that will help you figure out what your agency needs to do to become LGBT sensitive (http://www.hrc.org/topics/health-and-aging).

Want to learn more? Resources for healthcare providers:
- Joint Commission: (http://www.jointcommission.org/lgbt/). Comprehensive guide to making your office LGBT welcoming.

- GLMA: Health Professionals Advancing LGBT Equality: Has an annual conference with continuing education credits and offers much information on a website (www.glma.org). You might consider being listed in their provider directory as a welcoming provider.
- Lavender Health: A website with information for consumers and providers of healthcare (http://lavenderhealth.org/).
- Institute on Medicine (2011). *The health of LGBT people: Building a foundation for better understanding.* New York: National Academies Press.
- Linda Bacon (2010). Health At Every Size. This book and website is not specific to lesbian and bisexual women, but provides scientific evidence of the dangers of dieting and offers alternatives. (http://haescommunity.org/)

Written by Mickey Eliason, San Francisco State University, for Doing It For Ourselves, a health education and support program (http://difobayarea.org). See the website for more resources.

What you should know about me

My name: _____

I identify as: _____. You may record this on my medical records.

My significant other(s)_____. This is who I want involved in my care.

We

      ___are legally married

      ___are domestic partners

      ___ have power of attorney for healthcare decision-making

      ___ have other legal documents you should know about: (listed below)

Information about my children/family:

Other critical information:

Chapter 17: Nutrition and Eating Patterns

Anyone who has ever been to a lesbian/bisexual women's potluck gathering or brunch knows that we have more vegetarians, vegans, gluten-freeks, lactose-intolerants, food allergies, hypoglycemics, paleo eaters, and other dietary variations than the general population. As a group, lesbian and bisexual women may be more attuned to the need for nutritional guidance, but our stressful, busy lives and the sheer burden of trying to sort through thousands of messages about nutrition in the media and on the internet, make getting good advice very challenging. There are a few research studies that show that lesbian/bisexual women are more likely to use complementary and alternative health practices than heterosexual women, including acupuncture, herbal supplements, and meditation. Many lesbian/bisexual women value these mind, body, spirit resources, thus may be particularly suited to mindful eating approaches to health and nutrition. This section addresses nutrition from that mindfulness spin, and provides information that will be helpful for individual behavior change as well as broader awareness of food justice and nutrition education.

This section addresses nutrition in a general way. There is no one best "diet" for all people, and in fact, the one thing we know with certainty is that calorie restriction or deprivation diets do not work. In fact, we highly recommend that you do not diet. Over 95% of people who lose weight on a diet will gain it back and then some. Dieting and emphasis on weight loss has caused many of us to lose the ability to recognize our own internal cues about hunger and being full. Instead, this section provides information about food based on extensive research findings rather than fads or trends, and is based on a few general principles:

1. Much of our problem with nutrition stems from mindless eating. If we pay more attention and track what we eat, how we feel when we eat, and how we shop, our nutrition (and health) improves.
2. Common sense. If we shop with an eye to whole foods, fresh fruits and vegetables, and avoid highly processed stuff, we will get healthier!
3. Food justice is a lesbian/bisexual women's concern. As members of the human race, our health depends on making the food systems more healthy and accessible to all. Food justice is closely tied to animal rights movements, human health and wellbeing, and earth-centered justice and spiritual systems, all movements that many lesbian and bisexual women embrace.

RESEARCH ON WEIGHT LOSS

As noted in Chapter 5 and elsewhere, lesbian and bisexual women tend to be larger, as a group, than heterosexual women, and so some research has focused on weight reduction issues. But nutrition is a much larger issue than just weight loss, and all lesbian and bisexual women can benefit from understanding nutrition and eating healthier. So although this chapter begins with a review of the literature on weight loss efforts, the bulk of the chapter is about general tips for nutrition. There is no one best eating plan for everyone, so no "diets" or specific plans are recommended. Instead, the process called Intuitive Eating is explained in detail, so that you can identify the healthiest choices for yourself.

Effectiveness of Weight Reduction Strategies

Research over the past 30 years is clear: diets do not work, at least calorie restriction or deprivation diets. Changes in lifestyle patterns of diet and exercise are notoriously difficult to change, because weight is a product of more than just individual willpower and behavior. In the general biomedical literature on obesity treatment and prevention, most single-minded approaches (psychological interventions, nutrition education, exercise programs, commercial weight loss programs, etc) have had limited success in the short-term because they focus only on the individual and not the larger social contexts. There is some encouraging news for those who want to lose weight: psychological interventions (behavioral, cognitive-behavioral, motivational interviewing) when combined with diet and exercise can have moderate success (Corbalan, Morales, Cantras, et al, 2009; Shaw, et al, 2009). In particular, acceptance-based approaches that address eating in response to emotions and thoughts have been helpful for some women (Niemeier et al, 2012), and may be applicable to lesbian/bisexual women as responses to minority stress. Acceptance-based, or mindfulness approaches, aim not to change thoughts or emotions, but to accept them. Because lesbian/bisexual women appear to be more open to these alternative health interventions (Smith et al, 2010; Matthews et al, 2005), they may be highly effective components of any health program. Most studies are targeted at the general population and have not tested any particular approaches with lesbian and bisexual women. Approaches that are culturally specific may have greater chances of success, but even within lesbian/bisexual communities, there are potential differences in cultural norms about weight and body ideals based on race/ethnicity, gender expression (Fogel, 2010) and age (Roberts, 2010) that must be addressed.

In addition, we need to take heed of feminist critiques of the "war on obesity" that echo the comments of some lesbians our own and other research studies. That is, many lesbians define health much more broadly than just a number on a scale. Some think that the emphasis in most of biomedicine on weight reduction may be a violation of human rights and dignity whereas a focus on health is more acceptable and responsible (O'Hara & Gregg, 2012). So the purpose of this chapter is to focus on healthy eating, not dieting or weight loss.

As Brown-Saracino (2011) noted, lesbian/bisexual women value "ambient communities" based on safety, inclusion, shared identities and interests, thus are invested in the development of community rather than fitting into existing community resources not designed with our needs in mind. This may include community agencies that serve gay and bisexual men or transgender individuals; some lesbian/bisexual women may not be comfortable sharing facilities with other sexual and gender minority individuals whose needs are perceived as different. We may have the greatest success in shifting our behavior to healthier patterns when we make these changes in the context of a supportive, safe community.

Weight Reduction among Lesbian/Bisexual Women

Very little research has examined the effectiveness of specific types of weight-related strategies, or any health interventions for that matter, among sexual minority women. The little we know is summarized in this section. In a study of long-term breast cancer survivors (Boehmer et al, 2011), lesbian/bisexual women were more likely to improve weight-related behaviors after cancer treatment than heterosexual women, suggesting that when motivation is present, lesbian/bisexual women can and will engage in weight reduction activities. We don't know if those positive gains were maintained over time, though.

The Mautner Project in Washington D.C. produced a report on lesbian/bisexual women and weight concerns (2011) that included the results of an online survey of 242 respondents from across the U.S. and Canada. Of this sample, 68% had been advised by a health care provider to improve her health, and most were actively attempting to exercise more and lose weight. When asked what would support them in losing weight, 46% wanted more partner and peer support; 46% wanted a buddy or coach and 38% expressed an interest in a lesbian/bisexual-specific support group. So lesbian/bisexual women wanted to make changes with support of the people in their lives, not go it alone. Fogel, Young, and McPherson (2009) conducted focus groups with 14 self identified overweight lesbians to explore their experiences with weight loss, finding that most women had a long history of feeling shame about their bodies and fear about weight loss attempts . They felt that most weight loss programs in the general public were not safe for lesbians and they felt no sense of connection to other participants (a community level factor).

Roberts and colleagues (2010) conducted focus groups with 25 women who were at risk for heart disease. The age range was wide, from 22 to 60, allowing them to identify some generational differences in attitudes. Younger lesbian's attitudes about body size were similar to heterosexual women, whereas older lesbians reported being more influenced by feminist ideas of the body and rejecting heterosexual female imperatives to be thin. Among the older generation of lesbians, some were "fat positive" proponents, whereas other older lesbians felt that they had to lose weight to be healthier. In regards to interventions to reduce weight, Roberts and coauthors found that many lesbians of all ages were dissatisfied with the emphasis on reducing BMI or pounds, and were more concerned about overall health than losing weight per se. In addition, many reported barriers to getting healthy, such as the lack of accessible and inclusive gyms where they could work out with their partners and qualify for family memberships, having places where they are not the only overweight person working out, and finding workout gear that was comfortable. Many respondents agreed that they wanted health programs designed specifically for lesbians, and some wanted age-group specific programs because of generational differences. Brittain and colleagues (2006) reported that lack of lesbian-specific exercise groups and family gym memberships for same-sex couples/families (community level) were major barriers to exercising more.

Finally, in one of the few studies to directly examine lesbians in a weight reduction program, Sarah Fogel and colleagues (2012) studied 31 lesbians who were enrolled in a lesbian group of Weight Watchers. They had attempted many different types of weight loss strategies over the years prior to this program. Over the course of the group from enrollment to six-month follow-up, they did report lowered BMIs, but most of the weight loss occurred before they started the lesbian group. They did report a higher frequency of exercise from baseline to follow-up. Six months is a short time for follow-up, so we cannot learn too much from this study, beyond knowing that an increase in exercise is potentially a great outcome. The rest of this chapter focuses on ideas for getting healthier through food choices and finding out how food affects your body. We begin with a little introduction to the idea that some food causes or contributes to disease through the process of inflammation.

GENERAL NUTRITION INFORMATION

Inflammation and Food

There is considerable consensus now among scientists that inflammation causes most chronic diseases and is responsible for a lot of chronic pain. Inflammation is a normal and healthy process in our bodies that helps us deal with stress and traumas, but if the stress/trauma is chronic and ongoing, the system is overwhelmed and causes damage to organ systems. Inflammation comes from several different causes:

- o Injuries
- o Chronic stress (racism, sexism, heterosexism, and basic human stresses)
- o Air pollution
- o Lack of sleep
- o Lack of physical activity
- o Foods

Here is the typical process. A trigger (stress for example) in the environment stimulates cells in the amygdala. This starts two processes: 1) it activates the hypothalamus, which signals the pituitary gland to produce cortisol; and 2) it turns on the sympathetic nervous system which shuts down digestive processes and increases heart rate. The combination of higher heart rate and elevated cortisol leads to increases in blood sugar and blood pressure. We are ready for fight or flight.

In the short term, this system helps us deal with stress, and our systems return to normal quickly when the stressor is gone. But over time, with chronic exposures to stress-producing circumstances, the cortisol and elevated blood sugars do not return to normal quickly and end up damaging organ systems. Cortisol increases our craving for energy dense foods that can be converted quickly to energy (high fat, high sugar foods) and eating itself becomes a way to cope with the stress (emotional eating; comfort foods; soothing behaviors). Those energy dense foods are inflammatory as well because they raise sugar levels even higher, and can damage organ systems through the prolonged exposure to high blood sugar. Diabetes is one consequence, but heart disease, cancer, joint pain and arthritis, and auto-immune disorders can also result. The immune system becomes less effective and we are more vulnerable to all kinds of illnesses. The way to know if you have inflammatory damage occurring in the body before the symptoms of these disorders start to manifest, is through symptoms of metabolic syndrome (see Chapter 6) .

Everyone is different, so you will need to experiment with different foods for yourself to determine what affects you negatively. The lists below are foods that are often inflammation producers or inhibitors for many people and there is research to back up most of the foods on these lists. The majority of the inflammation producers work through rapidly increasing circulating blood sugar. It's important to note that we do need sugar—it is an essential nutrient. The problem is all the excess sugar in processed foods produces problems. Since we have moved from eating natural foods to a diet of highly processed foods, our food supply now has far more sugar than our bodies need. But we have become addicted to the taste of these processed foods with their combinations of fat, salt, sugar, and sometimes caffeine that make them so appealing. They are also widely available almost everywhere we go, and often at low cost.

Inflammatory Foods	Foods that Decrease Inflammation
Trans fats and many vegetable oils	Olive Oil (extra virgin), coconut oil
Sugar in any form	High fiber foods
White stuff (bread, pasta, potatoes)	Oily fish (wild salmon, tuna because of the omega 3 oils and Vitamin D) (warning: farmed salmon may not be very healthy)
Alcohol (mostly because of the sugar)	Brightly colored fruits and vegetables
Dairy	Freshly brewed teas (unsweetened)
MSG	Spices like turmeric (curcumin) and ginger
Gluten (wheat)	Dark chocolate in small amounts (the darker the chocolate, the lower the sugar content)

You can check out websites such as Dr. Andrew Weil's for more information about inflammation potential of foods, but because everyone is different, do track for yourself what foods feel good in your body, and which ones increase pain, stiffness, fatigue, or bad moods. Many of the foods on the inflammatory list are there because they produce excess levels of sugar. Our body needs sugar to survive, but most of us get far more than we need, and it is that excess sugar that causes problems. Another good resource is the Sugar Science website of the University of California, San Francisco.

High Fructose Corn Syrup (HFCS) and Other Sweeteners

HFCS is a chemical mixture of fructose and glucose, two forms of sugar. It is produced by separating cornstarch from the kernel of corn, mixing it with hydrochloric acid, pressurizing and heating it to break down the starch, then adding another chemical that changes it to glucose. Then it is exposed to another chemical that changes part of the glucose to fructose. So this is a highly processed chemical substance, not a natural food. It was introduced into the U.S. food market in 1967 (Wallinga, 2009) and now is the sweetener of choice in processed foods. Around 1970, 1% of foods were sweetened with HFCS, and now nearly half of processed foods have HFCS. At this point in time, the average U.S. citizen consumes about 12 teaspoons of HFCS each day, about the twice the recommended daily amount of sugar. HFCS is in many of the processed foods we eat: ketchup, cereals, granola bars, soft drinks, salad dressings, and yogurt, for example. Because the food lobbyists marketed it as a food substance, it never had to undergo any FDA approval process to prove that is was safe.

Why is HFCS so widespread in our food supply? It turns out that energy-dense foods (high sugar and fat content) are cheaper to make and more filling. HFCS gives food a longer shelf life. U.S. government subsidies favor the big corporate corn producers and so these products are cheap. Research on HFCS has been scant, but the animal studies show that HFCS decreases levels of insulin and leptin in the blood stream, leading to faster weight gain. In rats, HFCS contributed to greater abdominal fat and spikes in triglycerides (both symptoms of metabolic syndrome). So are other sweeteners safer? Is it better to eat pure sugar than chemically processed sweeteners? Unfortunately, there is no completely safe artificial sweetener, and no added sugar that is good for our bodies. The amount and type of sugar we get from whole foods is adequate to meet our bodies needs. All artificial sweeteners increase one's craving for sugar and contribute to weight gain and metabolic syndrome.

MINDFUL EATING APPROACHES

Mindful eating is the process of getting back in touch with the relationships between our mind, body, and spirit in relation to food. "Mindful" is a blanket term for all approaches that focus on paying attention to one's body and mind, but there are actually at least two different broad philosophies about mindfulness. In the more spiritual realm, mindfulness comes from Buddhist practices of viewing one's thoughts with compassion and non-judgment, so it focuses on the mind, and using meditation practices to increase awareness about our own behavior and thoughts. The idea that the body is a temple and what we eat can become part of a spiritual practice comes from this more spiritual meaning of the term. For example, Buddhism promotes vegetarianism in its respect for the rights of animals.

Mindfulness can also be viewed as separate from spirituality, and more as a science-based method for reducing stress and altering behaviors. Intuitive eating uses this science-based version of mindfulness, but also comes from studies on the biology and evolution of eating behaviors and physiological processes. It addresses the negative messages about food and our bodies from the media and culture around us. The two approaches to mindfulness share the component of paying attention to the body and our thoughts. In this program, we will focus on the science-based types of mindfulness, but have great respect for the more spiritual forms as well, and highly recommend them to participants who want to go that route. A set of readings about spiritually-based mindful eating is included at the end of this chapter.

Mindful practices teach compassion for our own thoughts and behaviors, and help us to suspend judgments. Lifestyle changes are notoriously difficult, otherwise everyone would eat right and get plenty of exercise. There are multiple obstacles to getting healthier, and if we beat ourselves up about our "failures," we set ourselves up for guilt and shame.

Why Mindful Eating?

Most of our eating is "mindless," meaning that we don't really pay attention. Brian Wansink, in a book on the psychology of eating called *Mindless Eating: Why we eat more than we think,* had this to say:

> *"Most of us are blissfully unaware of what influences how much we eat...we overeat not because of hunger but because of family and friends, packages and plates, names and numbers, labels and lights, colors and candles, shapes and smells, distractions and distances, cupboards and containers"* (p. 1).

Wansink noted that we make over 200 decisions about food every single day, most of them unthinking or automatic. Two research studies highlight the dangers of not paying attention when you eat:

- In the first, people were given a mineral drink to consume under relaxing conditions and then the absorption of the minerals was measured. People absorbed nearly 100% of the main nutrients. Then they were asked to drink the solution again, but this time, two different people talked to them at the same time; one in each ear. Under these stressful conditions, the participants did not absorb any of the nutrients from the drink (Barclay and colleagues, 1987). What does this say about emotional eating? No wonder we never feel satisfied with the food we eat when experiencing stress or high emotions.

- The second study measured digestion in people who ate before a movie or ate while watching a movie. All the measures of digestive functioning: saliva production, digestive enzymes, contractions of the stomach and intestines, blood flow to the stomach, were reduced when people ate while watching a movie (Giduck and colleagues, 1987). So what does this say about eating in front of the TV?

All of the approaches that we discuss here will help you to pay attention to both actual eating behaviors and making food choices, so that you do not act automatically, but purposefully. We will return to Wansink's research a little later, but first, here is a detailed plan for trying out Intuitive Eating. Before starting, please consider your reactions to this introduction.

- Are you a mindful or a mindless eater? What would you like to change in terms of your actual eating behaviors?

Intuitive Eating

This section summarizes two excellent books: Linda Bacon's, *Health At Every Size*, and Evelyn Tribole and Elyse Resch's *Intuitive Eating*. They both offer detailed instruction about Intuitive Eating, a plan to help restore your body's natural ability to feel hunger and fullness, and select the foods with the nutrients your body needs.

Intuitive Eating is based on the biological concept of homeostasis, or the balance in the body that is needed to maintain our bodies. In terms of nutrition, homeostasis means taking in the right nutrients, in the right amounts to sustain and nourish our bodies. The body has a dynamic interaction between hormones, proteins, neurotransmitters in the brain, thoughts and the external environment to tell us when to eat and when to stop eating. The body has been programmed to help us survive and prevent starvation. That is what makes weight loss so very difficult. As lesbian and bisexual women, we have also experienced a psychological form of homeostasis. When we can live in the external world who we are on the inside, we are happier. Being out keeps us in emotional balance and more resilient. In the same way, we need biological homeostasis. When our psychological balance is off, our physical balance is challenged as well. In DIFO, we explore some of the ways that being older women and having a minority sexual identification, can affect our psychological balance, and therefore, our physical health.

For most of our lives, we have been told that dieting is the only way to control our weight, and that we should want to control our weight. We either adopt a dieting way of life, or we feel that we are bad or irresponsible if we do not want to diet. Few of us escape this cultural message that women must diet. When we diet or restrain our eating behaviors, we interfere with homeostasis and over time, we lose the ability to recognize when our bodies are hungry or full. Lots of research has shown that dieting can actually cause harmful weight gain by increasing the release of hormones that are meant to prevent starvation.

Does this sound familiar? Some of us may have experienced a similar deprivation cycle in regards to same-sex attractions. If we recognized them, but tried to resist them, we restrained our fantasy lives and tried to deny our true natures. This strategy probably didn't work too well for you. Most people are happier and healthier when they are in touch with their true natures and listen to their bodies needs. Our bodies seek that balance in mind, body, spirit, and we learned we cannot deny our sexual attractions any more than our hunger for food. Food, sex, and intimacy are all deep human needs. Dieting is kind of like ex-gay religious conversion therapies. We can change our behavior in the short-term if we try very hard, but eventually our innate drive to survive and be our authentic selves will win out. How much damage do we do to our bodies, minds, and spirits when we resist our natural body instincts?

In *Health at Any Size* (2010), Linda Bacon proposed a new approach to eating that is supported by research, called Intuitive Eating. In 2005, Bacon and colleagues conducted a study that compared Intuitive Eating (IE) to a more traditional weight loss (WL) focused program. 78 women were randomly assigned to six months of either IE or WL program, and then the women were followed for two years. More of the WL group members dropped out of their program in frustration (42%) than the IE group members (8% dropped out). The women in the WL program lost some weight at first, but most gained it back by the end of the study. The IE women had stable weight throughout the two year period, but by the end had higher self-esteem, lowered their bad cholesterol, lowered their blood pressure, had fewer signs of disordered eating, were more satisfied with their bodies, and had increased their physical activity more than the WL group. In other words, they were healthier at a larger size. This finding of greater health benefits of IE has been found in several studies now (Cole & Horacek, 2010; Denny et al, 2013; Madden et al, 2012; Provencher and colleagues, 2009). Among young adults, intuitive eaters had lower body mass indexes than chronic dieters or binge eaters, and it appeared that intuitive eating protected young adults from eating disorders (Denny and colleagues, 2012). A study of mid-life women in New Zealand also found that those who were intuitive eaters had lower BMI (Madden and colleagues, 2012). The rest of this section gives you suggestions to trigger your own intuitive eating. Each section includes discussion questions. You can use these for journaling, reflecting on, or discussing with others. You can choose to do one section per week, or select out the parts that feel most relevant to you. The DIFO manual at the end of this book outlines a 12 week plan for introducing Intuitive Eating that may be helpful to you.

Reject the Diet Mentality

"There is an easy way to win the war against fat and reclaim your pleasure in eating: Just give up.....Stop fighting. Instead, turn to science." (Linda Bacon, p. 161)

The first step to Intuitive Eating is to stop dieting if you are currently restraining your eating. Dieting has been shown to cause at least five different kinds of harm:

- It upsets homeostasis, the body's balance mechanisms.
- It produces chemicals that inflame the liver and may even increase the risk for cancer.
- If we diet using high protein, low carb diets, we might be increasing risk for hypertension and heart disease.
- Any kind of dieting causes psychological harms, such as emotional distress, shame, and guilt, because ultimately, dieting sets us up for failure.
- Yo-yo dieting, or losing and regaining the same 20 or more pounds over and over, is much harder on the body than a slow steady weight gain, or staying at a higher weight over time.

Dieting is often the trigger for overeating, not a "lack of willpower." You can stop counting calories or carbs, stop eating only "fat-free" foods, or eating at only certain times of the day. You have permission to stop punishing yourself for eating "bad" foods, within limits of course. If you are diabetic, have food allergies, or have other health problems that require avoiding certain foods, please do not go off of those eating plans. You will still have great freedom to explore and diversify your eating plan.

It may be helpful in this stage to give up sodas of all kinds: diet or sugar. Diet sodas have been found to upset the ability to gauge our own bodily cues and to increase cravings for sweets. In one large study, regular drinkers of diet soda had a higher risk for diabetes than those who drank sugar-sweetened soda or non-sweetened beverages. This does not mean that you should switch to sugar sodas, though. Pay close attention to the sugar content of what you are drinking. Water is the healthiest beverage and can be made more interesting by adding fruits, cucumbers, mint, or whatever natural flavorings you like.

Tribole and Resch offered four steps to achieving this principle of giving up the diet mentality:

Step 1: Recognize and acknowledge that dieting is harmful to the body. If you are not already convinced, read their book or Linda Bacon's book, or other resources posed on the website. Another good resource is to subscribe to the HAES blog and consider the comments of people who have been working on intuitive eating for a long time. Go to this site to sign up:

http://healthateverysizeblog.org/

Step 2: Give up the diet mentality. It is one thing to acknowledge at one level that dieting is harmful, but another thing entirely to truly believe it and give up all the myths we have been taught for most of our lives. We need to accept that:

- Willpower has nothing to do with losing weight. You cannot fight your body's urge to survive. Calorie restriction goes against our evolution.
- Trying to follow some strict rules of any diet plan is nearly impossible. We lesbian and bisexual women are even more rebellious at heart than heterosexual women and we do not like to have others tell us what to do (or eat). When we feel hemmed in, we rebel. Sometimes we create those rules for ourselves and become our own worst enemy. Nobody, not even Dr. Oz, knows what is best for our own bodies, so give up letting anyone else tell you what to do. In addition, start tracking whenever you tell yourself what you "should" or "should not" eat. Once you re-calibrate your hunger and fullness cues, you can make healthier choices without guilt.

Step 3: Get rid of the dieting tools. No scales, no charts to count carbs, no BMI measurements are needed. Many of us are tempted to check in regularly and weigh ourselves, but weight fluctuates tremendously depending on whether we are retaining or sweating out water. It's not a reliable marker of anything. It will be much better in the long run to learn to trust how your body feels. We do recommend that you track your behavior to increase your awareness of your own body's needs, but not as a means of punishing yourself. Track your energy, your lung capacity, whether you feel bloated, and other concrete sensations rather than a number on a scale. Instead of tracking numbers on the scale, focus on setting goals that are concrete and define the change you want to see in your body. Maybe you want to walk up a flight of stairs without panting. Maybe you want less pain in your knees when you walk, or to feel less indigestion. Perhaps you want to lower your cholesterol levels.

Step 4: Compassion. Finally, cut yourself some slack. You have been absorbing these messages about the body and weight all of your life. Be gentle with yourself while you are re-learning your own body's cues and learning to love your physical container. You will be gauging your progress in this program not by a number on a scale or feeling full of willpower. Instead, you will be successful when you start feeling better in your own body; when you can trust your body to guide you to good choices (for you) in food and physical activity/movement.

Honoring Your Hunger

A dieting body is a starving body, and one that makes you obsessed with food. The second stage is to allow yourself to eat until you feel full. Practice paying close attention to your body while you eat so that you can regain the ability to detect when your body is full and not let your mind get in the way. You can never feel full if you are eating because of emotional reasons. Pay attention to how different foods make you feel. What gives you energy? Makes you feel sleepy? Gives you a stomach ache? Bloats or gives you indigestion? You will start identifying the foods that are the healthiest for you. You will likely discover that highly processed foods cause more negative sensations and do not satisfy hunger as well as higher quality, real foods. Think of Michael Pollan's suggestions for shopping for food: if you cannot pronounce an ingredient, you might not want to eat it. If it never spoils, it's a highly processed item, not real food. These processed items contain more chemicals than nutrients.

The body needs protein, carbohydrates, and fat to function properly, but not all sources of these nutrients are equal. Carbohydrates have been trashed in the dieting world, but your body needs carbs…just be mindful about the sugar content of what you are eating. Complex carbs release sugars in slower, healthier ways, whereas simple carbs are like consuming spoonfuls of processed sugar. The sugar that is in fruit is less damaging to your body, because it comes packaged in fiber which slows down the breakdown of the sugar. If you are diabetic, you need to pay closer attention to your sugar intake during this phase of learning about your own hunger. Some of us have dieted so long that we don't even recognize the signs of being hungry versus full. If you have difficulty sorting out the physical sensations of hunger from emotional and other cues, try tracking hunger cues for a few days, using the chart below.

Time	Hunger Rating Before	What I Ate	Hunger Rating After

Use a 0 to 10 scale for hunger, where 5 is the middle point or neutral (not hungry or full). A 0 to 1 means "starving." A 2-3 means ravenous or really hungry, and a 4 is mild hunger pangs (stomach gurgles, growls). On the other side of the scale, a 6 means satisfied, a 7, full, but 8-9 means stuffed and 10 means feeling sick because of overeating If you find that after eating a large meal with all the nutrients you need that you are still hungry, it is probably not physical hunger. Now you can start identifying the different kinds of hungers that you experience.

One of those is taste hunger, or wanting something because we anticipate it will taste good (dark chocolate, French fries), or because it's a special occasion (birthday cake, pride celebration). It's ok to indulge taste hunger and trust our bodies to eat just enough to satisfy the hunger. Then there's practical hunger. Let's say that you have a long meeting ahead of you and you know that by the middle of it, you will be hungry and

155

cranky. So you may decide to eat something before the meeting, even though you are not hungry. There is nothing wrong with this, as it may head off overeating after the meeting when you are ravenous. Another type of hunger that is harder to deal with is emotional hunger, or eating to sooth negative emotions. We will talk more about this later.

Making Peace with Food

If you make any particular food taboo or off limits, what usually happens? In most cases, that will be the very food that you crave the most. We all want the forbidden goodies. When you deprive yourself, you set up the high likelihood of rebound-eating. When you do give in to the temptation, you will eat much more of this item than if you had not made it off limits.

Tribole and Resch described a phenomenon that they call "Last Supper Eating." If you decide that starting tomorrow, you are no longer going to eat bread, tonight you might eat a whole loaf of olive herb bread. If you decide to go on a major calorie restriction diet on Monday morning, on Sunday night you might eat two cartons of the Ben and Jerry's ice cream in your freezer. For some of us, food insecurity may be the trigger for this Last Supper Eating. If we grew up in households where we were not always sure when we would get our next meal, we may fear the famine to come, and overeat when food is available. Another factor in Last Supper Eating is the "what the hell" effect. If you feel you have already violated your diet, or had a few bites of the forbidden food, your irrational brain says, "What the hell, I've blown it anyway so I might as well eat the entire pizza." When we do finally stop eating, stuffed and uncomfortable, guilt sets in and sets up the self-blame cycle.

With Intuitive Eating, you do not need to diet or make any foods taboo (within reason…if you are diabetic, you will have to watch the sugar content of what you eat; if you have celiac disorder, you will still suffer if you eat those breadsticks). But the philosophy of Intuitive Eating is that if you do not deprive yourself and you relearn your bodily cues, you can eat small portions of whatever you like without overeating. Your tastes can change, and if you don't deprive yourself you won't have intense cravings. Tribole and Resch provide five steps to making peace with food to try out this week.

Step 1: Pay attention: Write a list of foods that are appealing to you (include the things that you tend to deprive yourself of, or overeat when you have them available).

Step 2: Put a checkmark by the foods that you actually eat regularly and circle the ones that you put on the "forbidden" or "bad food" list.

Step 3: Give yourself permission to eat one food on the circled list this week. Go out and get some or order it at a restaurant.

Step 4: Eat it slowly and mindfully, enjoying every bite. Taste the flavors, smell it, bite down and experience its textures. Does it taste as good as you imagined? If you really love it and it tastes and smells as wonderful as you hoped, give yourself permission to have it again someday soon. If it doesn't, maybe taking it off the forbidden list helps reduce its appeal to you.

Step 5: If it was truly wonderful, keep some of this item in your kitchen so you know you could have it anytime you want (so you won't feel deprived), or give yourself permission to order it again when you go out to eat.

You can repeat this process until you have tried all the taboo items on your list and sorted out whether they really are among your favorite foods, or if you have created a monster out of the forbidden fruit. If you only eat when you are hungry, and you stop when you are full, you cannot do much damage by eating those treats on occasion.

The Voices Within

Many things influence how we feel about food and our own eating behaviors. Some of the voices in our heads come from our childhood, or the authorative voices in the media, or from health care providers. Some of these voices have become internalized into our own judgmental self-critic. We focus on the internal voice here, but the messages are echoed in the world around us. We are all exposed to many conflicting voices about our food choices and eating behaviors that can make life miserable at times. One of the loudest ones, that comes from all around us and becomes an internal voice as well, is the Food Police. The Food Police is an inner judge that sets the food rules, monitors our every move, and punishes us with guilt and remorse for our choices. But the Food Police is supported by other voices as well.

The Nutrition Informant may pretend to be about health, but it really is a self-critic. It may tell you to count calories, count points, weigh foods, eat only fat-free stuff, or check your weight on the scale twice a day. The Nutrition Informant is just the Food Police disguised as a supposed health advocate. But with mindful tracking of eating patterns and thoughts about eating, you can turn the Nutrition Informant into a Nutrition Ally. This voice reminds you about what foods make you feel bloated, gassy, uncomfortable, hyper, or gives you indigestion, and what foods make you crave other foods. In other words, it can become a guilt-free helper.

Another voice is the Diet Rebel. It chafes against the rules and wants to be bad. We lesbian/bisexual women often consider ourselves as rebels against society, so it's easy for the rebel voice to sneak in around our eating patterns as well. You can tell the Diet Rebel to lay off the negative comments about your body and the judgments about eating. If you eat something just to be a rebel, who are you hurting? Instead, you can apply that rebel voice to external forces: it can remind you that being a rebel can mean embracing food justice and studying the politics of food. Love and respect yourself but rebel against social injustice!

The Food Anthropologist is a neutral observer of your own behavior. If you notice when you are full and when you are hungry, what you eat when, and how it makes you feel, you learn about your own bodily needs. For some of us, this is an exotic new land that we have not explored, at least not since early childhood. Be curious, without being judgmental and track or journal about your discoveries.

The Nurturer is a very important voice that too often gets overshadowed by the louder Diet Rebel and Food Police. It is a soft and soothing voice that comes from your own gut. It knows what you need to feel comfortable, healthy, and safe. All of us need to pay more attention to our inner nurturing spirits and listen to our internal body wisdom. The nurturer helped us to come out and embrace our woman-loving spirit. We love other women, but do we love our own woman's body?

Once you have tracked your behavior, discovered your own body needs, and got back in touch with cues of hunger and fullness, you have become an Intuitive Eater. The Food Anthropologist and Nurturer have taken over center stage and relegated the Food Police and Diet Rebel voices to the background. Your Nutrition Informant has turned into an Ally. It all starts by paying attention to those voices.

- What do you tell yourself about food? What voices are loudest or most troublesome for you?

Feeling Your Fullness

This week it's time to give up the "clean up your plate" mentality and start to relearn when you are full. In the past, you may have felt that your eating got "out of control" because you waited to eat until you were ravenous. Or maybe your parents ingrained the guilt trip of eating everything on your plate. Perhaps you were over-eating for emotional reasons, not because of physical hunger. As you start to experiment with feeling your fullness, you will have to pay very close attention to your body when you are eating. There is some variability in how people describe feeling full, so there may be individual differences in this sensation. Some describe feeling neutral; not hungry, and not stuffed. Others describe a subtle feeling of the stomach being full. Others notice that they start to slow down their eating.

So if you are at that weekly lesbian potluck, put a smaller amount of food than usual on your plate and eat mindfully. Pay attention to your body's cues and stop when you feel that sensation of being satisfied or mildly full. If you feel stuffed, think back to notice if there was a point or a sensation just before you got that point that could indicate your tank is full. Be compassionate with yourself during this process. It took a long time to lose your intuitive eating voice, so it will take a while to get it back. Feeling your fullness relies on conscious, or mindful, eating. Tribole and Resch recommend two steps in developing this mindfulness:

Step 1: Pause in the middle of a meal to check in with your body. Ask yourself these questions:
- How does it taste? If you are not enjoying this meal or snack, you can stop now. Are you eating it just because it is there?
- Am I still hungry? If so, keep eating, or choose something else to eat.

Step 2: Pause again at the end of the meal to assess your level of fullness. Remember that it is ok to leave food on your plate, or eat it all. Your cue is whether your stomach is full, not the food or the plate. You can use the following scale to track fullness for a while, until you can feel your own hunger and fullness naturally.

Time	What I am eating	Fullness rating

Use a 0 to 10 scale of fullness, where 0 equals feeling completely empty, 1-2 is ravenously hungry, 3-4 is hunger pangs, 5 is neutral or not feeling hungry or full, 6-7 is satisfied, 8-9 is stuffed and 10 is sick.

Here are some other suggestions for being more mindful or aware of your own body cues of hunger and fullness:

1. Eat without distractions. Avoid eating in front of the TV, computer, newspaper, or whatever else takes your mind off of eating. Focus on the taste, the textures, the aromas, and your body's responses to the food.
2. Reinforce your conscious decision to stop eating. How often do you continue to pick away at a meal just because the food is still in front of you? Put away leftovers or leave the table.
3. Practice saying "no thank you" when you are offered food when you are not hungry. You have no obligation to eat every moment at a party or to be pressured by a friend to eat a dessert or appetizer that you really don't want.

There has been some research on what predicts overeating, and a few of those factors include:

- The amount of time since you last ate. The longer you wait, the hungrier you will be and your body will want to gorge. Nibblers who eat small frequent meals tend to have fewer binges.
- The kind of food you eat. High fiber, protein-packed foods (lean meats, beans, tuna, cheese, nonfat yogurt, whole grain breads and crackers) tend to keep you full longer than greens, fruits, or vegetables. "Air" foods like low calory snacks (rice cakes, celery, diet sodas) do not make you feel full or last for long.
- The amount of food left in your stomach. If you wait until your stomach is completely empty, you will be more likely to overeat.
- How hungry you felt when you started to eat. If you are at the point of ravenous, you will probably eat more.
- If you are with others. Eating with a social group is usually associated with a longer duration of a meal, and more food in general, unless you have a dieter's mentality that leads you to eat less if you think others are watching you.

Getting Satisfaction From Food

Deep satisfaction is happiness. Eating should bring happiness, not guilt, remorse, or a sense of duty. If you are moderately hungry, you will enjoy a meal more than if you are ravenous or not hungry. If you are emotional, you will enjoy it less. It's hard to digest when you are angry with your mother or irritated with your partner. The key to satisfaction is finding the food that "hits the spot" and delights the senses. Here are five steps to a satisfying culinary experience.

Step 1. What do you really want to eat? Don't eat something just because it is there, or because you think you should eat it. Figure out what you really want and eat it in a mindful way. If you constantly say, "I don't know what I want to eat," you may need to repeat some of the earlier activities, like making lists of favorite foods, paying attention to your body, and committing to eating what you really want.

Step 2. Focus on the sensual experiences of eating. Mindful eating means being aware of the taste, aroma, texture, temperature, appearance, and volume of the food you are eating. Find out what really gives you pleasure and makes you feel satisfied (full), without painful after effects.

Step3. Savor your food. Make time for your meals; at least 15 minutes to sit down and do nothing but eat. Eat slowly so that you can fully engage your taste buds. Put down your fork every few minutes to feel your body. Track when you are getting full and stop before reaching "stuffed." If possible, have a variety of foods on your plate to provide different nutrients and different sensory experiences.

Step 4. "If you don't love it, don't eat it, and if you love it, savor it." This is self-explanatory!

Step 5. Check in regularly to see if foods still taste good. If you eat a lot of the same food, over time it may lose its appeal. Researchers call this "sensory-specific satiety." Once it stops giving you pleasure, maybe you only want to eat that first pleasurable bite and then stop. Or replace it with a new food experience.

Coping with Emotions without Food

Emotional eating begins very early in life, from the time we are offered the breast or bottle when we are crying, to being offered a cookie when we fall and bump our heads, or were given an ice cream cone to celebrate getting an A on a test. We are practicing emotional eating when we "clean our plates" to please a parent or partner. We learn to associate the comfort of a loving family with the food we eat, as well as the distress of a dysfunctional family with the traumas of family meals. Food is offered as evidence of love, a reward, or a means of comforting all sorts of ills (feed a cold!). For some of us, eating became a way of coping with unwanted or feared sexual feelings. We had no one we felt safe with to talk about our attractions to girls, so we stuffed our fears and guilt with food. Emotions are so wrapped up with eating that we often no longer recognize when we are eating to sooth an emotion rather than a physical hunger. For the next two weeks, we will work on the issues of emotional eating. Eating itself can become emotional. Can you fill in the blank in this statement:

"I felt guilty because I ate_____."

If so, you had an emotional response to eating. It's time to give up the guilt and show yourself some compassion. Tribole and Resch suggest that emotional eating is on a continuum from pleasurable eating to punishing eating. See if you can ease yourself up toward the pleasure end of the continuum.

Sensory gratification (eating for the pleasure and satisfaction)
Comfort eating (mild emotions)
Distracted eating (eating to avoid feeling something like boredom or anxiety)
Sedation (eating yourself into a near coma)
Punishing eating (a pattern of overeating followed by severe guilt)

We may have different experiences with different emotions; some may cause eating and others not so much. Start by checking your own awareness of the relationship between eating and emotions by filling out the following survey.

I often eat when	Never	Rarely	Sometimes	Often
I feel bored				
I want to procrastinate				
I need to bribe myself to do something				
I want to reward myself				
I feel excited				
I need to feel comfort/soothing				
I want to show or receive love				
I am frustrated				
I am angry				
I feel stressed				
I feel anxious				
I feel depressed or sad				
I want to feel connected				
I want to lose control				
Other reasons I eat:				

Discussion questions:
- Try filling out the emotional eating scale everyday for a week to see what emotions come up for you, or use the daily tracking tool with the DIFO manual.
- Is there a pattern? What can you do to begin to break the pattern?

Here is another activity to track emotional eating. Consider four steps every time you think of eating something.

Step 1. Ask yourself, "Am I physically hungry?" If yes, eat. If no, go on to step 2.

Step 2. "What am I feeling?" See if you can identify the feeling: write about it, call a friend and talk it out, talk to a therapist, sit with the feelings and experience them.

Step 3. Identify what you need. What are the unmet needs or unaddressed issues that make this feeling keep coming up for you? Is there a common pattern? Is it mostly frustration, mostly anger, mostly sadness, or a wide variety of feelings? What events in the external world bring these feelings up?

Step 4. Take an action to relieve the emotion. Ask for help, make requests for changes in the behavior of people around you, or change your own behavior. Emotions pass quickly, unless we latch on to them. If you just experience it, the emotion is often gone in a matter of seconds or a few minutes. If you have attached yourself to the emotion, you might be able to de-tach by using another coping behavior:
- Get more rest (nap, go to bed 15 minutes earlier)
- Get more sensual pleasures (take a hot bath, get a massage, have more sex…)
- Express the feeling instead of bottling it up or denying/repressing/distracting (have a BMW session: 5 minutes when you let yourself bitch, moan, and whine)
- Feel that you are heard and understood (ask a friend or partner to listen to you BMW without offering solutions or commentary)

- Do something creative or stimulating (read a book, dance, take a walk, enjoy some music, do a crossword puzzle, go to a movie)
- Put on some music and dance for 5 minutes
- Receive comfort and warmth (pet your cat, walk the dog, tend to your garden, get yourself flowers)
- Meditate

Add to this list the things that you know give you pleasure, and try doing more of them each day.

Another activity to consider this week is to divide a piece of paper in half and on one side, list the benefits you received from emotional eating (it numbed you to pain, the food tasted good, it was a distraction from stress, etc), and on the other side, list the problems that emotional eating caused for you (maybe it numbed the joys of life as well as the pain, perhaps it caused high blood pressure, or knee problems, or made you feel uncomfortable in your own skin, or guilty, etc). Seeing it laid out this way may prompt some ideas for dealing the emotion better.

Keep in mind that if you stop emotional eating, you may have to face and experience the emotions that you were numbing or distracting yourself from. If these are too intense, you might want to consider counseling or doing some serious self-care activities until you have established healthier coping strategies as a habit. It will not be uncommon to have some "relapses" back to emotional eating when stress gets too high. We all resort to earlier habits sometimes. The key is to not beat yourself up about it; just get back on track as soon as you are able.

Respecting Your Body

How's your body image? What do you like about your body? What do you love? Or do you focus only on the "problem" areas? Making peace with food is nearly impossible unless you also work on making peace with your body. A first step is to avoid telling yourself any negative stories about your body—no "fat talk" or putting yourself down. Start finding the positives and give gratitude for what your body can do for you. Did it take you for a nice walk in the woods this week? Did it get you to work? Did it have fun on the dance floor? Did you use those arms to wrap around your girlfriend? Did you draw in breath and smell those beautiful flowers in your garden?

Body respect is a major challenge in our culture, with constant messages all around us to look younger, thinner, more muscular, a different shape, more grace, more athletic…the list goes on and on. If you look at so-called women's magazines, you will see hundreds of messages about the need to change your body. Cover up the blemishes, erase the wrinkles, get rid of cellulite, dye your hair, beautify those feet, remove that facial or leg hair, fade those age spots. If you really tried to meet all the expectations for women in our society, you would spend all of your waking hours on self-improvement activities (and most of them would not work anyway!).

Thankfully, many lesbian and bisexual women have rejected some of the messages about how women are supposed to look, but that does not mean we are totally immune to the messages from dominant society. In addition, we may have pressures from our communities, our partners, or maybe we just think we know what we are supposed to look like to be desirable lesbian or bisexual women in our local communities. In most research, lesbians are more accepting of larger bodies than heterosexual women. Our own expectations can be unrealistic and we might project our anxieties on community norms. In your lesbian/bisexual women's community, what have you learned about the acceptability of larger bodies? Do you identify as butch, femme, or somewhere in the middle? Has your personal gender expression changed over time? For some women, there was pressure to "look like a lesbian" when they first came out to be more readily identifiable, but over time, they develop their own style. Was this true for you?

Another way that lesbian communities have been positive about the physical body is the greater acceptance of aging. Lesbian/bisexual women are more likely to be considered as desirable for dating and relationships at much older ages than heterosexual women. What experiences have you had as you age?

Julia Cameron's The Writing Diet

If you read through the Intuitive Eating plan and are not ready to go that route yet, here's another plan to consider. This one is for people who enjoy writing. You could possibly do this plan by just thinking about the questions and issues or discussing them with a friend, but it will work better if you put pen to paper or fingers to keyboard.

One of the oldest practices for changing one's behavior is to track patterns through writing or journaling. Julia Cameron, author of *The Artist's Way* and many other books, noticed that many of her students lost weight once they started to write regularly. She suggested that "weight loss is a frequent by-product of creative recovery. Overeating blocks our creativity. The flip side is also true: we can use creativity to block our overeating" (Cameron, 2007, pg xv). Some readers may find her focus on weight loss off-putting, but the bottom line is that journaling about our health may be beneficial to tracking and identifying unhealthy patterns and triggers, and monitoring our attempts to be healthier. The writing exercises that Julia Cameron recommends may be useful as a part of a comprehensive health program for those who enjoy the writing process. Tracking, whether in a journal or other forms, is a type of mindfulness practice that can be applied to health. Cameron's book lays out several "tools" for using writing to address your health. I've adapted them to our DIFO program here. You might want to try one tool per week and see what works best for you. There are seven tools. Her book also gives much practical advice on where we might encounter resistance and underlying issues that affect our daily health choices.

Week 1: Morning Pages
One of the first and major suggestions that Cameron proposes is to unblock our creativity using "morning pages." Every morning before you do anything else (ok, you can go to the bathroom first), write three pages. Write whatever comes into your head without any editing or thinking or censoring. This is a means of "getting current" with your feelings and what is working you. Morning pages allow you to purge the negative and mundane and clear your mind. Now you can notice the patterns, see how every day is full of "choice points" where we make decisions that impact health and wellbeing. For example, when I was upset by a homophobic remark from one of my siblings, did I choose to go for a walk, or to plunk myself on the sofa to draft an angry email in response? What would be the healthiest choice for me?

You can choose to keep your morning pages, or discard them. The point is to purge on paper, not to write the great lesbian romance novel. Some people find that they have insights into what's really bothering them when they review their morning pages, but others find them to be just rubbish!

Week 2: Keep a Food/Activity Journal
Another tool is to keep a food journal. This is not the place to record frustration about your homophobic boss or sexist neighbor, but to focus on nutrition. Here you can record what you eat, how you felt during and after eating it, what emotions or thoughts or triggers in the environment were associated with eating, what you craved, and so on. After a few weeks of recording these thoughts, you can start reconnecting your mind and body. You might notice that when you eat lunch at your desk, you are hungry again in an hour because your mind did not pay attention to the process of eating and you are out of touch with bodily cues for hunger and fullness. You could use the DIFO tracking tool, with additional blank pages added to create your own journal or create your own journal to track issues that are relevant to you.

In addition to recording food and associated emotions and thoughts, you could try writing prompts related to food, such as:

I eat when I _____.
I crave _____ when I feel _____.
When I over eat, I feel _____.
When I eat a healthy meal, I feel _____.

Regular writing, like regular meditation, yoga, walking (or sex), can put us back in touch with thoughts, feelings, and align them with the body. If you really want to be serious about this, carry a small journal/notebook with you all day, and every time you feel hungry or reach for something to eat, stop for a moment and write about the experience. Try it for just one day and see if it's useful.

- How does your body feel? (are you actually hungry or is there some other sensation?)
- What are you feeling emotionally? (bored, nervous, angry, neutral, etc)
- What are you thinking? (need a break from work, looked at the clock and are thinking it's time for lunch, processing a conversation you had with your partner, etc)
- What choices do you have available to address your bodily sensations, thoughts, and feelings? Do you need to eat now? Can you choose a healthy snack or meal?

You might notice that you love the first bite or two of that French vanilla ice cream, but start to feel a little bloated by the fifth or sixth bite. You could keep a container in your refrigerator and have just two bites a day--that way you get the pleasure without the pain! No two people are alike, so you will need to experiment to find the foods that satisfy your hunger and give you pleasure without pain an hour later. Intuitive eating is a great approach to doing just that.

Week 3: Walking

For those who are able, walking can be a form of writing in one's head, a way to problem-solve, a stress reliever, a muscle relaxer, a form of spiritual practice, or a social event. Whether you go for a slow, deliberate walking meditation in nature, power walk to the post office, or go for a stroll with friends, walking is good for the body, mind and spirit.

For problem solving, think about the issue that is bugging you right now, whether it is a relationship problem, a nagging boss, or a concern about your health, then go for a walk by yourself and see what bubbles up. You may have to clear your mind of other issues first by focusing on your breathing or the rhythm of your footsteps, then put the problem before you in your mind.

Daily walks of only 20 minutes are beneficial to your health and can lower cholesterol, decrease symptoms of depression, and relieve stress. Walking by yourself in nature settings can foster the sense of connection to the land, sea, sky, trees, and wildlife whereas walking with others can strengthen your social bonds and deepen connection with community. In San Francisco, you can join the SF Walking Dykes, who stroll for 60-90 minutes in mostly flat, easy trails in Golden Gate Park. Meet at the Conservatory of Flowers at 11 am any Saturday to find this community of walkers. There are also Gay and Lesbian Sierrans for those who want more vigorous hikes. If these are not options, just a 10-15 walk in your own neighborhood can strengthen your connection to the place and make it more like "home."

Week 4: Working with 4 Questions

This week you may take up the food journal again, if you stopped using it, and this time address four very simple questions every time you reach for something to eat. These questions work well with the Intuitive Eating plan to help you reconnect to your body's wisdom. Ask yourself (and/or write about):

- Am I physically hungry? (or is it something else I'm feeling)
- Is this what I feel like eating?
- Is this what I feel like eating right now?
- Is there something else I could eat instead? (if my first choice is not very healthy...although maybe my answer is yes, this is what I want to eat right now. So then, eat it with intention and no guilt).

What you want to do with this final question, is to avoid eating something that you don't really want, just because it's there when you are in a mood. The point is to be mindful about your bodily sensations and what you choose to eat, not to be judgmental. If you start criticizing yourself or engaging in negative body talk in the journal, you may be becoming your own worst enemy. Track your behavior like the Food Anthropologist---objectively, factually, without judgment or criticism. If you have been keeping a journal for a while, you might want to review it for times when you have been too hard on yourself or made negative comments about your own body. From now on, try a more positive, nurturing approach to journaling.

Week 5: A Culinary Artist's Date
In Cameron's first book, the Artist's Way, she talks about treating oneself to an art gallery, a film, a coffee shop or restaurant with one's notebook or laptop to write, a trip to a bookstore, or anything else that inspires creativity. In the Culinary Artist's date, you may decide to go to a farmer's market in a different part of town, take a cooking class, go to a used bookstore and browse cook books, eat at your favorite restaurant, or try something brand new. The point is that you are treating yourself to something related to food that gives you pleasure. If you decide to have a banana split, be sure that you savor every single bite of it. If you decide to have a spinach salad, be sure that you savor every single bite of it. Enjoy your meal and record the details here in this journal. The point is to make an event out of it—a treat for your senses. Record how it looked, how it smelled, how it tasted, and how much you enjoyed the experience—but write about the experience after you have finished eating so that you are mindful while eating.

Week 6: HALT
HALT stands for "don't get too Hungry, Angry, Lonely, or Tired," and comes from the alcohol recovery world. These are emotional states and physical states that make us vulnerable to temptation and making poor choices, like overeating or eating something that makes us feel bad later, drinking, smoking, or lying on the sofa instead of moving around. Maybe we experience only one of them regularly, or maybe all four are our demons. If you track your bodily sensations, thoughts, and feelings regularly, though, you can start to identify them before they take over. If you eat before you get too hungry, intervene before your anger gets out of control, take a social action before loneliness sets in, and rest before you drop from exhaustion, you will take care of your body in healthier ways. You might journal about HALT for a week to see which of these emotional states turn up most often for you, and how you usually respond. At the end of the week, assess your experience and record your findings in your journal. Or use a brief tracking tool, like the one below.

How often did I overeat or eat unhealthy items today because of:

Emotional State:	Never	Sometimes	Often	Very Often
Hunger				
Anger				
Loneliness				
Being Tired				

Week 7: Find a Body Buddy
A body buddy is an objective observer; someone you can be painfully honest with, who will not engage in negative body talk, shame, or guilt-trip you. Your body buddy can be the person you check in with daily, or call/text when you are tempted or feeling powerless. If you do not have someone in your personal life who can be the buddy, contact another DIFO member, or consider joining the Health at Every Size community in the bay area or online. Find someone who can help you stay positive while supporting you to be healthier. Ideally, what qualities would you like to have in a body buddy? Is there someone in your life now who would be willing to help you?

Weeks 8 to whenever: Practice Your Favorites
For the rest of the program, you can choose the tools that worked the best for you, and explore them in more depth. Or maybe you will want to blend two of them: walk with a body buddy twice a week; take Artists Culinary Dates for breakfast and do your morning pages. Pay attention to what works for you, and why. Which of these tools or practices can you sustain over a long period of time, until they become habits?

OTHER MINDFULNESS APPROACHES

Intuitive Eating is mainly about paying attention to what you eat and how you feel when you eat. Brian Wansick's book, *Mindless Eating*, is all about the psychology of food and eating, and shows just how much we are influenced by the context, the people we are with, the containers, and even the descriptions of the food we eat. That is, how we eat, rather than why. Here are some of the interesting findings from his research:

The Psychology of Eating

Changing our food environment is a double-pronged process. We have a social responsibility to vote for food conscious politicians, support campaigns for local causes like getting farmer's markets in our neighborhoods, voting against government subsidies to fast food, and creating demand for organic produce. At the individual level, we can change our own personal food environments to reduce those mindless extra bites that add unnecessary calories. Be sure to personalize these suggestions to your own environment and needs:

1. Use smaller plates and bowls. The bigger the plate, the more we pack on food. You can always go back for seconds if you are still hungry.
2. Tall slender glasses are better than short squat ones if you want to limit certain kinds of beverages. And do not "supersize" when eating out.
3. Prepare less food to begin with.
4. "Out of sight": keep the tempting foods for special occasions (the dark chocolate, ice cream, etc), farther back in the cupboard or refrigeration and put the healthier options up front and center.
5. Slow down when you eat. Use chopsticks for a while to force yourself to slow down. This allows your stomach to catch up and notice fullness cues. Chewing more between bites aids digestion and slows you down. Your brain registers the taste and texture better as well when you focus on eating and chewing.
6. Convenience foods like cookies, granola, chips and so on are better if wrapped individually, than if you eat right out of a bag. Take just one serving out of the cupboard at once, not the whole bag. If you go back for another, you have to do it more mindfully.
7. When you serve a meal, put the vegetables and fruits on the table, but leave the meat and carbohydrates on the counter so you are more likely to eat seconds on the healthier options.
8. When you have a snack, whether its popcorn, nuts, or chips, put them in a small bowl rather than eating out of a large container.

Eating out with others can be tricky. In one study, if people ate out with one other person, they ate 35% more than if they ate alone. When with a group of seven or more, they ate 96% more (that's twice as much food as eating alone). But this is not always true. Some people who fear criticism from others actually eat less in a group than when alone. Figure out what is true for you. If you eat more with a group, trying pacing yourself with the slowest eater in the group. Make a plan for altering your own food environment and track how it works for you:

Eating Whole Foods

Another mindfulness practice is to pay attention to the quality of what you eat, not the quantity. Many experts think that the highly processed foods, full of unnatural chemicals, are what causes a lot of human illnesses. Returning to more natural foods can help you get back to basics and get more nutritional value (and pleasure) from eating. This section comes from Michael Pollan's writing about food.

"Eat Food. Not too much. Mostly plants."

These words begin an essay by Michael Pollan examining our culture's shift from food as a part of culture and life to food as science (particularly chemistry!). After spending years researching the food industry and how food companies develop and market products, Michael Pollan developed "9 Principles of Healthy Eating:"

1. **Eat Food:** We have forgotten what food is and what it looks like. Much of what we eat comes boxed, shrink-wrapped or frozen. Most of the things in the grocery department are not 'food' -- they are really products developed by companies and marketed to you. Food is found only in the produce, meat, fish and dairy departments. A basic rule is that if the item didn't exist in the 1800s, it probably isn't food. Food goes bad. Food spoils.

2. **Avoid Health Claims:** Any item that has a health claim on the package is being marketed to you. When foods are processed, many of the nutrients are removed from them. Food products that advertise added vitamins and minerals are often replacing natural nutrients that were removed during processing. Avoid 'products' that make claims and stick to eating food. If you want extra vitamins, eat more fruit and vegetables.

3. **Choose Food With Familiar Ingredients:** Food labels have a tremendous amount of information. Don't be distracted by all the numbers. Look to the ingredient list. The shorter the better. If you don't know what something is on that ingredient list, put it back. Better yet, buy things without labels, such as produce, fish and meat.

4. **Go to the Farmer's Market:** Almost everything sold there is fresh and local. Find a farmer's market near you and become a regular. The temptations of the supermarket aren't there and the food is more nutritious because it is freshly picked.

5. **Pay More, Eat Less:** Organic fresh foods cost more. Food from the farmer's market often (but not always) costs more. But, buying healthy ingredients still costs less than eating out. When you are meeting your nutritional needs with these fresh foods, you will need to eat less overall and be less likely to buy expensive snacks. Your food bill will probably even out in the end and you will be healthier.

6. **Eat Mostly Plants, Especially Leaves:** Plants are good for us. Eating more plants brings health benefits. If we fill ourselves up on plants, then we eat less of unhealthy foods. Plants have antioxidants, omega-3 fatty acids and fiber (anti-inflammatory agents). Vegetarians have better heart health than meat eaters. Flexatarians (occasional meat eaters) have much better health statistics than regular meat eaters. The more vegetables you eat, the healthier you'll be.

7. **Follow the French Example:** The French live well and live long because they are eating food, not products. The rich meals served in French restaurants in the U.S. are not typical of the daily meal of the French (and still have more nutrients than the average fast food hamburger). Some principles of French eating include: eat small portions, do not eat seconds, do not snack between meals, eat with people, and take pleasure in your food (be mindful while you eat).

8. **Cook:** Cooking is a great way to get in touch with your nutritional needs. You will learn about how foods interact, how to create great tastes, and how to get more pleasure in your eating. Cooking is a fabulous pastime and could add years to your life. So buy food, mostly plants, and cook them.

9. **Choose a Variety of Foods:** The more variety you have in your diet, the greater chances of meeting all your nutritional needs. Try new vegetables. Vitamins, minerals and other nutrients are all available from nature -- you just have to eat different things to attain a good balance.

Discussion Points:
- Which of the nine principles would be the easiest for you to incorporate in your daily life and why?
- Which ones are most challenging?

The nine principles are a good start to adopting intuitive eating. Our bodies evolved to recognize fullness and hunger based on real foods. When we eat highly processed foodstuff, the chemicals and unnatural ingredients like high fructose corn syrup confuse our bodies and we no longer recognize that we are full. Going back to real food will help our bodies readjust…then we can have occasional treats if we still want them.

WATER

How much water do you need each day? Your water needs depend on many factors, including your health, how active you are and where you live. Although no single formula fits everyone, knowing more about your body's need for fluids will help you estimate how much water to drink each day.

Health benefits of water

Water makes up about 60% of your body weight and is the largest element of the human body. Every system in your body depends on water. For example, water flushes toxins out of vital organs, carries nutrients to your cells, and provides a moist environment for ear, nose and throat tissues. Water keeps you lubricated when sexual desire strikes. Lack of water can lead to dehydration, a condition that occurs when you don't have enough water in your body to carry out normal functions. Even mild dehydration can drain your energy and make you tired.

How much water do you need?

Every day you lose water through your breath, perspiration, urine and bowel movements. For your body to function properly, you must replenish water by consuming beverages and foods that contain water. So how much fluid does the average, healthy adult living in a temperate climate need? The Institute of Medicine determined that an adequate intake for women is 2.2 liters (about 9 cups) of total beverages a day.

Factors that influence water needs

You may need to modify your total fluid intake depending on:

- **Exercise.** If you exercise or engage in activity that makes you sweat, you need extra water to compensate for the fluid loss. An extra 400 to 600 milliliters (about 1.5 to 2.5 cups) of water should replace the water you lose for short bouts of exercise, but intense exercise lasting more than an hour (for example, running a marathon) requires more fluid intake. How much additional fluid you need depends on how much you sweat during exercise, and the duration and type of exercise. During long bouts of intense exercise, it's best to use a sports drink that contains sodium, as this will help replace sodium lost in sweat and reduce the chances of developing hyponatremia, which can be life-threatening. Also, continue to replace fluids after you're finished exercising.
- **Environment.** Hot or humid weather can make you sweat more and requires additional intake of fluid. Heated indoor air also can cause your skin to lose moisture during wintertime. Altitudes greater than 8,200 feet (2,500 meters) may trigger increased urination and more rapid breathing, which use up more of your fluid reserves. If you are traveling to the mountains, increase your water intake.
- **Illnesses or health conditions.** When you have fever, vomiting or diarrhea, your body loses additional fluids. In these cases, you should drink more water. Sometimes, your doctor may recommend oral rehydration solutions, such as Gatorade, Powerade or CeraLyte. Also, you may need increased fluid intake if you develop certain conditions, including bladder infections or urinary tract stones. On the other hand, some conditions such as heart failure and some types of kidney, liver and adrenal diseases may impair excretion of water and even require that you limit your fluid intake.

Sources of water

You don't need to rely only on what you drink to meet your fluid needs. On average, food provides about 20 percent of total water intake. Many fruits and vegetables, such as watermelon and tomatoes, are 90% or more water by weight. Beverages such as milk and juice are composed mostly of water. Even beer, wine and caffeinated beverages — such as coffee, tea or soda — can contribute, but these should not be a major portion of your daily total fluid intake. Water is still your best bet because it's calorie-free, inexpensive and readily available.

Staying hydrated

Generally if you drink enough fluid so that you rarely feel thirsty and produce 1.5 liters (6.3 cups) or more of colorless or light yellow urine a day, your fluid intake is probably adequate. If your urine is dark yellow and cloudy, you probably need more water. Although uncommon, it is possible to drink too much water. When your kidneys are unable to excrete the excess water, the electrolyte (mineral) content of the blood is diluted, resulting in low sodium levels in the blood, a condition called hyponatremia. Endurance athletes, such as marathon runners, who drink large amounts of water, are at higher risk of hyponatremia. In general, though, drinking too much water is rare in healthy adults who eat an average American diet.

REFERENCES

Books and articles on Intuitive Eating

Bacon, L. (2010). *Health at every size*. Dallas, TX: Benbella Books.

Cole, R. & Horacek, T. (2010). Effectiveness of the My Body Knows When intuitive eating pilot program. *American Journal of Health Behavior, 34*(3), 286-297.

Denny, K., Loth, K., Eisenberg, M., & Neumark-Sztainer, D. (2013). Intuitive eating in young adults. Who is doing it, and how is it related to disordered eating behaviors? *Appetite, 60*(1), 13-19.

Madden, C., Leong, S., Gray, A., & Horwath, C. (2012). Eating in response to hunger and satiety signals is related to BMI in a nationwide sample of 1601 mid-age New Zealand women. *Public Health Nutrition, 15*(12), 2272-2279.

Provencher, V., Begin, C., & Tremblay, A (2009). Health at every size and eating behaviors: 1 year followup results of a size acceptance intervention. *Journal of the American Dietetic Association, 109*(11): 1854-1861.

Tribole, E. & Resch, E. (2012). *Intuitive Eating: A revolutionary program that works*. New York, St Martin's Griffin Press.

Books on Mindful Eating from a Spiritual Perspective

Jan Chozen Bays (2009). *Mindful eating: A guide to rediscovering a healthy and joyful relationship with food*. Boston: Shambala Press.

Thich Nhat Hanh and Lillian Cheung (2010). *Savor: Mindful eating, mindful life*. New York: Harper Collins Publishers.

Julia Cameron (2008). *The Writing Diet*. NY: Jeremy Tarcher/Penguin.

Other books on mindful eating

Pollan, Michael (2013). *Food Rules*. NY: Penguin.

Wansick, Brian (2010). *Mindless eating: Why we eat more than we think*. New York: Bantam Books

Other References:

Boehmer, U., Mertz, M., Timm, A., Glickman, M., Sullivan, M., & Potter, J. (2011). Overweight and obesity in long-term breast cancer survivors: How does sexual orientation impact BMI? *Cancer Investigation, 29*(3), 220-228.

Bowen, D., Balsam, K., Diergaarde, B., Russo, M., & Escamilla, G. (2006). Healthy eating, exercise, and weight: impressions of sexual minority women. *Women and Health, 44,* 79-93.

Brittain, D., Baillergeon, T., McElroy, M., Aaron, D., & Gyuraski, N. (2006). Barriers to moderate physical activity in adult lesbians. *Women and Health, 43,* 75-92.

Brown-Saracino, J. (2011). From the lesbian ghetto to ambient community: The perceived costs and benefits of integration for community. *Social Problems, 58* (3), 361-388.

Corbalan, M., Morales, E., Cantras, M., et al. (2009). Effectiveness of cognitive behavioral therapy based on the Mediterranean diet for treatment of obesity. *Nutrition, 25,* 861-869.

Fogel, S., Young, L., Dietrich, M., & Blakemore, D. (2012). Weight loss and related behavior changes among lesbians, *Journal of Homosexuality, 59,* 689-702.

Fogel, S., Young, L., & McPherson, J. B. (2009). The experience of group weight loss efforts among lesbians. *Women and Health,* 540-554.

Matthews, A. K., Hughes, T. L., Osterman, G. P., & Kodl, M. M. (2005). Complementary medicine practices in a community-based sample of lesbian and heterosexual women. *Health Care for Women International, 26(5):* 430-47.

Mautner Project (2011). Lesbian overweight and obesity research. "Tackling the lesbian obesity epidemic" messages and images report. Washington, D.C.

Niemeier, H. M., Leahy, T., Reed, K. P., Brown, R., & Wing, R., (2012). An acceptance-based behavioral intervention for weight loss: A pilot study. *Behavioral Therapy, 43,* 427-437.

O'Hara, L., & Gregg, J. (2012). Human rights casualities from the 'war on obesity': why focusing on body weight is inconsistent with a human rights approach to health, *Fat Studies, 1(1),* 32-46.

Roberts, S. J., Stuart-Shor, E. M., & Oppenheimer, R. A. (2010). Lesbians' attitudes and beliefs regarding overweight and weight reduction. *Journal of Clinical Nursing, 19,* 1986-1994.

Shaw, K., O'Rourke, P., DelMar, C., & Kenardy, J. (2009). Psychological interventions for overweight or obesity (Review). *Cochrane Database of Systematic Review, 1,* NO. CD000381.

Smith, H., Matthews, A., Markovic, N., Youk, A., Danielson, M., & Talbott, E. (2010). A comparative study of complementary and alternative medicine use among heterosexually and lesbian-identified women: data from the ESTHER project. *Journal of Alternative and Complementary Medicine, 16(11),* 1161-1170.

Chapter 18: Physical Activity: Moving For Our Health

This chapter describes the physical activity components of DIFO, and is meant to supplement the video, Moving For Our Health. We recognize that every woman has a unique body and has different needs and preferences for physical movement, so we offer a wide menu of ideas here and let you design your own program. **Moving For Our Health** is a video demonstrating a gentle, but very powerful movement and breathing routine that can be done in 15-20 minutes if you do the whole thing. Almost all women are able to do most of the activities here, and even though they seem simple, they could benefit even the most serious athlete, as they focus on the core and on stress-relieving breath work. It's not "exercise" so much as learning to track the physical body and get in touch with body cues. This chapter and the video was developed by our two physical movement experts: Penny Sablove whose background in martial arts and physical therapy, and Wini Linguvic, a fitness coach and yoga teacher extraordinaire. They designed the activity which includes core strengthening, body mindfulness and stress reduction. Project manager Deborah Craig shot video and still photos, edited the video, and created the script at the end of this chapter.

PHYSICAL MOVEMENT: A POWERFUL PROTECTIVE FACTOR

Are you concerned about getting a chronic physical health problem like diabetes or heart disease as you age? Do you already have a chronic health problem, mental or physical, that affects your quality of life? Research is showing that one of the most powerful risk reducing activities you can do is to increase the amount of time each day that you move your body. A sedentary lifestyle may be as harmful to one's health as smoking, so in this manual, we encourage you to move more, and move better. We focus on gentle activities that strengthen the core and help us to relax and reduce stress. These activities are central to maintaining independent living as we age, and focus on being able to get out of our chairs, turn to look behind us, and reach for objects safely. These are activities that everyone, regardless of health status and ability level, can do safely. We also provide tips for those who want more vigorous activities.

Health Benefits of Movement

Overcoming fears of and barriers to physical activity is important, because some studies find that physical activity promotes health whether or not you lose weight (Shaw et al, 2009). Physical activity also decreases symptoms of dementia and mental health disorders. Research has shown that exercise is an effective but often underused treatment for mild to moderate depression. In many studies, physical activity worked better than medications in reducing symptoms of sadness and increasing feelings of wellbeing. When people move, the body releases chemicals called endorphins. These endorphins interact with the receptors in the brain that reduce feelings of pain and increase self-esteem. The feeling that follows a run or workout is often described as "euphoric." A "runner's high," can create a positive outlook on life. Endorphins are analgesics, which means they decrease pain. They also act as sedatives. They are manufactured in the brain, spinal cord, and other parts of the body and are released in response to brain chemicals called neurotransmitters. Endorphins bind to receptors in the body the same way that some pain medicines do. However, unlike morphine, the activation of these receptors by the body's endorphins rarely leads to addiction or dependence.

Regular physical activity has been shown to:
- Reduce stress
- Ward off anxiety and feelings of depression
- Boost self-esteem
- Improve sleep
- Strengthen the heart
- Increase energy levels
- Lower blood pressure
- Improve muscle tone and strength
- Strengthen and build bones

- Help reduce body fat and build muscle

Lesbian/Bisexual Women's Barriers to Physical Activity

A few research studies have explored the challenges to getting enough physical activity for lesbian and bisexual women (Brittain et al., 2006, 2008; Fogel et al, 2009; Roberts et al, 2010). These studies found that the reasons could be divided into general factors that apply to all women, such as feeling shame about how one's body looks, lack of time, local gym/rec center/parks that are not safe for women, and difficulty finding appropriate workout clothes that fit and look ok. All women experience some changes in their abilities to engage in physical activity as they age.

Lesbian/bisexual women specific factors have been found in several research studies (Boehmer et al, 2013; Brittain et al, 2006, 2008, 2013; Kelly, 2007; Roberts et al, 2010; Yancey et al, 2003), such as:

- For those who were not "out" in public: An expectation that one had to be "out" to participate on a lesbian sports team and concerns about being seen exercising with a lesbian partner.
- Feeling self-conscious in locker rooms with heterosexual women.
- Lack of ability to get family membership at gyms with partners/family.
- Few lesbian/bisexual women's specific recreational opportunities, especially for older women and those who are not "sporty dykes." Many women reported wanting to find a buddy or group of lesbian/bisexual women to exercise with.
- Pressure to conform to a "lesbian standard" of athletic and androgynous.
- Pressure to not "look like a lesbian" or "too fat to get a man."
- Gender expression: those who were tomboys and/or athletes, and more "butch" may be more likely to engage in certain types of physical activities that result in moderate to vigorous exercise than those who are more feminine.
- Body size and shape: some heavier lesbian/bisexual women report feeling self-conscious or uncomfortable at gyms, pools, rec centers.

The research on whether lesbian/bisexual women get more, less, or the same amount of exercise compared to heterosexual women is pretty mixed. Most of the studies find no differences or find that lesbian/bisexual women get a little more exercise. But the studies are pretty limited. There are lots of factors that cause women to become more sedentary and move their bodies less than is optimal.

- What are the major barriers for you personally? What keeps you from moving?

Tips for Choosing Physical Activities

Pick Activities You Enjoy! You will be more motivated if you are doing something that you are truly interested in—something that brings you joy. What if you enjoyed dancing in the past but never enjoyed exercise where you didn't interact with others? Even if you can no longer dance the way you used to, maybe you can do chair dancing instead? What if you used to enjoy walking but chronic plantar fasciitis now keeps you from doing that? If you like being in water, you might enjoy water walking or deep water walking. It's less important to do something that you feel would be "good for" you—like yoga or swimming or pilates—and more important to seek out what you enjoy and brings you pleasure. And of course if you like yoga, that's great!

- List activities that you used to enjoy in your journal. Why don't you do it now? Can it be modified so you can still enjoy it?
- Now list activities that you have not done in the past, but would like to try.

Be Safe. If you have any medical problems or physical limitations, check with your primary care provider before you start anything new. And start slow and small even if you have no physical limitations or disorders. One way to stop your progress on your goal is to over do it and hurt yourself.

Get Out Of the House. We recommend that you consider finding an activity that takes you out of your house and into another realm. A class that you must commit to; a walking partner that makes you accountable; a social group that encourages you is more likely to be successful than staying at home with your usual hard-to-break routines. However, we recognize that sometimes it is not realistic to take a class or get outside. In that case, you can commit to activities that increase your physical movement at home.

Designing Your Personal Movement Plan

Step 1. Find a Place: Once you have an idea of what type of activity might appeal to you, call or go online to check out programs at accessible venues near you - senior centers, swimming pools, the YMCA, etc. This is the first step to developing a fitness program. If you opt to stay at home, consider where in your house/apartment you can do the activity most effectively. The chair dancing, home stretching routine, increased frequency of sex with your partner, or walking around your own block might be just as good as going to a gym, and probably much less expensive. Anything that gets you moving even a little more each day is great.

Step 2. Try a Class or New Activity: Second step - try out something that appeals to you. Or try a video, try setting aside 15 minutes for dancing in front of your stereo, get a yoga mat and try some gentle movements. Mine your list of activities from above. When you find something you like, go to Step 3.

Step 3. Make a Manageable Commitment: make a one month commitment to attend the program or do the activity regularly (preferably you do something daily). After a month, reassess and think about whether the program or activity is a good fit for you. Also make a commitment to do something everyday. If you take a yoga class once a week, practice at least one of the activities you learn every day, even if just for 5 minutes. Daily practice is critical to creating new habits.

Step 4. either go back to step #1 with a new activity, or continue with your month-to-month commitment. Sustaining a program is like any relationship: It isn't always exciting and rewarding in the moment, but overall, it's worth it. Many people are able to stick to a movement plan more easily after a number of months because the positive health effects are so evident.

Frequency or How Often Must I Exercise?
BE REALISTIC, not idealistic. To successfully meet your goal, consider carefully how many times a week (1-3 times for a class is more realistic than every day) you will be able to do the activity you plan, taking into consideration transportation, time of day, etc. It's much better to plan to swim twice a week and succeed than to aim for 5 times a week and not hit that target. But you can do something every day. Take that swim aerobics class twice a week, but commit to walking 15 minutes the other days, or use the DIFO video in between swimming sessions.

Duration or For How Long?
You might want to spend one week or so really keeping track of what you are currently doing. For each day, how much activity do you get? Try to calculate the number of minutes and plot them below. List what you did, including housework, running errands, doing laundry. You might download a pedometer app for your phone and track your steps for a week. Anything that takes some energy counts. Make a the chart like the one on the following page to track your physical activity for at least one week. What patterns do you notice?

Day	What I did	For how long?	How I felt physically and mentally after.
Sunday			
Monday			
Tuesday			
Wednesday			
Thursday			
Friday			
Saturday			

Once you know how much time you are putting into activities now, you can make goals that slowly increase your duration of activity. Maybe just 5 minutes of walking the first day, 10 minutes of swimming, 10 minutes of chair dancing. The point is to start doing something, even if just for a few minutes. As your body adapts and you start to get more energy, you can increase frequency and duration if you choose.

Another alternative is to track the amount of time you spend sitting or sedentary each day and slowly reduce that number. Here's a sample chart for doing that.

Day	Hours sitting daytime	Hours sitting evening	How I felt today
Sunday			
Monday			
Tuesday			
Wednesday			
Thursday			
Friday			
Saturday			

Three Key Components To A Physical Activity Plan

There are three components to consider when developing an effective and appropriate personalized physical activity routine.

- **Consistency**
- **Intensity**
- **Tracking**

Consistency refers to adding in movement on a frequent and regular basis. If you are just starting a new activity, like tai chi, once a week might be a realistic goal that you can change after a few weeks. Focus on consistency first, even if you feel the activity is not enough to make a difference. The difference is that you are developing a routine of taking care of your health on a regular basis. Much of the research on creating new habits shows that you need daily practice for about 3 months to lay down the new pathways in your brain.

Intensity refers to how easy or hard you are working and is critical on both ends of the spectrum. When first starting out, it is optimal to start very gently especially if you haven't exercised in a while. Working harder is not always the best choice, because over-doing can put your body out of whack and imbalances happen. Remember this a process of integrating new healthy habits and we want to find a level of effort that serves your goals. Later on you can consider whether and how to raise intensity levels while keeping the activity safe and appropriate for your needs. Lots of research shows that as we age, lower intensity activities are just as good as high intensity, and maybe even better. Several studies are showing that walking has more health benefits and less risks than running, for example. Swimming is easier on the body, but more effective in producing health benefits than tennis. The whole goal of increasing your physical movement is to feel better in your body, not to focus on "no pain no gain" types of activities. Slow, gentle, but regular activity is best for most of us.

Tracking. Track what you do. If you are walking, use a pedometer or an app for your phone to record your steps. Just the process of paying attention to how many steps you walk each day will make you more mindful of your physical activity. If you want more information, check out devices like FitBit that give you more information like heart rates and calories burned and monitor your sleep cycles. Keep a fitness journal until your new habits are well-established.

The rest of this chapter provides text and pictures to go along with the video, Moving For Our Health, which you can view on our website for free anytime:

http://difobayarea.org

The instructions below include notes to facilitators. A facilitator is anyone who is watching others perform these movements, or someone who is leading the group. We cannot always know if we are doing movements correctly without a mirror, so having someone observe us is very helpful in getting the most benefit from the movements. The movements in this section and in the video, were selected because they are gentle and can be done by women with a wide range of health. They are deceptively simple, but quite powerful ways to strengthen your core, stay living independently, and relieve your stress.

MOVING FOR OUR HEALTH

Part 1: "Grounding"

1.1 Trunk Mobility

Note: VERY IMPORTANT: The movements in this section are designed to improve how people move, and in that way create greater capacity. Positive changes result when the brain senses that the movement feels good and then adopts that way of moving. If the movement creates strain, it will not change how a person moves. In this section, make sure to emphasize that movements should be very small, at least to start with, and always done slowly. Monitor yourself closely and stop the moment you feel any strain or pain. Sometimes it's helpful to monitor what you are feeling—for example, "Do you feel movement in the low back with the cycle of the breath?" Always pause after posing a question, and feel what is happening in the body.

Three Movements of the Spine
There are three basic movements that the spine and torso can make: 1) rounding and arching, 2) sidebending, and 3) rotating. We need to have capacity to move in all three of these directions and the exercises in this section will help with that.

1.1.1 Breathing

- Sit at the front of the chair, feet firmly planted on the floor.
- Wiggle a little bit to feel the sitting bones.
- Can you feel your sitting bones? You don't need to use muscles to sit upright. When you are sitting on your sitting bones, the vertebrae of the spine are naturally supported.
- Put one hand on the lower belly and the other on the lower back and breathe deeply.
- Can you feel movement in the lower back area? Notice the movement of the back, how it arches a little bit with the inhale and rounds a little with the exhale, as shown in Figure 1.
- Repeat for five breath cycles.

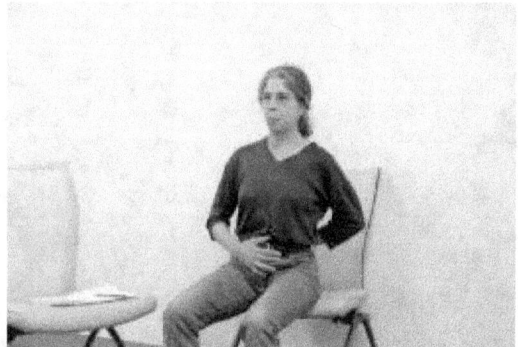

Figure 1: Breathing and opening/closing the trunk

1.1.2   Rounding & Arching with the Breath

Note: These exercises need to be done very gently. Make the movements small and slow, staying within your range of comfort.

Facilitator Note: CAUTION: Make sure that people make small, gentle movements with the head and neck, and are not exaggerating, especially not the movement of looking upwards. If moving the neck seems painful for some participants, encourage them to just roll their eyes upwards.

- Just a few times, gently look up towards the ceiling and see how far you can look **easily**, without strain.
- Begin rolling the sitting bones backwards a bit to round the spine a little as you exhale. The pelvis will tilt back; the spine will round forwards. The head will also bend forward naturally as the spine rounds with the exhale, as shown in Figure 2. This happens in one smooth motion. Make the movement small, nothing exaggerated. When you roll the sitting bones back, you take away the support for the spine and the whole spine rounds naturally. It's like taking away the foundation of a house: the house collapses.
- Next, allow the pelvis to rock forward, the spine to arch a bit, and the head to tilt back a bit, as shown in Figure 3. This happens in a sequence, with the pelvis rocking forward, then the chest coming forward, and LAST, the head looking upwards as the chin moves away from the throat a little bit and the eyes roll upwards, in a wave type motion. **Do not lead with the head!** The head should be the last body part to move. If it is difficult to move the head, just allow the eyes to roll upwards in the sockets.
- End in a neutral position.
- Did you notice how you are breathing, when you tend to inhale and when you tend to exhale?
- Repeat for five breath cycles. End in a neutral position, looking straight ahead, neither rounded or arched.

- Sitting on your sitting bones, once again just look upwards and notice how far you can see easily. Has anything changed?

Facilitator Notes: Ask the group at what point they exhaled or inhaled. Then demonstrate that exhaling tends to make the spine round, and inhaling tends to arch the spine. Notice that the pelvis rocks forwards towards the pubic bone as you inhale, and backwards towards the tailbone as you exhale. If you were sitting on the face of a clock, your pelvis would rock in a line between 12 o'clock as you inhale and 6 o'clock as you exhale.

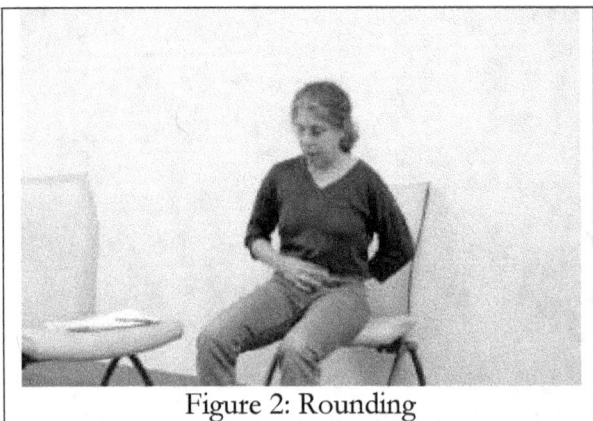

Figure 2: Rounding

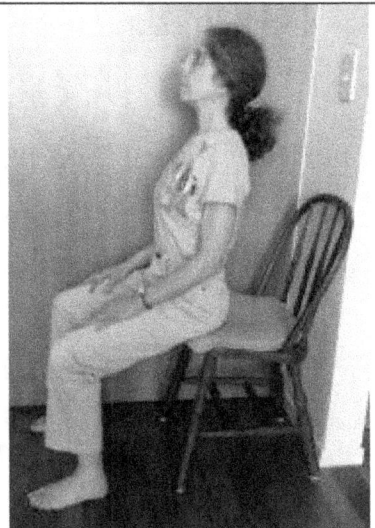

Figure 3: Arching

Adding the Arms (Optional)
- Let your arms hang down, palms facing the outside of each thigh, as shown in Figure 4.
- As you inhale and arch, open the arms out to the side and turn the palms upwards (Figure 5).
- As you exhale and round the spine, allow the arms to come back to hanging by the sides, as in Figure 6.
- Repeat for five breath cycles. Again, do not exaggerate any body part, including the movement of the arms.

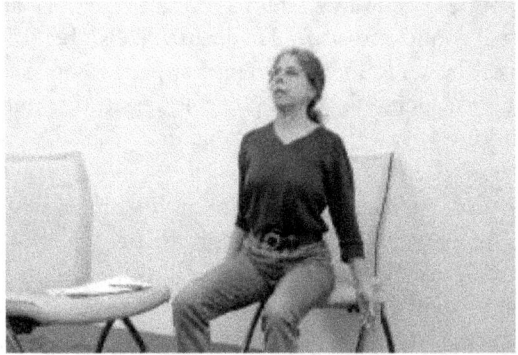

Figure 4: Neutral

176

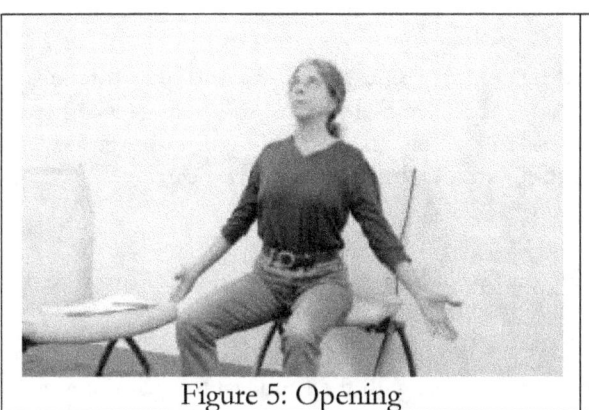
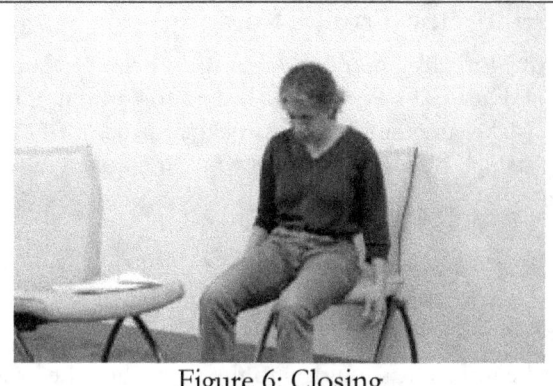

Figure 5: Opening | Figure 6: Closing

1.1.3 The C-Shape (side-bending)

Facilitator Notes: There are two ways to reach out to the side: one is to lean over as a tree being felled. Although some women will do it this way, this is **not** the movement being described here. The other way is to make a C shape with the spine as described below. This is what we are aiming for. CAUTION: Make sure that people do not exaggerate the movement of reaching.

- Sit at the front of the chair with your feet firmly planted, sitting on the sit bones so the spine is supported in a neutral position.
- Tilt the head, right ear to the right shoulder, open the left side of the ribcage, reach up and out to the left with the left arm, as if to reach for a piece of fruit from a tree. The right buttock will lighten from the seat of the chair, the ribcage will open on the left and fold on the right, the spine assumes the shape of the letter C, as shown in Figure 7.

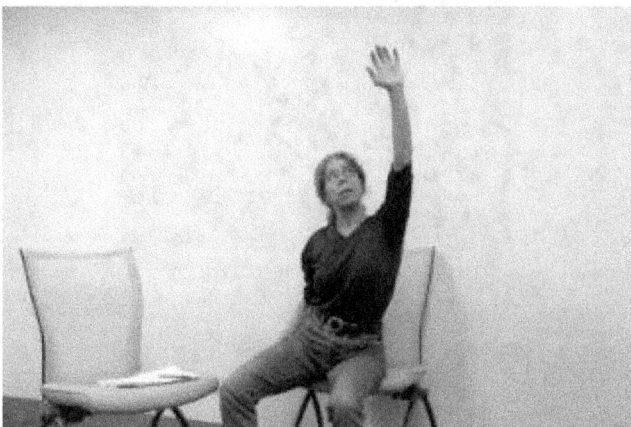

Figure 7: The C shape

- Return to neutral; repeat on the left side three times.
- Repeat on the opposite side three times.
- Breathe normally (not coordinated in a particular pattern with the movement).

Note: Notice that your pelvis rocks over towards the right hip as you reach to the right and towards the left hip as you reach towards the left. If you were sitting on the face of a clock, your pelvis would roll in a line between 3 o'clock and 9 o'clock.

1.1.4 Turning the Trunk (Rotating)

Facilitator Note: Tell people to scan with their eyes in the direction they're turning and avoid over-rotating the neck and head. If someone has discomfort turning the head, encourage them to just roll their eyes in that direction. Make sure that no one turns their head in an exaggerated fashion. In a moment you will turn to look to your right. Only go as far as you can comfortably, without strain. Notice how far you can see comfortably.

- Sit at the front of the chair, feet firmly planted, sitting on the sit bones so that the spine is supported in a neutral position.
- Shift the left side of your pelvis forward so the left knee moves forward in space.
- Then turn the shoulders to the right, then the head, in that order, with the head last (or just the eyes if the neck is painful), as shown in Figures 8, 9 and 10.
- Do this three times. **Pause.**
- Now, once again, just turn to look to your right. How far do you see now? Is there a difference?
- Do the same on the opposite side three times.

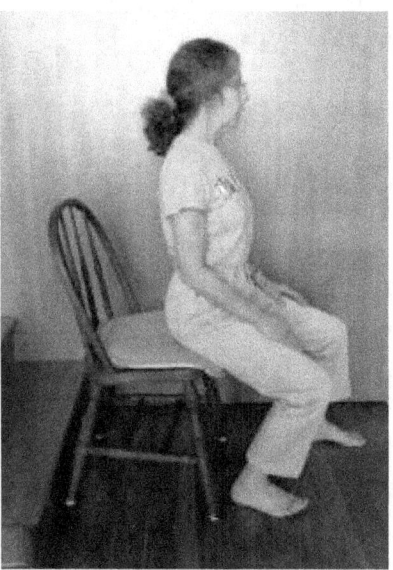

Figure 8: Pelvis turning

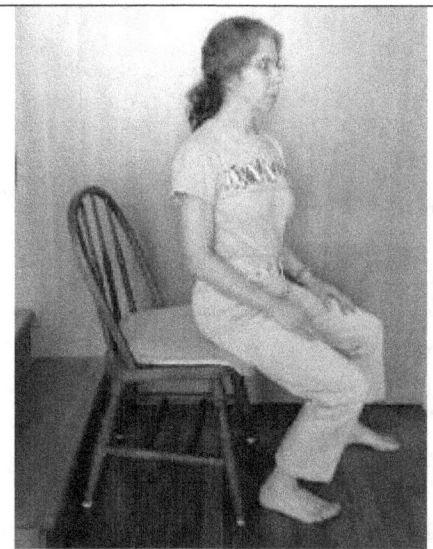
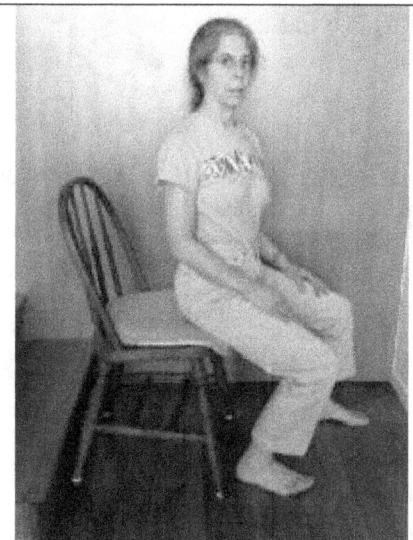

| Figure 9: Pelvis plus shoulders turning | Figure 10: Pelvis, shoulders and head turning |

1.2 Core Strengthening

1.2.1 Activating the Core

- Sit at the front of the chair, feet firmly planted, sitting on the sit bones so that the spine is comfortably supported in a neutral position.
- Put one hand on the lower belly and the other on top of one thigh, as in Figure 11.
- Tighten the abdominals. Notice that the thigh also contracts and the foot presses lightly into the floor. It may be difficult to contract the abdomen, so you can tighten the thigh and press the foot lightly into the floor, noticing that the abdominal muscles will also contract.
- Repeat three times.

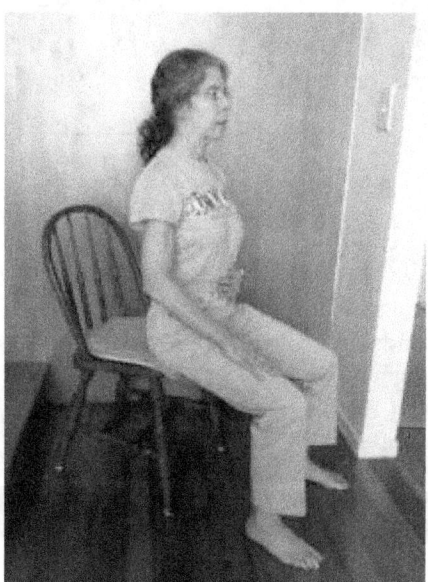

Figure 11: Activating the core

1.2.2 Reaching Overhead

Facilitator Note: Now we're going to strengthen the core—the abdominals—but challenging them to stay contracted as we move the arms and legs. Moving the arms and legs makes it harder to keep the abdominals contracted.

- Sit at the front of the chair, feet firmly planted, on the sit bones.
- Contract the abdominals again and keep them turned on while you lift one or both arms overhead, as shown in Figures 12 and 13.
- Make sure to monitor the contraction of your abdominals and only lift your arm(s) as far as you can without losing the contraction.
- Repeat three times. (Your movement need not be coordinated with your breath. Just breathe naturally.).

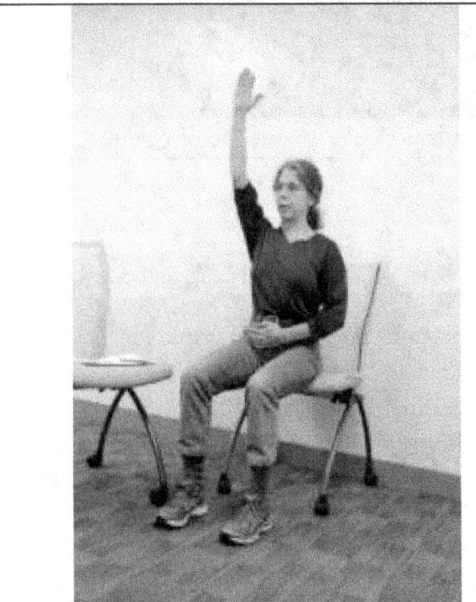

Figure 12: Reaching overhead (traction) with one arm

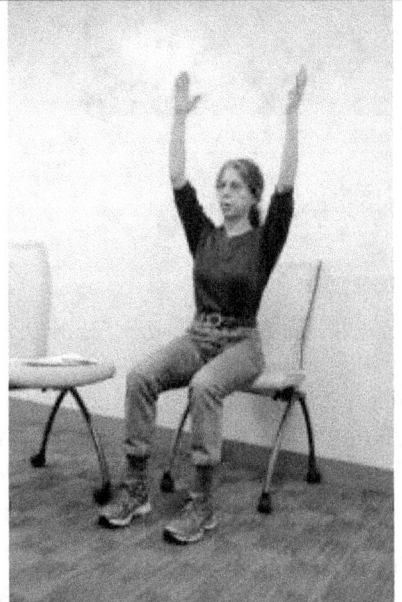

Figure 13: Reach overhead (traction) with both arms

1.2.3 Lifting a Leg

- Sit at the front of the chair, feet firmly planted, on the sit bones.
- Contract and hold the abdominals. Continue to hold the contraction while lifting a leg, as shown in Figure 14. Hold for 2-3 seconds. If it is too difficult to lift the leg, just lift the heel so that the toe remains on the floor, as in Figure 15.
- After you lower the leg back down, relax the abdominals before beginning the next repetition.
- Repeat three times for each leg.

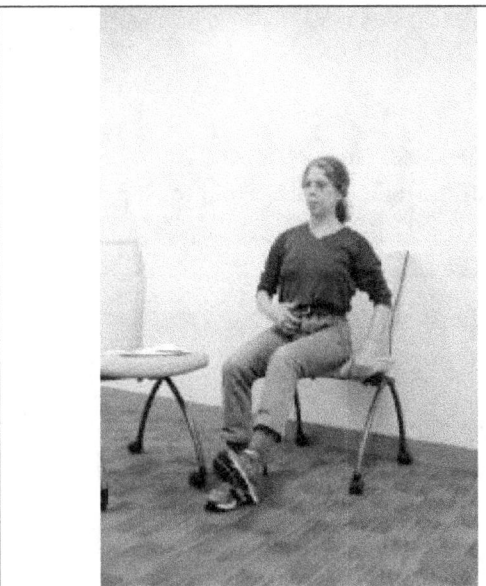

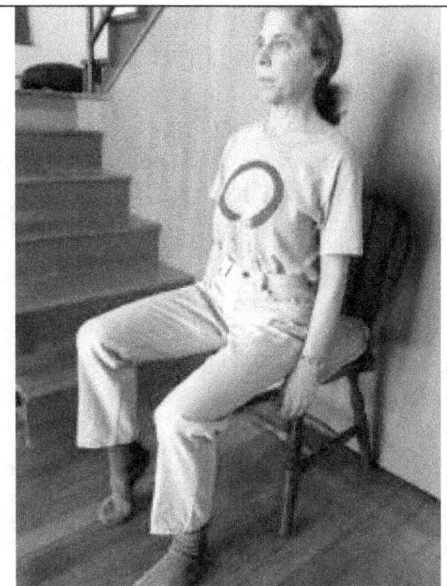

Figure 14: Lifting a leg	Figure 15: Lifting just the heel

1.2.4 Lifting Leg and Opposite Arm (Added Challenge)

- Again contract the abdominals and then lift a leg and opposite arm together, as shown in Figure 16. If this is too difficult, continue lifting either a leg or an arm but not both.
- Repeat two times for each side.

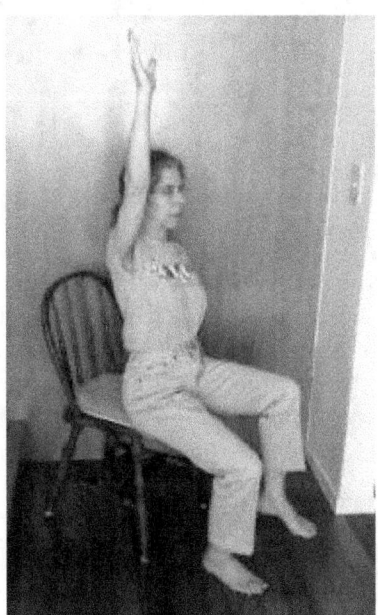

Figure 16: Lifting a leg and adding opposite arm

1.3 Hip Strengthening

- Sit at the front of the chair, feet firmly planted, on the sit bones.
- **Abduction (or resist spreading of the thighs):**
  - o Place hands on outside of thighs, right on the right, left on left (Figure 17).

181

        o   Apply pressure inwards with the hands, resist with the legs so that they stay in place and are not moved inwards. Hold for 3-5 seconds.

        o   Repeat two times.

- **Adduction (or resist closing of the thighs):**
  - o   Place hands on the inside of the thighs and press outwards (Figure 18).
  - o   Resist with the legs so that they stay in place, are not moved outward. Hold for 3-5 seconds.
  - o   Repeat two times.

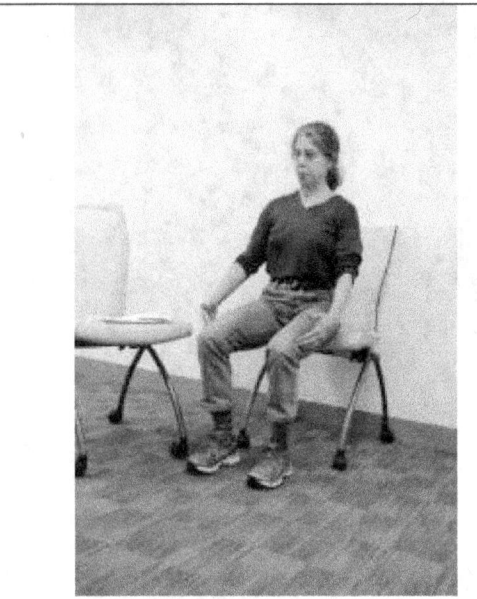 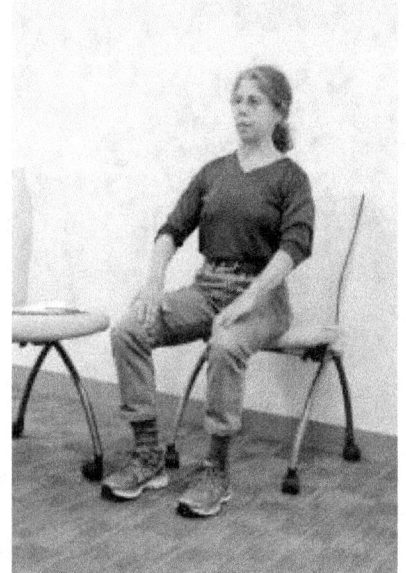

| Figure 17: Resist spreading of the thighs (abduction) | Figure 18: Resist closing of the thighs (adduction) |

1.4 Leg Strengthening

1.4.1 Up/Down From a Chair

Facilitator Notes: The guiding principle of this exercise is that in getting up, you first tilt downward: Your head goes down as your butt goes up, like a seesaw. It is harder to get up if you move upward first, instead of downward, whether you are getting out of a regular chair, a wheelchair, etc. The key concept is that we need to move to get our weight into our feet first before standing up. If some women don't find sliding the hands useful or possible, it doesn't matter as long as their head moves down and their butt up. For women who are unable to get up from sitting, there is a seated alternative below for leg strengthening.

- Sit at the front of the chair, hands on your thighs, and begin to massage your hands down the front of your legs. Your butt should lighten a bit as you reach down and more weight comes into your feet, as shown in Figure 19.

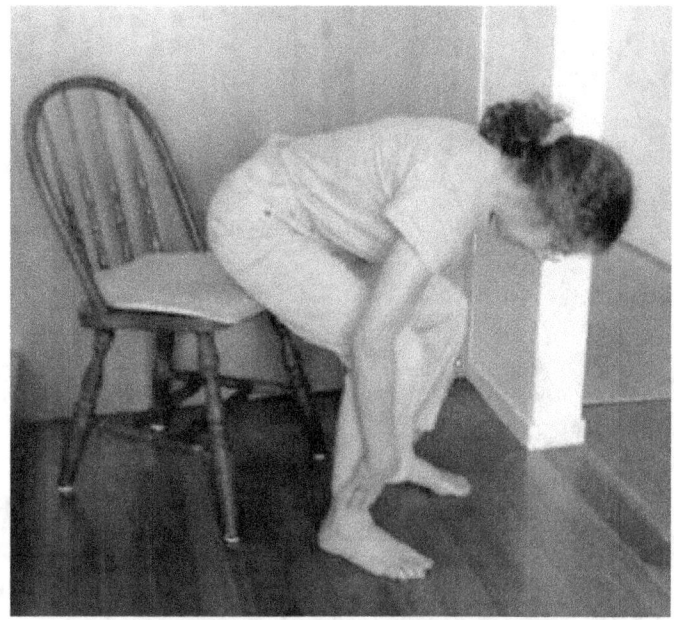
Figure 19: Sliding hands down legs

- Extend one hand out as if holding an imaginary ice cream cone a few feet away, and continue to slide your other hand down your shin (Figure 20).

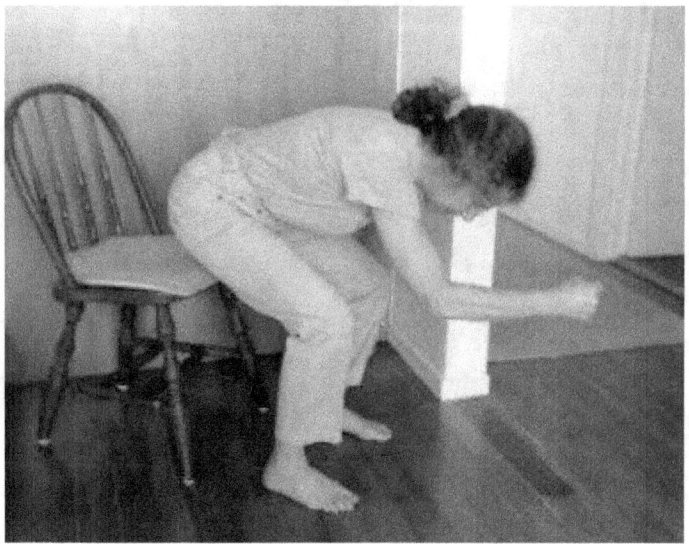
Figure 20: Getting up from chair

- As your hand slides down your shin, your butt will lift and more weight will transfer into your feet. **Hold the ice cream cone about a foot away from you** to start with. Now pretend to lick the melting ice cream from the bottom of the cone to the top, and come up into standing (Figure 21).
- Repeat three times.

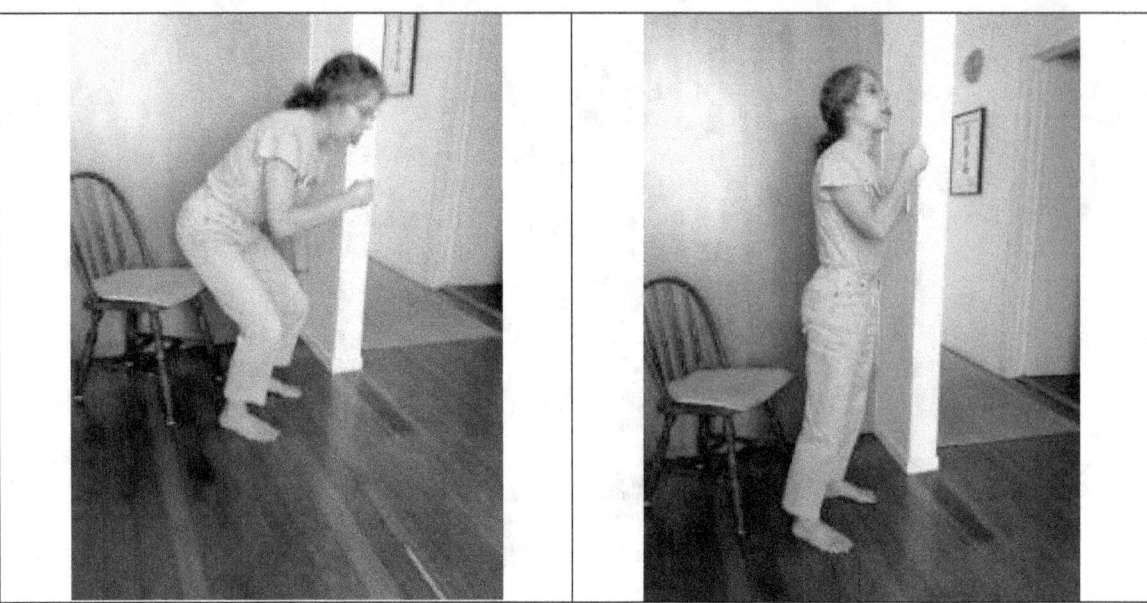

Figure 21: Coming up to standing

1.4.2 Leg Strengthening in a Chair (Seated Alternative)

If the previous exercise feels too difficult, you can try this seated alternative:

- Sit in a chair so that your feet are on the floor and your back is supported.
- Extend one leg out at the knee as straight as is comfortable, hold for 3-5 seconds, and then lower it, as in Figure 22.
- Repeat three times for each leg.

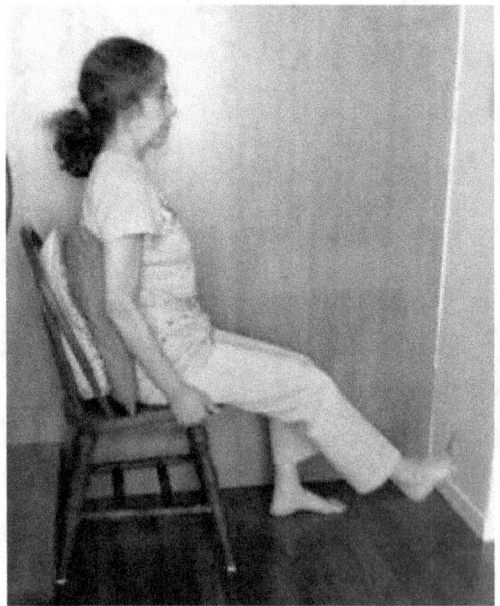

Figure 22: Leg strengthening (seated alternative)

1.5 Strengthening the Arms

Facilitator Note: For women who are unable to do the standing wall press ups, there are two seated alternatives below.

1.5.1 Wall Press Ups

- Stand facing the wall, an arm's length away.
- Place your hands on the wall directly in front of your shoulders, your elbows should be fully extended, not bent. You can place your hands flat or make them into fists, if that feels better.
- Keeping your body in a line like a wooden board, allow your elbows to bend so that your face comes closer to the wall, and then push back so that the arms are straight again, as shown in Figure 23 (fists) and 24 (flat hands). Do **not** let the body sag as you dip towards the wall, and do **not** disturb the straight line of the body as you push back to the starting position.
- Repeat three to five times.

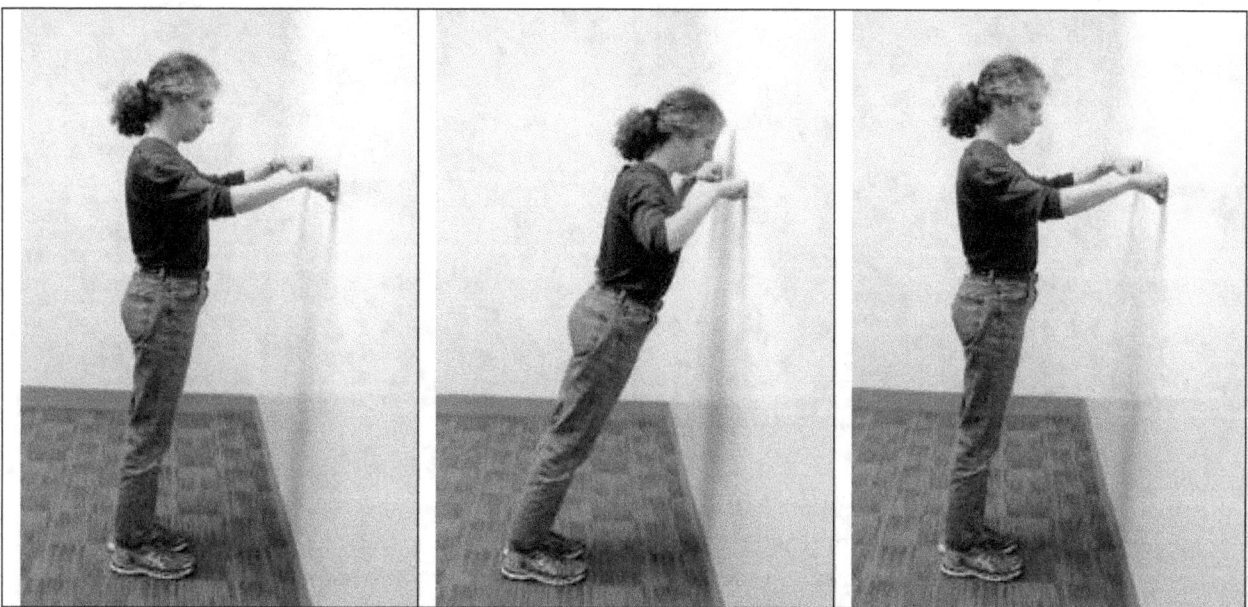

Figure 23: Wall press ups with fists

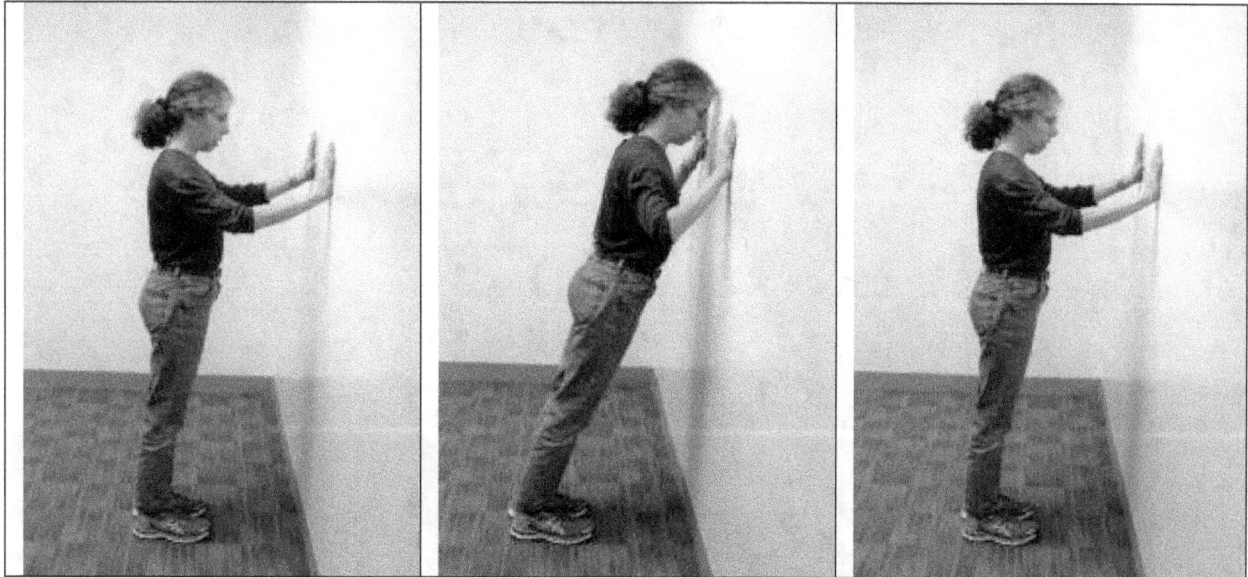

Figure 24: Wall press ups with flat hands

1.5.2 Press Ups at Table (Seated Alternative)

If the previous exercise feels too difficult, you can try this seated alternative:

- Sit at the edge of your chair, feet planted, hands resting arms length away on a flat surface such as a table or a counter top.
- Keeping your upper body aligned and straight, allow your elbows to bend so that your chest moves towards the table top, as shown in Figure 25. Keep the upper body straight; do not allow it to sag.
- Push back to the starting position.
- Repeat three to five times. You can build up to ten times.

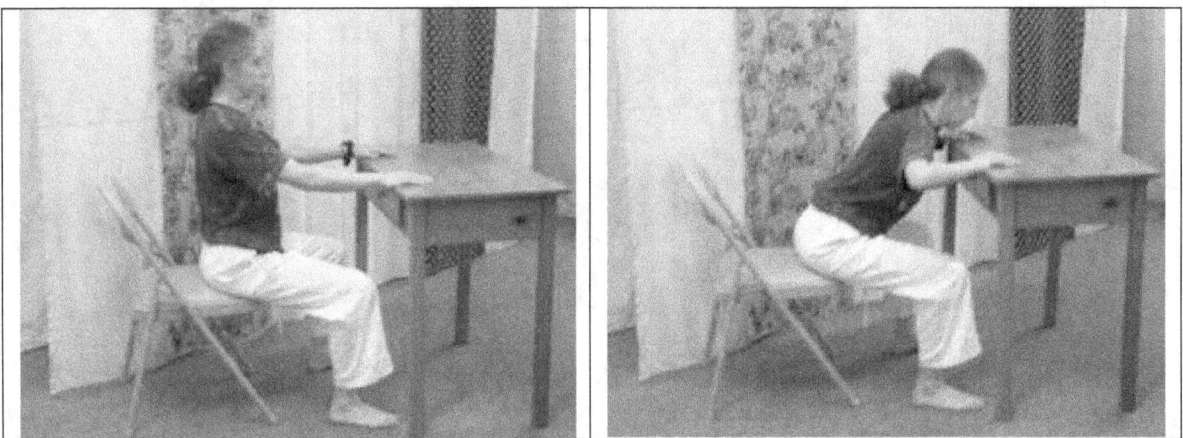

Figure 25: Press ups at table (seated alternative)

1.5.3 "Stick 'Em Up" (Seated Alternative)

If the previous exercise is also too difficult, you can try this other seated alternative:

- Put the palm of one hand on your breast bone with the thumb pointing up and the fingers pointing towards your other shoulder. Bring the other arm into a "stick 'em up" position, as shown in Figure 26.

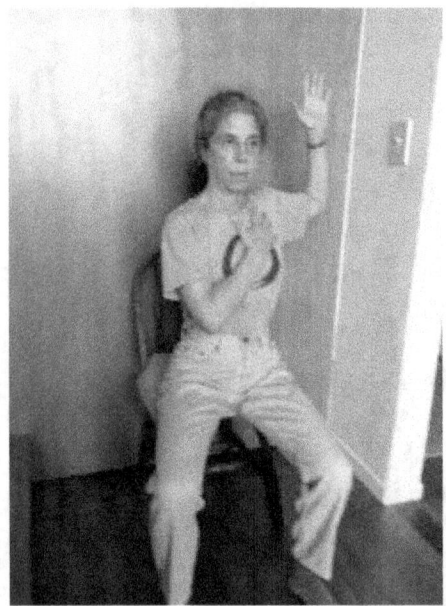

Figure 26: Arm strengthening (seated alternative)

- Press your arm forwards, feeling the muscle with the hand on the chest. This is the muscle you are working to strengthen (Figure 27).

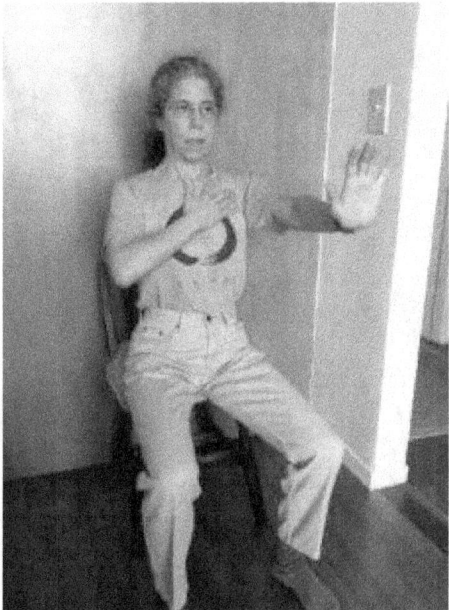

Figure 27: Arm strengthening (seated alternative)

- Place hands in front of you, palms touching. Resist with the hand behind as you press forwards with the closer hand. (Figure 28.)
- Repeat five times.

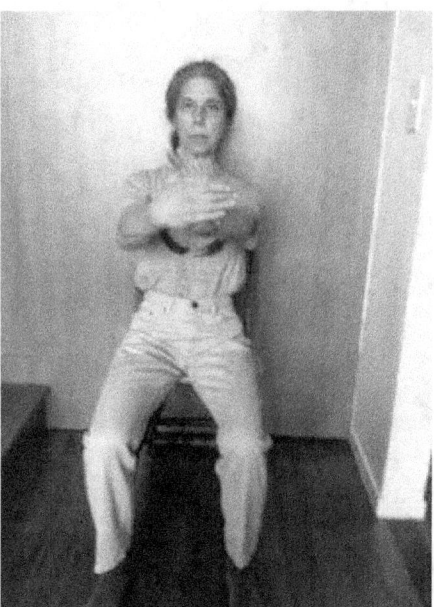

Figure 28: Arm strengthening (seated alternative)

Part 2: "Extending"

Facilitator Notes: When first learning to teach these poses, it's fine to read the instructions out loud line by line. It's important to speak calmly and with authority. As you grow more comfortable with the activities, find the voice that works for you. Also, it's best to focus on what to **do** rather than what not to do. For example, instead of saying "don't slouch," instead suggest "lift the chest and breathe fully."

2.1.1 Mountain Pose

Facilitator Notes: For women who are unable to do the standing versions of mountain pose, there is a seated alternative below. Also, suggest that they press their inner heels towards the floor and feel their feet in their shoes. Bring their awareness to their back body and see if they can feel their back ribs expand with teach exhale. Suggest that they relax their face, relax their jaw, and observe the spaces between their breaths.

- Stand with your feet hips width apart.
- Bring arms by your sides.
- Straighten your arms and legs.
- Lift your chin slightly.
- Look straight ahead, as shown in Figure 29.
- Hold this pose for five slow breaths.

Facilitator Note: Slow down your narration and make sure to count out the breaths in a slow, even pace. You can count your own breaths to make sure participants are practicing the pose for the correct amount of time.

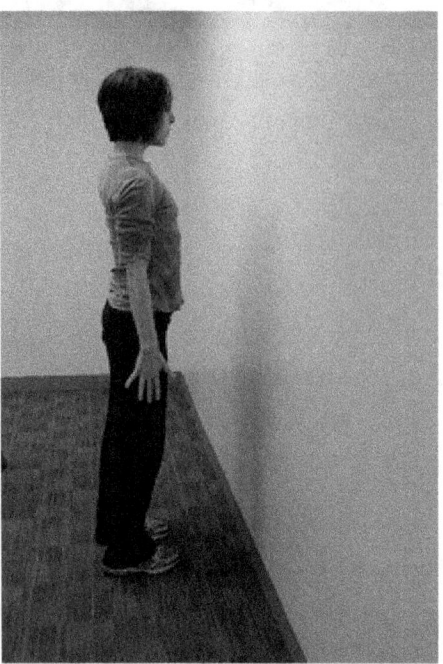

Figure 29: Mountain pose

2.1.2 Mountain Pose with Arms Up

Facilitator Notes: Most women learn to see how small they can get, but it's a nice feeling to be tall and strong. Suggest to participants that they can take up a lot of room and make their presence known. Tell women if it hurts to reach their arms out to the side and up, they can reach forward and up. If raising their arms overhead causes discomfort, offer them the option of simply standing in mountain pose with their arms at their sides.

- Stand with your feet hips width apart.

- Reach your arms over your head in line with your shoulders.
- Draw your shoulder blades down your back, as shown in Figure 30.

Facilitator Note: Tell participants to observe that they can breathe more deeply with their arms up. Tell them to try breathing into the back of their body, the part so many of us forget about.

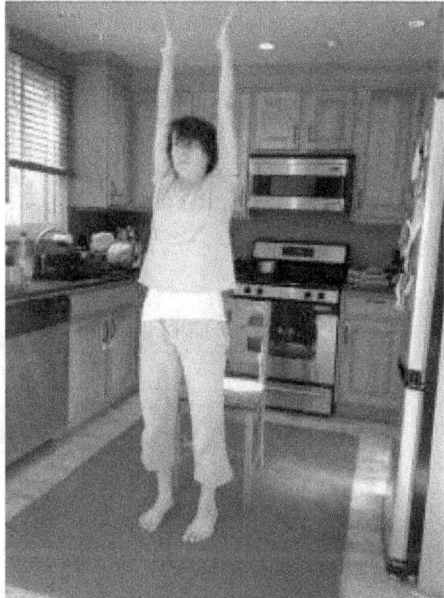

Figure 30: Mountain pose with arms overhead

2.1.3 Seated Mountain Pose (Seated Alternative)

Facilitator Note: The tips from the previous mountain poses apply to this one as well. If women are in a wheelchair, you may want to suggest that they find length from their hips to their shoulders. Remind them to breathe fully and deeply.

If the previous exercise is too difficult, you can try this seated alternative:
- Sit on a chair with your feet hips width apart.
- Find length in your spine by drawing in the navel.
- Press your inner heels into the floor. (See Figure 31.)

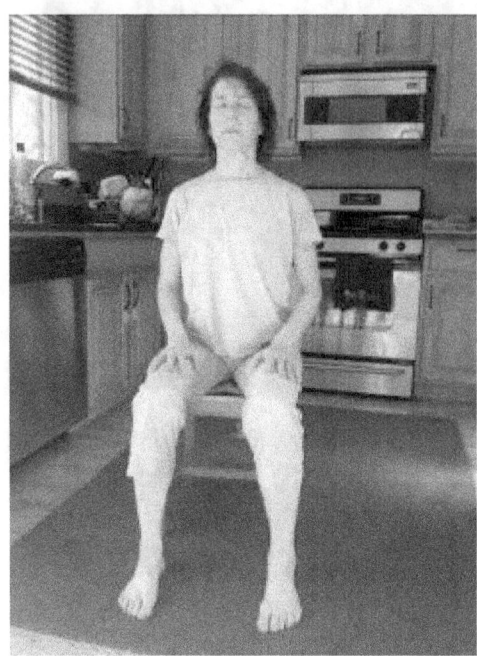
Figure 31: Seated mountain pose

Do It For Yourself Tips:

- Observe your breath. Notice whether the inhale or exhale is easier.
- Distribute the weight evenly on the feet.
- Observe any tendency to lean forward, back or to the side.
- Press the inner heels down.
- Firm the thighs by lifting the kneecaps.

2.2.1 Leaning Mountain

Facilitator Notes: For women who are unable to do the standing versions of this pose, there is a seated alternative below. Advanced option: After participants have done this exercise for at least a few weeks, try telling them to find space between their right ribs and right hip when leaning to the left. When they switch and lean to the right, they can look for length between their left ribs and left hip.

- Step one arm's length from the wall.
- Press your left hand firmly into the wall in line with your shoulder.
- Extend your right arm up and stretch toward the left
- Stretch your right hand away from your right foot.
- Hold for five slow breaths.
- Repeat on the other side.

2.2.2 Standing Side Stretch (Easier Version of Leaning Mountain)

Facilitator Note: Tell participants to bring their attention to the side that's closest to the wall and make it as long as their other side. Tell them to breathe into both sets of ribs evenly and to try to also breathe into the back of their ribs.

- Again step one arm's length from the wall.
- Press your left hand firmly into the wall in line with your shoulder.
- Extend your right arm upwards. Reach directly up instead of sideways, as shown in Figure 32.

190

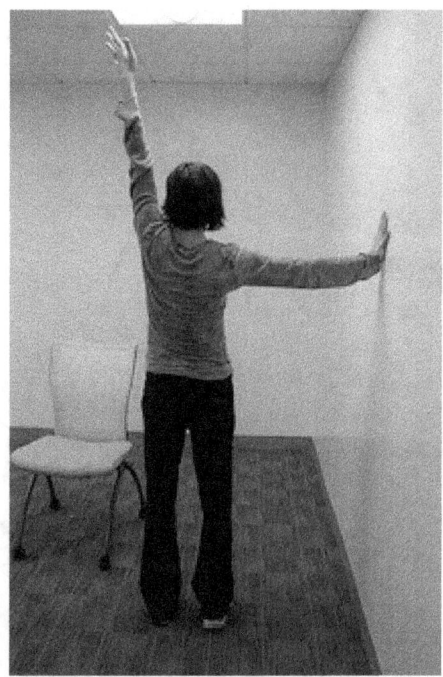
Figure 32: Standing side stretch

Do It For Yourself Tips:
- Observe your breath. Notice where you might be gripping.
- Distribute the weight evenly on the feet.
- Observe any tendency to lean forward, back or to the side.
- Press the inner heels down, lengthen the tailbone down and soften your ribs.
- Firm the thighs by lifting the kneecaps.

2.2.3 Seated Side Stretch (Seated Alternative)

If the previous exercise is too difficult, you can try this seated alternative:
- Sit tall in your chair with your feet firm on the floor or on some support.
- Lean your right hand onto your right thigh
- Extend your left arm up and stretch toward the right
- Stretch your left hand away from your left hip
- Hold for five slow breaths
- Repeat on the other side
- Press your inner heels into the floor and lengthen your spine.
- Reach up and slightly to each side, anchoring the hips down in the chair, as shown in Figure 33.

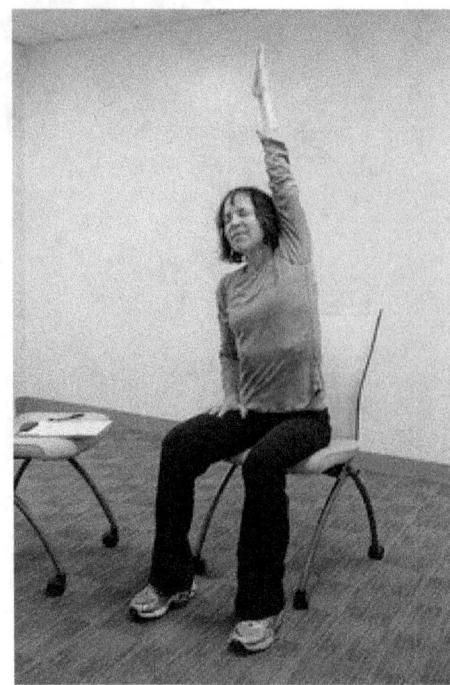
Figure 33: Seated side stretch

Do It For Yourself Tips:
- Press the feet firmly into the floor to engage the legs.
- Gently draw the tailbone down and low belly in.
- Move the base of the sternum inward as you lift the chest.
- Find length in all directions, especially on the side of the body closest to the wall.

2.3.1 Triangle Pose, Hand on Chair

Facilitator Note: Triangle pose with hand on chair is easier than the next variation, where you put your hand on your thigh. For participants who might feel challenged, you can recommend that they repeat this pose instead of going on to the next triangle pose.

Facilitator Note: Read out the directions below and suggest that participants lengthen their torso away from the hips. Once participants are in the pose, tell them to breathe into the back of their body, letting the breath fill out the shape of the pose.

- Stand behind a chair.
- Step your legs slightly wider than your shoulders.
- Turn your right foot out to 3 o'clock and left foot in to 1 o'clock.
- Place your right hand on top of the chair.
- Bend your right knee so that knee is in line with your ankle.
- Keep your left leg straight, drawing your inner thigh up into your outer thigh.
- Reach your left arm up and towards right, keeping your waist long as shown in Figure 34.
- Hold for five slow breaths.
- Repeat on the other side.

Facilitator Note: If anyone has trouble reaching their arm over their head for any of the triangle poses, tell them it is fine to put their hand on their hip.

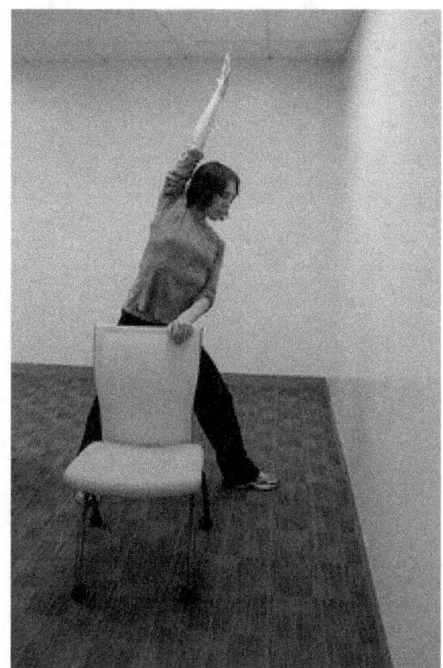

Figure 34: Triangle pose hand on chair

2.3.2 Triangle Pose, Hand on Thigh

- Stand behind a chair.
- Step your legs slightly wider than your shoulders.
- Turn your right foot out to 3 o'clock and left foot in to 1 o'clock.
- Place your right hand on top of your thigh to increase the depth of the pose, shown in Figure 35.
- Bend your right knee so that knee is in line with your ankle.
- Keep your left leg straight, drawing the inner thigh up into the outer thigh.
- Reach your left arm up and towards right, keeping waist long as shown in Figure 34.
- Hold for five slow breaths.
- Repeat on the other side.

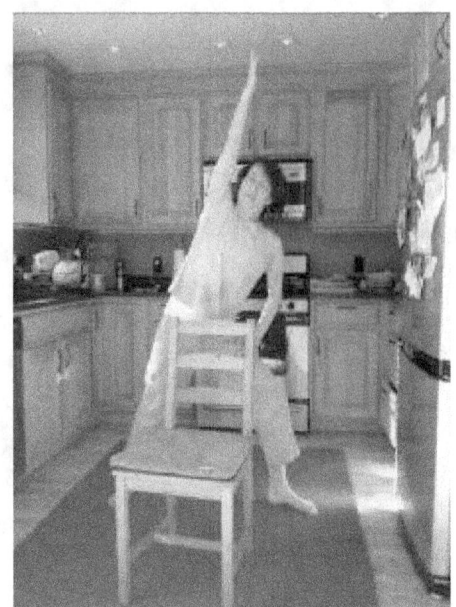

Figure 35: Triangle pose hand on thigh

Do It For Yourself Tips:

- Observe your breath. As you breathe deeply, allow the breath to saturate the pose.
- Press the feet into the floor and work towards stretching the floor with the feet to turn on all the lights in the legs
- Press the inner heels down, lengthen your tailbone down, and soften your ribs.

2.3.3 Seated Triangle Pose (Seated Alternative)

If the previous exercise is too difficult, you can try this seated alternative:

- Sit on the edge of a chair, your feet about hip's distance apart.
- Turn your right foot out and your left foot in.
- Place your right hand on your right thigh, reach your left arm up overhead, and lean towards the right (Figure 36).

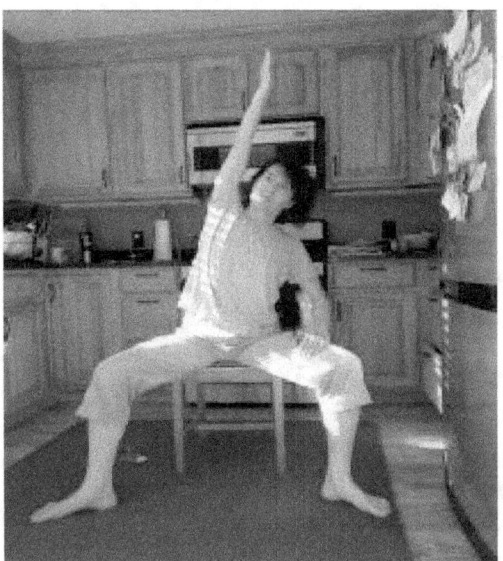

Figure 36: Seated triangle pose

2.4.1 Standing Twist

- Stand sideways facing a chair in mountain pose.
- Activate your legs by pressing your inner heels into the floor.
- Draw your belly up and in and lengthen your tailbone down.
- Place your right hand on top of the chair and gently rotate to the left, as shown in Figure 37.
- Hold for five slow breaths. Repeat on the other side.

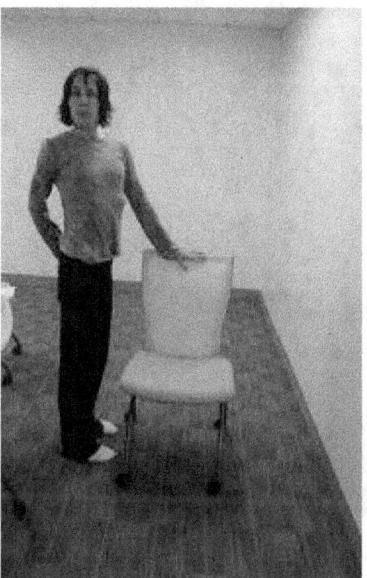

Figure 37: Standing twist

2.4.2 Standing Twist with Foot Up

- Stand to the left of a chair.
- Place your right foot on the seat of the chair.
- Anchor your left heel into the floor and place your left hand on the outside of the right knee.

Facilitator Note: Tell participants that they can put their left hand on top of their right thigh if it's not comfortable for them to put it outside the right knee. Also suggest that they try lifting their ribs away from their hips and breathing to expand their ribs.

- Lengthen your spine and rotate towards the right, as shown in Figure 38.
- Hold for five slow breaths
- Repeat on the other side.

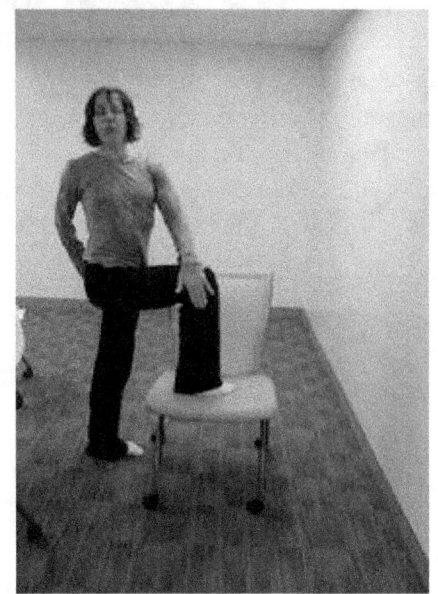

Figure 38: Standing twist with foot up

Do It For Yourself Tips:

- Observe your breath. With each inhale work towards lengthening the spine. With each exhale work towards pressing the feet into the floor.
- The key to healthy spinal rotation is finding length first. Imagine a balloon on your sternum that is creating length. Inhale to get longer, exhale to go deeper.
- Press the inner heels down on both feet and draw the shoulder blades toward each other.

2.5.1 Puppy Dog

Facilitator Note: Tell participants to feel free to step closer to the wall and bend less if that will feel better and safer for their back. Have them pivot from their hips and not their waist (this is a common mistake)

- Stand tall in mountain pose about one leg's length away from the wall.
- Bend forward from your hips 5 to 10 degrees—whatever is comfortable.
- Press your hands into the wall in line with your shoulders
- Activate arms and push hands in and down, as shown in Figure 39.
- Breathe deeply for 5 breaths.

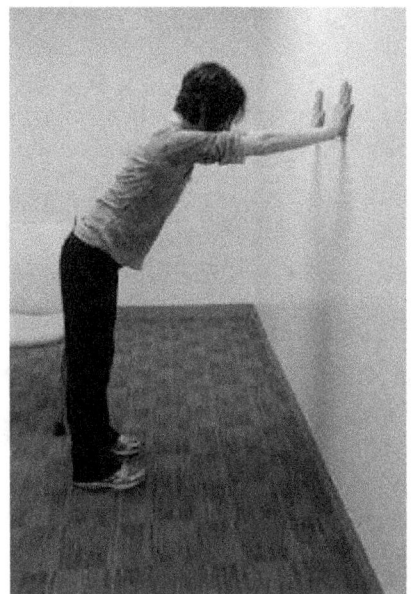
Figure 39: Puppy dog

2.5.2 Seated Puppy Dog (Seated Alternative)

Facilitator Note: Suggest that they expand the chest on every inhale, and draw in the navel and lengthen the lower back on every exhale.

If the previous exercise is too difficult, you can try this seated alternative:

- Sit in a chair with your feet about hip's width apart.
- Lean over in the chair with your spine extended.
- Relax your neck and shoulders (see Figure 40).

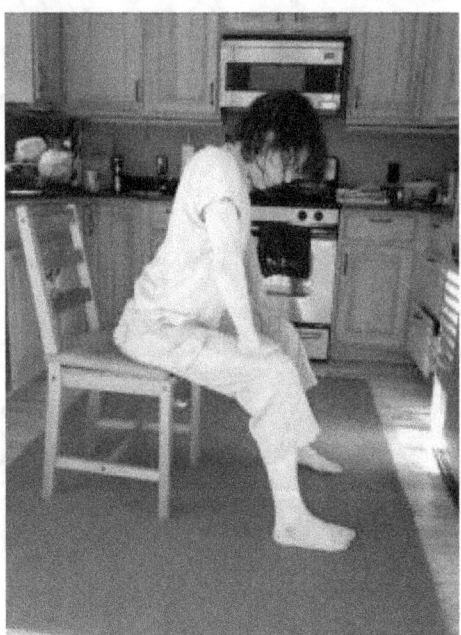
Figure 40: Seated puppy dog

Part 3: "Balancing"

Facilitator Note: Make sure you take the time to do the five breaths with the participants in each movement. In other words, make sure to guide them by reading the script so they can follow along with you.

3.1 Three-Step Breathing

In three-step breathing each inhale is followed a brief pause.

- Find a comfortable seated position.
- Close your eyes, keeping eyes soft.
- Relax your hands, staying receptive (Figure 41).
- Gently exhale and then inhale 5 times observing the length of each breath.
- Begin three step breathing:
    - Inhale for two to three seconds.
    - Pause for two seconds.
    - Take another sip of air.
    - Let the breath settle.
    - Take another sip of air.
    - Pause for two seconds.
    - Slowly exhale.

Facilitator Note: Read through the previous script for each breath cycle. For example, the first week, read through the script five times. Then gradually build up to ten times.

- (Repeat for 5 - 10 cycles of breath.)

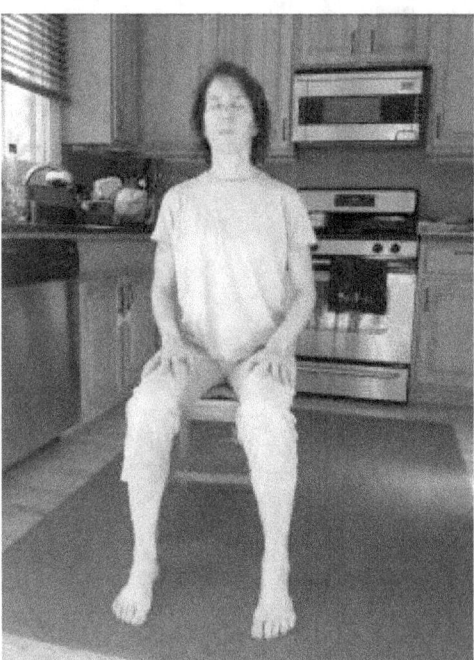

Figure 41: Three-step breathing

Do It For Yourself Tips:
- Always go according to your comfort. Do not strain at all.
- Find a comfortable length of inhale and pause that works for you today.

198

- Take a shorter inhale and shorter pause if necessary.
- Build up to ten rounds of breath over time.
- Instead of counting rounds you can set a timer for one to five minutes.
- Experiment with this breathing exercise when you feel stressed.
- After you complete your breathing practice, sit quietly for 1-5 minutes.

3.2 Alternate Nostril Breathing

Facilitator Note: Go through the following instructions as a script for every cycle of breath. Talk the participants through each breath. For the first week, read through the whole script five times. Then gradually build up to ten times.

- With your right hand make a yogi peace sign with your index and middle fingers.
- Place your index and middle fingers on the area between the eyebrows, as shown in Figure 42. Then follow these steps:
    o Step One: Use your right thumb to close off your right nostril.
    o Step Two: Inhale slowly through the left nostril.
    o Step Three: Pause for a moment.
    o Step Four: Close your left nostril with your ring finger and release your thumb from the right nostril.
    o Step Five: Exhale through the right nostril.
    o Step Six: Inhale through the right nostril.
    o Step Seven: Pause for a moment.
    o Step Eight: Use your thumb to close off the right nostril.
    o Step Nine: Breathe out through the left nostril.
- This is one round. You can build up to five to ten rounds over time.

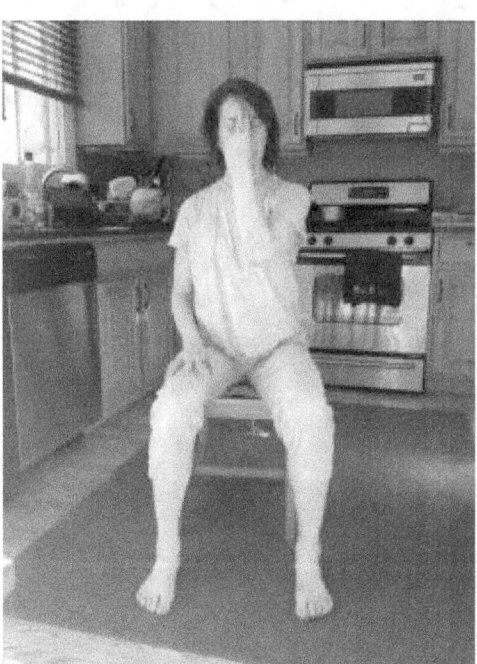

Figure 42: Alternate Nostril Breathing

Do It For Yourself Tips:
- Always go according to your comfort. Do not strain at all.

- Find a comfortable length of breath and pause that works for you today.
- Take a shorter inhale and shorter pause if necessary.
- Build up to ten rounds over time.
- Instead of counting rounds you can set a timer for one to five minutes
- Experiment with this breathing exercise when you feel unbalanced.
- After you complete your breathing practice, sit quietly for 1-5 minutes.

Conclusion

This chapter has presented ideas for developing physical activity goals, and addressing the barriers to physical activity. The bulk of the chapter outlined a gentle, but quite effective physical activity routine designed to strengthen the core, increase mindful awareness of the body, and teach stress-relieving breath work. This program requires no special equipment, no particular clothing, and no fees to the gym. You can do it at home for free!

REFERENCES

Boehmer, U., Mertz, M., Timm, A., Glickman, M., Sullivan, M., & Potter, J. (2011). Overweight and obesity in long-term breast cancer survivors: How does sexual orientation impact BMI? *Cancer Investigation, 29(*3), 220-228.

Brittain, D., & Dinger, M.K. (2013). BE-PALS: An innovative theory-based intervention to promote moderate physical activity among adult lesbians. *Journal of Women's Health,*

Brittain, D., Gyurscik, N., & McElroy, M. (2008). Perceived barriers to physical activity among adult lesbians. *Women in Sport and Physical Activity Journal, 17,* 68-79.

Fogel, S., Young, L., Dietrich, M., & Blakemore, D. (2012). Weight loss and related behavior changes among lesbians, *Journal of Homosexuality, 59,* 689-702.

Fogel, S., Young, L., & McPherson, J. B. (2009). The experience of group weight loss efforts among lesbians. *Women and Health,* 540-554.

Kelly, L. (2007). Lesbian body image perception. The context of body silence. *Qualitative Health Research, 17,* 873-883

Shaw, K., O'Rourke, P., DelMar, C., & Kenardy, J. (2009). Psychological interventions for overweight or obesity (Review). *Cochrane Database of Systematic Review, 1,* NO. CD000381.

Yancey, A.K., Cochran, S.D., Corliss, H.L., & Mays, V.M. (2003). Correlates of overweight and obesity among lesbian and bisexual women. *Preventive Medicine, 26*(6), 676-68.

Chapter 19: Conclusions and Future Directions

This book is a work in progress. As new research becomes available, we will update it. As you have seen through-out this book there is so much that we do not know about lesbian and bisexual women's health, and more research is needed to fill in those gaps. In the meantime, we can apply some tried and true methods to improve our health; the information that you found in the last few chapters that were more action-oriented. We need research to show whether lesbian/bisexual women respond to health programs and health information in the same way that heterosexual women do. Our DIFO research has shown that many older lesbian/bisexual yearn for communities from which to work on health, but have many challenges in creating that space on their own.

We do have some findings from our project, and more detailed findings will be posted on the DIFO website as it becomes available. So far, about 115 women have participated in one of 12 DIFO groups in several Bay Area locations. They were an average of 61 years old, ranging from 42 to 83! Almost 40% reported that they had a significant disability that limited their ability to perform activities of daily living. The women were mostly highly educated, but most had limited finances and some were living below the federal poverty level. About 85% were white women, and the remainder represented many racial/ethnic groups. To summarize some of the benefits that women experienced from the 12 week program, we found that:

- Women showed modest gains in quality of life, and reported feeling more content with their lives
- Women showed more robust changes in mindfulness about eating, a first start in changing long-term eating patterns. They were more aware of what they were eating and starting to make links between emotions and eating. Mindfulness increased to increase for 4 months after the program ended.
- Physical activity increased while women were in the program, but started to decline after the group support ended
- Most importantly, many women reported that they felt a strong sense of community and cherished the time spent with other women with similar backgrounds, shared experiences, and the same goal of getting healthier. They reported that they could be vulnerable and talk about hard topics in their groups.

The Future

Lesbian and bisexual women's communities have been creative in developing local resources for their communities, but must not be expected to "go it alone" without support of health care institutions and policy makers to address the community and structural barriers to better health. So we urge you to stay in touch with local resources, do what you can as an individual to stay as healthy as you can, but do not ever lose the activist spirit to improve the world for generations to come! "We are the ones we've been waiting for." Lesbian and bisexual women have had to be advocates for their own rights, and the right to good health. We cannot give up yet, because our health needs are even greater as we age.

Please let us know what you think of the content of this book: what was helpful, what was missing, what was misleading or unclear. This is truly a collective project and each new edition, like the Our Bodies, Ourselves books, will get more accurate and more practical over time.

So you have reached the end of the information part of the book. If you are so inclined, you can now go on to the manual for the group work. DIFO is a group education and support program. If you are in the San Francisco Bay Area, you may be able to find an existing group. If you live elsewhere, you have a couple of options. You can start your own group, using these materials and the website. We are happy to support you as much as we can, so be in touch. Or you can do the workbook on your own or with a few good friends. Whatever you choose, best wishes in becoming your healthiest self!

Part IV:
DIFO Workbook

Now that we have presented all the information about health, this part of the book outlines an action plan for actually implementing the information into your own life. You can do this on your own, but for maximum effectiveness, it was designed to be done in groups. Groups support and encourage, share resources, improve social capital, and generally make us feel more connected to something outside of ourselves. We start with a short section on facilitating a DIFO group, for those who would like to host and conduct a group, and then outline a 12 week program. You are welcome to make modifications to the format and topics. As part of the research study, we started with 12 consecutive weeks of session lasting for 2 hours per session. We found that some groups wanted to meet for longer periods of time per session, and three hours worked well for those groups. You can adjust the format in any way that best suits your group.

Facilitating a DIFO Group

To be successful, groups must be facilitated. DIFO was set up to be a peer-to-peer program, so you do not need any professional or academic credential or qualifications to be a facilitator. This section presents some general guidelines for facilitation that we have found helpful in past DIFO groups. You can choose whether to have one person be the facilitator for each and every session; to have a team of facilitators; or to share facilitation so that everyone in the group facilitates at least one session. Everyone who facilitates should read this section.

The Target Group

The target population of older lesbian/bisexual women may contain some who are transphobic and biphobic as a by-product of some early lesbian feminist philosophies that came from white, middle class feminist philosophies of women-only spaces (Alimahomed, 2010). Facilitators may need to gently help participants to be as welcoming and inclusive as possible. The groups will also likely include some participants with visible disabilities and some with invisible disabilities. As a community, sometimes lesbian/bisexual women with disabilities have been rendered invisible because of lack of physical access or lack of welcome at lesbian community events (Wadle & O'Toole, 2010). Sometimes women of color have also felt less welcome in LGBTQ communities that are dominated by white people with unexamined racism (Nadle, 2013). In DIFO, we want everyone to feel welcome and included. We include discussion questions to highlight those issues of being included and validated in several sessions.

Because many lesbian and bisexual women are women of size, we will also need to deal with the stigma of larger bodies. Our society is fat-phobic, and sometimes this extends to lesbian/bisexual women's communities. Larger women have more trouble getting and advancing in jobs and are treated with derision and scorn, often resulting in shame, guilt, and depression. This program welcomes those women of greater size. The manual is aimed at an older and larger lesbian/bisexual audience. You will need to assess community norms and labels and use language that is common to your target population. Those labels might include queer or gender queer for younger populations or two spirit, same-gender-loving, or gay for other communities. In addition, some women in the groups will embrace the term "fat" as a positive term, and others will be offended by it. Open discussion of terms will help to make the group a safe place to explore a fat-positive, body-positive philosophy.

General Considerations for Facilitating Groups

Some things to consider before deciding whether to facilitate a DIFO group include personal issues and group dynamics. On a personal level, ask yourself these questions:

1. Have you fully embraced your own sexuality and physical body? This program is about accepting oneself on all levels: your sexuality, gender expression, body size and shape, age, ethnicity, physical ability level, and so on.

2. Are you committed to a "healthy at any size, shape and ability level" approach? This program will not focus on losing weight or changing one's body size, but instead, emphasizes being healthier in body, mind, and spirit. Some participants will lose weight as they make changes in their choices and behaviors, but the program will not apply any pressure to lose weight or alter one's body. We will equally support those who want to lose weight, shed inches, or be healthier at the size and shape they are already in.

3. Are you yourself committed to a healthy lifestyle? You will be a role model. You do not have to be perfect, but motivated to keep working on yourself. However, do not assume that participants will have the same experiences or need the same plan that you used to get healthier. In other words, don't give unsolicited advice that implies everyone should use the same plan you used to get healthier.

4. Are you sensitive to the diversity among the lesbian/bisexual population? The program is meant to be inclusive of women across a wide variety of ethnicities, social class backgrounds, religions, disabilities, genders, and other forms of diversity. We ask that you make no assumptions about any

participants in the groups, and if group members make such assumptions, or make comments that might be offensive or seem insensitive, you address them. If you as facilitator ignore insensitive comments, some participants will feel unsafe.

In terms of working with groups, consider your experience facilitating groups in the past. If you have never facilitated a group before, think about groups you have participated in, and what made the group work well. In DIFO, we strive to create a welcoming, inclusive, and safe environment for women who may have experienced ableism, sexism, homophobia, gender normativity, biphobia, transphobia, fat phobia, racism or other forms of oppression. The forms of oppression that women have experienced may have kept some of the women from accessing health care services in the past, or from using mainstream group health programs, such as smoking cessation classes, or from benefiting from gyms and recreation center programs. To create trust and safety, you will need to spend some time in the first session talking about ground rules and then be mindful to enforce them. Think about how you handle conflict—what will you do as facilitator if two or more group members get into an unproductive argument or conflict? Can you mediate and resolve conflict?

You are a facilitator of the group, not the teacher or leader. That means you are there to provide structure, be the guardian of the ground rules, and introduce topics and discussion questions. You may need to intervene if certain group members monopolize conversations, but hopefully group participants will do more talking than you will. You are the resource person, the cheerleader for the health promotion team, but also a full and engaged participant.

Overall Considerations for Conducting DIFO Group Sessions:

Group size: We recommend group sizes of 8 to 12 participants, but this may depend on the space available to you. If you have a larger group, break into pairs or groups of 3 for some of the discussion questions so everyone gets to share.

Location: Some women may be sensitive to the history and geography of the place you choose to hold groups. Make sure that they are LGBT and/or women-inclusive sites where participants can be comfortable being themselves. The location must be accessible for women with physical disabilities.

Room set-up: Circles are best for discussion because they encourage everyone to feel a part of the group, and foster participation. Try to find chairs without arms that can accommodate larger women more comfortably. If possible, bring colorful tablecloths or other items to make the space warm and inviting. As women arrive for the session, have them put on a name tag to facilitate getting to know everyone's names. Be available to greet women as they arrive to create a welcoming environment. After the first week, you may ask a participant to serve as greeter each week.

Snacks: If you choose to have food available, model healthy food choices by providing vegetables, fruits, tea, and non-processed foods. Please do not provide soft drinks of any type or sugar-sweetened or artificially-sweetened beverages. Water is the easiest and can be "jazzed up" by slicing up a cucumber, lemons, or adding a few sprigs of mint to it.

Equipment/Supplies: None is needed, but a flip chart may be helpful to focus discussions if your location does not already have a white or blackboard. Name tags, pens and paper, napkins, markers may be useful.

The remainder of this section of the manual provides a script for each of the 12 sessions. The weekly sessions are a blend of three major activities/topics:

1. Physical movement and meditation. We recommend a very gentle practice that can be done anywhere, anytime, by anyone with no special equipment or special clothes. This is outlined in Chapter 18, and there is a video version for free on our website (www.difobayarea.org). It's

gentle enough that everyone can do it, but it's also powerful enough that most participants will see results if they do this for a few days. This activity that we call DIFO Moving for Our Health will help participants make the shift from work, the commute, or daily life, to a quieter more reflective state for the remaining session. As the facilitator, please study the materials ahead of time so you can guide participants through the movement.

2. Intuitive eating. Instead of recommending any particular diet plans, we will teach a form of mindful eating that seeks to restore the body's natural ability to detect hunger and fullness and monitor the effect that different kinds of food have on energy level, wellbeing, and health. There is no one diet plan or nutritional information that is appropriate for everyone. Make sure that you are comfortable with this program before attempting to discuss it in group.

3. Stress reduction. Many factors cause or lessen stress related to being a woman, being a lesbian or bisexual person, being gender different, getting older, being a person of color, and so on. Many factors in our daily lives create the conditions for stress. In this program, we discuss many of those stressful factors and build community support to help us make changes in our individual responses to stress. We also put stress in perspective as a social justice issue. Finally, we provide guidance about stress reducing activities like increasing physical activity, meditating, and journaling. Just being in a group of like-minded women with a common goal is a potential stress reducer. s facilitator, it will be your job to make sure the group stays positive. If any members lapse into negativity, gently redirect them to focus on the positives and solutions.

REFERENCES

Alimahomed, S. (2010). Thinking outside the rainbow: women of color redefining queer politics and identity. *Social Identities, 16*(2), 151-168.

Nadal, K. (2013). *That's so gay! Microaggressions and the lesbian, gay, bisexual, and transgender community.* Washington, D.C.: American Psychological Association Press.

Wadle, D., & O'Toole, C. (2010). "I feel so vulnerable." Lesbians with disabilities. In Dibble, S., & Robertson, P. (editors). *Lesbian Health 101: A clinician's guide.* San Francisco: UCSF Nursing Press.

Welcome and Introduction to DIFO

The Doing It For Ourselves (DIFO) program was developed for, and by, lesbian and bisexual women with historic funding from the Office on Women's Health (OWH). OWH is an office of the U.S. Department of Health and Human Services that oversees research on women's health at all the other government agencies. They funded five projects across the United States to study the influence of health programs targeting lesbian/bisexual women over 40. In addition to DIFO, the OWH funded:

- WHAM (Women's Health and Mindfulness) through the Lyon Martin Clinic in San Francisco;
- SHE (Strong, Healthy, Engaged) in New York City;
- OPAH (Out, Proud, and Healthy) in St Louis and Columbia, Missouri;
- MOVE (Making Our Vitality Evident) in Washington, D.C.

Each of these projects collected data on participants before and after being involved, so many publications related to older lesbian/bisexual women's health are emerging from the research. Some of that research is reported in the book that accompanies this workbook.

The Doing It For Ourselves (DIFO) program captures the do-it-yourself spirit of many lesbian/bisexual women who value a balance between independence and community building and support of others. We designed this program to provide education and support, and hope that it will build a community of like-minded women seeking to improve their health or keep healthy as they age.

What Kind of Group Is This?

DIFO is primarily an educational group, with a bonus of group support. It is not a therapy group. The facilitators are peers, not mental health professionals. We encourage women who are recovering from traumas in their lives to seek help from professionals while doing this program. We will provide lots of information about mental and physical health, but this program is about education and support, not treatment. In addition, the groups are quite diverse, including women from many different backgrounds, life experiences, and belief systems. We strive to create a space to foster growth in all of us, through listening to each other's experiences and supporting others who have different goals.

Principles of DIFO. The principles that guide this program include:
- Body acceptance is a key to good health:
  - We embrace the idea that you can be healthy at any size, shape, and ability level;
  - We also acknowledge that body acceptance is on a continuum, and it's a difficult process to truly accept one's body.
- Paying attention and tracking the state of our bodies, minds, and spirits is critical to change:
  - We can change individual behaviors like eating patterns when we know our motivations and habits but we are often on automatic pilot and out of touch;
  - Some things are out of our control. We may blame ourselves if we do not pay attention to the community and societal level factors in the external world. These include social and political forces that affect women's health and community building;
  - This concept of paying attention is called "mindfulness." As women, we have learned to pay attention to our surroundings to stay safe. We can use those same skills to track and change health-related behaviors.
- Health is a holistic concept:
  - we define health as body, mind, and spirit wellbeing, and
  - health can be applied to communities as well as to individuals.
- Community supports health:
  - Group support and sense of belonging helps individuals to make changes and also promotes change at the larger community level;
  - As older lesbian and bisexual women, we may feel a need to create communities that focus on our particular needs and interests. We can "do it for ourselves" as we always have.

What Happens in Group Sessions?

The sessions are a blend of three major activities/topics related to education and group support:

1. Physical movement and breathing. We will teach participants a very gentle practice that can be done anywhere, anytime, by anyone with no special equipment or special clothes. But it's powerful enough that most participants will see results if they do this for a few days. This set of activities that we call *Moving For Our Health* will help participants make the shift from work, the commute, or daily life, to a quieter more reflective state for the remaining session. We hope you will practice it at home as well. The instructions are located in Chapter 18, and there is a free video on the website (www.difobayarea.org).

2. Intuitive eating. Instead of recommending any particular eating plans, we will teach a form of mindful eating that seeks to restore the body's natural ability to detect hunger and fullness and monitor the effect that different kinds of food have on energy level, wellbeing, pain, and health. There is no one eating plan or nutritional information that is appropriate for everyone. This is not a weight loss program, and we let every participant set their own goals. Some may choose to try to lose weight, and others will choose to get healthier without any weight loss goals. Intuitive eating comes from the Health At Every Size ™ approach.

3. Lesbian and Bisexual Woman-Centered Content. Many factors cause or lessen stress related to being a woman, being a lesbian or bisexual person, being gender different, getting older, being a person of color, having a physical or mental disability, and so on. Many factors in our daily lives, simply as human beings, create the conditions for stress. In this program, we discuss many of those stressful factors that are common to lesbian and bisexual women, and build community support to help us make changes in our individual responses to stress. We also put stress in perspective as a social justice issue. We provide guidance about stress reducing activities like increasing physical activity, meditating, and journaling. Just being in a group of like-minded women with a common goal is a potential stress reducer.

Every session includes time to check in about your progress and to share your experiences with other women in the group. To make our time together the most productive, we will ask everyone to use generative speaking.

DIFO Group Process: Generative Speaking

DIFO is primarily an educational group, but also can provide support for achieving better health. Each person comes to the group with her own background and very different experiences, but we do not have time to explore the life histories of each individual. All of the groups so far have included active listening as part of their group agreements, but what about guidelines for speaking? Consider using a process called generative speaking when in DIFO groups, so that each person gets the greatest possible value from the group experience.

Generative Speaking: When you are checking in, or responding to one of the discussion questions posed in the group, a generative response is one that leads to positive responses. For example, comments that:

*   Share an insight you had as a result of the program or about your health behaviors
*   Share a breakthrough that you had, like breaking an old habit
*   Pose a genuine question to the group, related to the topic of the session
*   Show present-forward problem solving—share a solution that worked for you

Examples:

- "This week I tracked my hunger cues and I found that I do most of my emotional eating in the evenings. I had never made the connection that during the day I could distract myself from stress, but in the evenings, all the stress of the day caught up to me."
- "I read the section on thin privilege and realized how much I bought into that concept and thought that thin people were superior to fat people. I am being more careful about the comments I make related to a person's appearance."
- "I have been tracking stress this week, and I've noticed that it's really hard for me to figure out whether stressful situations at work are related to me being a lesbian, or whether they stem from my own perfectionism. I'd love any feedback others have on figuring that out."
- "I tried out "my fitness pal" on line this week. I discovered that tracking food has helped me see how much more I was eating when I ate out than when I ate at home."
- "I walked to the gym yesterday to use the treadmill. I realized that I enjoyed the walk to the gym much more than the walk on the treadmill, and I decided to walk in a park instead of at the gym. It's cheaper and more pleasant. I discovered that I don't have to go to the gym to get healthier. If anyone would like to walk with me once a week, talk to me later."

Speaking that Gets Groups Off-Track: Some types of sharing actually get in the way of everyone moving forward and staying positive. These are more negative or dead-end comments. Consider not speaking if your intention is:
- To get attention or from a place of insufficiency (a "poor me" comment or putting yourself down)
- To tell a story (tell enough to give context to your comments, but a whole story can trigger other people's trauma, make people glaze over, not listen and miss the point)
- To dwell in the past (the past cannot be changed, so telling a story from the past keeps us from moving forward)
- To indulge an old pattern or an agenda (to get sympathy, to build a case against an ex or a family member)
- To give advice. Everyone's circumstances are different. You can share something that works for you, but do not tell anyone else what they should do.

These comments shut down conversation, or lead to people feeling pity, agreeing with you to make you feel better, rolling their eyes, not listening, or dismissing anything you say as irrelevant. When we speak with negativity or with an agenda, people become suspicious of us. We have learned patterns of negativity in our communications through our families, culture, and our needs to try to connect to others. But negative bonding can be more harmful than helpful in groups. You may find that this process of generative speaking may improve your relationships with partners and friends as well. We can avoid wearing out our significant others with negative talk.

Practice speaking with positivity, to generate solutions and move the discussions to community building and connection, not bonding over sad stories. Cross-cultural anthropologist Angeles Arrien, who developed this process of generative speaking in her group work, pointed out that indigenous people would find sharing stories of past wounds to be dishonorable. She described sharing a sob story as being like "backing up the dump truck and releasing all of your garbage on your friend." If you have a need to tell the stories (and sometimes it's useful to do so), see a therapist, join a therapy group, write in a journal or turn it into a written story. In DIFO meetings, share the essence of what you learned from the experience rather than the experience itself.

Tips for Getting the Most Out of DIFO
You will get the most out of the program if you fully engage and bring your full self to the program. We recommend that you:

- **Read.** Read the session assignments before you come to group, so that you will have thought about the discussion questions and content. The discussion will be richer. The suggested readings are listed at the beginning of each session.
- **Practice.** Do some of the action steps between sessions, think about the content, have discussions with others, and most of all, apply some of the suggestions to your own behavior. No change can come about without taking some action.
- **Track.** You will learn the most if you pay close attention to your own reactions to the materials, to what others in the group say or do, and to your own resistance and habits. We recommend journaling. You can use this workbook as a journal, or have a separate journal to track your progress. If writing does not float your boat, find a buddy to talk to about the discussion questions between sessions. A way to track as a group is to join one of the free fitness websites, such as myfitness pal, and set up a group to motivate each other. Just be sure it does not turn into a competition!
- **Participate.** Share in the group discussions, post on the blog site, bring resources to the group, and most of all, if someone says or does something that makes you uncomfortable, say something. We can all learn from those moments of discomfort when we get challenged to examine our own words and intentions. Don't wait until the next session. Learn to address discomfort when it happens to avoid building up resentments and misunderstandings. We have all been socialized in a society that is sexist, racist, ableist, body negative, and so on. We will be healthier if we can create spaces that are relatively free of those poisonous influences so they do not become internalized as stress and contribute to illnesses.

We hope your DIFO group will be a place of information, support, and space to share your own wisdom. You do not have to "do it yourself" all the time, but here in DIFO, we can work together as a community to get healthier habits as we age into our elder wisdom years.

Session 1: Defining Health and Getting Started

Suggested Readings:
Chapters 1 and 2
Welcome and Intro to DIFO (pp.

Breathing to Arrive: The facilitator will select a breathing activity from Chapter 18 to start the group. This form of meditation helps people with the transition from the day into a more reflective state of mind.

Check In: Getting Acquainted. Share your name and briefly, what brings you to this group. What do you hope to get out of the group?

Defining Health

Some experts consider health to be a multi-factored concept. In DIFO we will use several different ways to define health, but will start with one simple one today. Use the worksheet below to explore your current and ideal health in three categories: Physical Health, Emotional, Mental, and Psychological Health, and Spiritual Health. By spiritual health, we mean what or who you turn to when in turmoil, or what gives you inner peace, or helps you thrive and feel connected to the world.

In this program, we will discuss strategies for achieving your ideal, even within limitations. Spiritual teacher Angeles Arrien, as she developed some health challenges in the decade of her 70s, stated,

> *"My life is like a haiku; within the limitations, I have endless possibilities."*

If you are not familiar with haiku, it is a form of poetry with a very rigid structure. It has 3 lines, with lines 1 and 3 having 5 syllables and line 2 having 7 syllables. It must use a nature metaphor. But within that structure, there are limitless possibilities for creating beautiful poetry. Before we can explore possibilities, we have to assess our current state of being and uncover our assumptions or expectations about our ideal health.

Type of Health	Ideal	Current health and any challenges
Physical		
Emotional/ Psychological/ Mental		
Spiritual		

Discussion in small groups:

- How does your cultural upbringing or ethnicity affect how you define health?
- In what areas do you feel your health is the strongest? What have you been doing to achieve that good health?
- Where do you feel the most challenged or limited at this time? What are some ideas for addressing those perceived limitations?
- Is your ideal health realistic? Is it based on impossible standards or grounded in reality?
- How has aging impacted your thinking about your ideal health?

"Fat Talk" and other body negativity

Some women engage in talk that puts down their own bodies. They make jokes about old people, or label themselves as having a "senior moment." It's easy to buy into ageism when we are surrounded by it in all aspects of culture. One of the most pervasive ways that women in our society put ourselves down is through "fat talk." "Fat talk" has been found to increase body dissatisfaction and be "contagious"---that is, when one woman makes a negative comment about her body in a group, most of the time other women will also put themselves down. We don't know whether lesbian/bisexual women do this to the same extent, but we know that fat talk is harmful and violates the DIFO principles of positivity and body acceptance. Here are some examples of how language can be reframed to be more body positive:

Body Negative/Derogatory	More Positive/Constructive
My toes are ugly	I feel self-conscious about the way my toes look in sandals
I hate my flabby thighs	I am uncomfortable with how my thighs look in the mirror because they don't look the way I want them to.
I feel fat	I feel out of breath or my clothes feel too tight (or whatever concrete sensation you mean by "feeling fat")
Since I turned 50, I have turned into a fat cow	I have put on weight since I turned 50.
I have to lose weight!	My blood sugar level has been rising, and I need to bring it down. (but keep in mind that weight may have nothing to do with your blood sugar)

Pay attention to the language that you use about your body or aging. Reframing negative comments into thoughts or feelings will allow you to delve into the underlying feelings of being self-conscious, distressed, ashamed, guilty, uncomfortable, angry, and the whole gamut of emotions that we have been taught to have about our body parts and/or functions without putting down the body part! In DIFO groups, you can practice loving your own body and accepting all its parts, even as they are changing. Talking about dieting or weight loss can trigger other women's traumas, so carefully consider your words.

Establishing Group Agreements

Our next task is to decide how we want our groups to function. As a program, DIFO is committed to creating as much safety and inclusion as possible, and keeping information you hear in the group confidential. Each group can decide what other agreements they will have: how to make sure everyone's voice is heard, how to get the most value out of the time spent together, how to stay positive and remind each other of generative speaking and avoid negative stories of the past.

DIFO Program Agreements For All Groups:

1. Keep personal information shared in groups confidential. Please share materials and lessons learned with anyone you want, but not what an individual says in a group session.
2. Keep in mind that many women are survivors of trauma, and avoid sharing stories of past or current traumas. Stories can be triggering, so focus on the lessons you learned from past experiences rather than details of the traumas.
3. Stay positive about your body, age, or behavior, or the bodies or behaviors of others.

Note other group agreements here:

Action Steps

Each week, several action steps will be suggested. Choose the ones that best fit your own goals, or decide as a group which ones you will all do in between session. This week, consider:

- Develop a system for tracking your own health in all three aspects: physical, mental/emotional, and spiritual.
- Skim the DIFO book to become familiar with the contents.
- Watch the DIFO video on the website
- Begin thinking about what health behavior changes you might want to make
- Do the suggested reading for Sessions 1 and 2

Check Out: Introduce yourself again at the end, and say one word or phrase that describes how you are feeling at the end of this first session.

Session 2: Introduction to Intuitive Eating and Setting Goals

Suggested Reading:
Chapters 15 and 17 (skim)

Breathing Meditation

Introduction to Intuitive Eating

In this program, we will not be recommending any specific type of eating plan for any participants. Instead we will challenge some of the myths about weight and about food that we have been sold by the powerful food and weight loss industries in the United States. We have all heard that "obesity" is an epidemic in the U.S., and that obesity leads to diabetes, heart disease, cancer, and many other health problems. The message is that we have done this to ourselves by eating too much and not exercising enough. Recently the American Medical Association decided to label obesity as a disease, in spite of much opposition from scientists and activists. The real story about the relationship between weight and health is much more complicated than a simple epidemic of laziness and gluttony. It's a story of food politics, greed, medicalization of everyday experience, social justice issues, and changes in our modern lifestyles that make eating healthy and getting enough physical activity challenging.

In the 1970s, feminists were alarmed by the way that women were targeted for their appearance, especially related to weight. Two major scientific studies had shown that weight loss programs were almost totally ineffective—95% of people who lost weight on any kind of diet gained it back, and then some. The authors suggested that weight loss programs do more harm than good, and that there was no evidence that weight is a predictor of health problems. Feminists endorsed several grassroots movements including Size Acceptance (or fat positive, body positive) and Health At Every Size ®. These movements proposed that there has always been wide diversity in physical body size, shape, and ability levels, and that there is no one ideal body type. They pointed out the dangers of dieting and the fact that modern food production processes have disrupted the body's ability to recognize cues of hunger and being full. Lesbian and bisexual women have been very active in these movements, so many are knowledgeable about size acceptance.

A "healthy" weight will be different for each person, depending on unique body needs. In DIFO, we want to assist each woman to find the best foods that give the body pleasure and the right nutrients and do the least harm possible, find regular fun physical activities that are gentle on the body, and reduce stress.

We were born with a body that told us when we were hungry. When we were full, it told us to stop eating. The body can detect what nutrients we need and make us want those foods. Dieting and highly processed foods, as well as all the emotional messages we get about eating have disrupted our body's natural processes. DIFO will guide you through a process of rediscovering your body's natural ability to regulate itself, drawing heavily from the Health At Every Size® model.

Take a Break to Move (use some of the movements from Moving For Our Health or choose your own)

Goal Setting Activity

Next we will start identifying goals to work on in the DIFO program. Each woman can set her own goals, although we ask that you have one goal in each of three areas: nutrition, physical activity, and stress reduction. The first step is to think about your motivation to make changes in these three areas. To do this, we look at the stages of change model. Chapter 15 has more information on making changes in your behavior, and outlines a more complex process for identifying hidden mindsets that keep us from changing if you want to explore your own psyche more deeply.

Step 1: Stages of Change Model Applied to DIFO. How do people make big changes in their lives? One theory that has been useful in smoking cessation, drug and alcohol treatment, and changing nutrition habits is the transtheoretical stages of change model. It suggests that we all go through several steps before we make a change in our behavior relatively permanent. You have probably cycled through these stages many times in your life. Think about where you are now in terms of your nutrition, physical activity, and coping with stress.

Stage	What it means	Nutrition	Physical Activity	Stress
Pre-contemplation (not ready)	This is before you seriously started thinking about getting healthier. Once you have considered one aspect of being healthier, you can never go back to this stage.			
Contemplation (ready)	The process of thinking about getting healthier, but not yet doing anything. You started this program, so you are probably in contemplation on many health behaviors.			
Preparation	This is the step of making a plan to get healthier. You may have started looking into gyms, reading about healthier foods, looking for farmer's markets, or seeking a therapist.			
Action	In this stage, you try out your plan and see how it works. You may have to work out obstacles and challenges.			
Maintenance	Once you have a plan that works, you have to stay motivated to keep to the plan. Because there are temptations all around us, we need to monitor our behaviors. This means paying attention to your body, building in time to shop, cook, and getting physical activity every day.			
Slips	We will succumb to temptations now and then. Use a slip as a lesson—what do we learn about our triggers? What do we need to do differently? Or maybe just forgive ourselves and move back to the action phase and start again. A slip is not failure, it is merely being human. Community can help us get back on track.			

Any comments on your levels of motivation? In what areas would you like to be at a different stage?

Step 2. Brainstorming Goals. Now you need to figure out what goals you want to work on in this program. Start by drafting some ideas in each area. Note what kind of improvement you would like to see, not just a vague comment like "exercise more." Instead, a goal like "be able to walk a flight of stairs without getting out of breath" is more measurable and specific.

Nutrition Goal Ideas:

Physical Activity Goal Ideas:

Stress Reduction Goal Ideas:

Step 3 (Action step assignment for this week). Over the next week, select the one goal from each list that you want to focus on in DIFO, and write it so that it is SMART. That is, it is

- ☐ **S**pecific and Concrete
- ☐ **M**easureable
- ☐ **A**wesome (something you really want to do)
- ☐ **R**ealistic
- ☐ **T**ime-related (has a deadline)

When you have modified each goal to be "smart," record it on the chart at the end of this session.

Action steps:
- Keep tracking your health and decide what to focus on, and how you want to track it.
- Do Steps 3 and 4 on goal setting and decide if you want a different system for tracking than the chart above. Another example of a daily tracking tool is attached. You will be most successful if you come up with your own system to track your goals. You might want to use an existing program, like myfitnesspal or other web-based applications, or make a form of your own.
- Check out the Health At Every Size website and do more reading about Intuitive Eating (Chapter 17)

Check out: Are you ready to believe in Intuitive Eating? Why or why not?

Step 4 (Action step assignment): Tracking the Goals. Record each goal in the boxes below. This form will appear at the end of each session so that you can track your progress and note, in the most kind and compassionate way of course, what you are learning about yourself. If you did not work on your goal this week, contemplate what barriers kept you from doing this work. It's all evidence that will help you learn about your motivations, daily patterns, and barriers to changing health behaviors.

Goals	What I did this week:	Evidence: What I learned about this goal this week.
My physical activity goal:		
My nutrition goal:		
My stress reduction goal:		

Example of a Daily Diary Self-Tracking Tool

Date: _____

Morning I got up at _____ My sleep quality was ___good ____ fair ____ poor
What I ate for breakfast:_____

_____
Morning Snacks: _____
Physical activity: _____
How I felt physically: _____
How I felt emotionally: _____

Afternoon What I ate for lunch: _____

_____
Snacks:_____
Physical activity: _____
How I felt physically: _____
How I felt emotionally: _____

Evening What I ate for dinner:_____

_____
Snacks: _____
Physical activity: _____
How I felt physically: _____
How I felt emotionally: _____
I went to bed at: _____

Daily Summary

Today, my ___ was	Excellent	Very good	Good	Fair	Poor
Overall health					
Energy level					
Nutrition					
Pain					

Thinking about physical activity, how many minutes did I spend today on:

    Mild activity   _____ (did not break a sweat or breathe heavily)

    Moderate activity   _____ (some heavy breathing, but could talk)

    Vigorous activity   _____ (hot and heavy!)

What triggers or stresses did I have today and how did they affect my ability to make healthy choices?

What did I notice about the relationships between eating/nutrition, physical activity, mood, and my health today?

Sample Completed Daily Diary Self-Tracking Tool

Date: September 9, 2014

Morning   I got up at 6:45_ My sleep quality was __good _X__ fair ___ poor
                     What I ate for breakfast:_2 fried eggs and 3 strips of bacon, cup of tea
                     Morning Snacks: a cup of grapes around 11
                     Physical activity: walked 6 blocks from car of office
                     How I felt physically: sluggish, indigestion started around 10:30
                     How I felt emotionally: a little anxious about deadlines, stressed

Afternoon   What I ate for lunch: turkey sandwich, small bag of chips, iced tea around 12:30
                     Snacks: chocolate-covered almonds—a big bunch of them at 3:30
                     Physical activity: none: at my desk doing a big report all day
                     How I felt physically: indigestion continued in afternoon, back ache, sleepy at 4
                     How I felt emotionally: emotionally wrung out, stressed

Evening   What I ate for dinner: got home late and tired, so ate peanut butter and toast
                     Snacks: craving salt at bedtime so ate some peanuts (1/3 cup?)
                     Physical activity: hardly left the sofa in the evening
                     How I felt physically: still had some indigestion, headache, achy all over
                     How I felt emotionally: hard on myself for not getting enough done, still stressed
                     I went to bed at: 10:45

Daily Summary

Today, my ___ was	Excellent	Very good	Good	Fair	Poor
Overall health				X	
Energy level				X	
Nutrition			X		
Pain				X	

Thinking about physical activity, how many minutes did I spend today on:
   Mild activity   __15 min__(did not break a sweat or breathe heavily)
   Moderate activity   __0__ (some heavy breathing, but could talk)
   Vigorous activity   __0 (hot and heavy!)

What triggers or stresses did I have today and how did they affect my ability to make healthy choices?
Deadlines at work had me stressed out all day and kept me from taking a walk at lunch. I ate at my desk and didn't even notice what I was eating.

What did I notice about the relationships between eating/nutrition, physical activity, mood, and my health today?
Bacon! This was the second time I noticed having indigestion on a day when I ate bacon. I also had more back pain…wonder if it's related? Will track that. I noticed that stress kept me chained to my desk. If I had taken a short walk, I might have been more productive and felt better. Also, I realized that I often feel a slump around 3:30 or 5 and I crave caffeine or sweets at that time.

Session 3: Healthy at Any Size, Shape, Age, and Ability Level

Suggested Reading:
Chapter 5: Body Size/Shape and Health (skim)
Chapter 6: read the section on metabolic syndrome (64-44
Chapter 17: Nutrition. Read the sections on Inflammation (pages 150-151), and Rejecting Dieting (153-155)

Breathing Meditation: Start the session with a few minutes of breathing activities from the Moving For Our Health video/instructions. You may want to experiment with doing this breathing practice everyday. Many women find that just a few minutes of deep breathing can help relieve stress and/or reduce fatigue.

Check In
What did you learn from tracking your goals this week?

Lesbian and Bisexual Women in the Media
What hit show best represents our communities? The L Word? Orange is the New Black? Both shows sensationalize sex between women and do not show the wide range of real women's bodies or experiences. How does not seeing ourselves reflected in media affect us?

Stereotypes about Women's Bodies and Thin Privilege

- As a youth what did you learn about how your body was supposed to look?
  - How did those messages affect you personally? How were they enforced? By whom?
  - How do those lessons affect you now?

- What pressures do you experience now as a more mature adult?
  - Does your lesbian/bisexual women's community have unspoken norms about how women's bodies should look? How about your racial/ethnic communities? Your work community?
  - Are you pressured to look "less dyky" by colleagues or your family? Or more "dyky" by members of the gay community? What does it mean to "look like a lesbian?"

- What privileges come with being thin in our society?
  - How does thin privilege compare to other forms of unearned rewards in society, like white privilege, male privilege, and heterosexual privilege?

Stress: Media Attention to Weight and Health
Today we will discuss research findings about the link between weight and overall health. Biomedical studies supposedly find a link between heavier weight and health problems such as diabetes, heart disease, joint problems, asthma, and some cancers, but a growing number of researchers are suspicious of these findings. This movement is called the Obesity Paradox, and promotes the idea that you can be a large woman and be healthy. Those alternative voices suggest that health problems are not linked to weight, but to inflammation, metabolic syndrome and long-term dieting. That is, these 3 problems cause both an increase in weight and other health problems. In addition, there is no evidence that losing weight by dieting will make you healthier. In fact, it may make you unhealthy. Is this new information to you? Were you aware of the health dangers of dieting before?

Nutrition: Three Factors Related to Food and Health.

Metabolic Syndrome. This is a constellation of lab results and effects on the body that probably result from the other two factors: inflammation and dieting, but may also be related to genetics. These are the signs of metabolic syndrome. If you have 3 or more of these, you might be at risk for health problems:

- A waist measurement of more than 35 inches around.
- A fasting blood glucose level of 100 mg/dL or higher; or taking medication because you have high blood glucose levels.
- A triglyceride level at or above 150 mg/dL. Triglycerides are a form of fat in your blood, and are also a good measure of the effects of sugar on your body.
- An HDL cholesterol level (the "good" cholesterol) below 50 mg/dL; or taking medication to increase your HDL level.
- A blood pressure at or above 130 mm Hg systolic (the top number) or 85 mm Hg diastolic (the bottom number); or taking medication to treat high blood pressure.

Inflammation-Producing Foods: The cause of much chronic disease is inflammation. Things that inflame the body kick off the immune system response, but over time, our bodies wear out and cannot fight off the injuries or insults as well. That is when disease occurs. Some foods produce inflammation in the body, most notably, excess levels of sugar. See Chapter 17 for a list of inflammation producing foods, and some foods that help to reduce the effects of inflammation. If you hear someone in the media saying all that counts is the number of calories you eat each day, beware! There are major differences in the quality of the foods we eat, and that is more important than how many calories they contain.

Dieting. A major factor related to health problems is repeated dieting. Our bodies evolved to protect us from starvation and famine. Everything about the body's functioning is set up to resist losing weight. Studies show that people can lose weight in the short term, but that more than 95% will gain it back, and often end up heavier than before. This is because the body's set-point weight gets increased by chronic dieting attempts. Many people lose the same 20 pounds over and over, in a repeating pattern called weight-cycling. Linda Bacon, in Health at Every Size, reports that dieting:
1. Slows down your metabolism so it takes longer to burn calories
2. Makes you digest your food faster, so you feel hungry sooner
3. Increases craving for high fat foods
4. Increases appetite
5. Reduces energy levels (which discourages physical activity)
6. Lowers the body temperature
7. Reduces your ability to notice when you are hungry or full, making it easier to confuse hunger with emotional needs
8. Reduces muscle tissue
9. Increases the fat-storage enzymes and decreases the fat-release enzymes
10. Increases the set-point (the weight where your body stabilizes and resists changes)

Chronic dieting increases the risk for heart disease, may even double the risk of heart attack, cause headaches, menstrual cycle irregularities, fatigue, dry skin, and hair loss. There are also psychological consequences of dieting, such as disordered eating (bulimia, anorexia, binge eating), increased susceptibility to stress, feelings of failure, lower self-esteem, and greater social anxiety.

Take a break to move your body

Intuitive Eating: Dieting? Don't Do It!

Dieting is often the trigger for overeating, not a "lack of willpower." Intuitive eating asks you to stop counting calories or carbs, eating only "fat-free" foods, or eating at only certain times of the day. You have permission to stop punishing yourself for eating "bad" foods, within limits of course. If you are diabetic or have other health problems that require avoiding certain foods, please follow those plans. You will still have great freedom to explore and diversify your eating plan.

It may be helpful in this stage to try an experiment of eliminating certain foods for a short period of time so you can see how you feel with and without them. If you consume sodas, diet or regular, give them up for a week. Diet sodas upset the ability to gauge our own bodily cues and to increase cravings for sweets. Some recent studies have found a substantial link between diet sodas and heart disease. Regular soda contains an enormous amount of salt as well as sugar and increases your thirst so you drink more than you need (it never really quenches thirst). Robert Lustig (2013) reported that just one 12 ounce can of regular soda each day could lead to a major load of inflammatory processes in the body. The carbonation is not so good for us either. Pay attention to the sugar content of what you are drinking. Water is the healthiest beverage and can be made more interesting by adding fruits, cucumbers, mint, or whatever natural flavorings you like. Track how you feel for one week of no sodas. If this was a useful experiment, you might trying eliminating other foods for just a week, and track how you felt. This is an experiment, so be nonjudgmental and compassionate with yourself! The purpose is not to deprive yourself of something you love; just to try an experiment.

Physical Activity: The first step to increasing physical activity is to track what you are already doing. Have you started tracking yet? What do you need to do to get motivated to track your activity? Start with a non-judgmental assessment of your typical day. Note how you feel on days when you get more movement than on more sedentary days. Can you feel any difference in energy level, pain, mood?

Action Steps

- If you have not yet given up a dieting mentality, think about or journal on these questions:
  - What experiences have you had with dieting? How can you improve your nutrition without dieting? Do the worksheet about motivation to give up dieting.
- Check in with your buddy about intentions / challenges and tracking your goals.
- Read about inflammation and food on the website or do your own research.
- Check out the Health At Every Size blog… http://healthateverysizeblog.org/

Check Out: What about this session do you want to continue to think about this week?

Are You Motivated to Give up Dieting?

Use this page to explore your feelings about giving up dieting, if you have not done so already.

Are you convinced by the discussion of the harms of dieting? Why or why not?

What is keeping you from giving up dieting? Express those doubts here:

What steps can you take to move toward a diet-free lifestyle? List at least 3.

Tracking Goals

Goals	What I did this week:	Evidence: What I learned about this goal the past week.
Physical activity goal:		
Nutrition goal:		
Stress reduction goal:		

Session 4. Influence of Family, Friends, Significant Others, and Thoughts

Suggested Readings:
Chapter 11: Interpersonal Influences (skim)
Chapter 17: The Voices (page 157)

Breathing Meditation

Check In
What has been working for you this week? Any tips or insights gained from tracking your behavior?

Stress: Family of Origin, and Beliefs about Food
We have a long history with stress and health behaviors, stemming from our childhood, and sometimes old family patterns are hard to break.

- What did you learn about dealing with stress as a child? Has your family of origin continued to influence you as an adult?
- What did you learn about food from your ethnic group, country of origin, or family?

Even if our families rejected us when we came out, and even if we have no or limited contact with them now, we learned patterns of responding when we were children that affect us even now, unless we took action to change them. Some of us learned emotional eating from our families of origin. Did your parents or other relatives ever encourage you to eat to soothe your emotions, or manipulate you into eating out of guilt? Can you think of examples of things from your childhood that led to linking eating with emotions? Next, think about whether those behaviors are replicated in your current relationships with significant others, family, or close friends.

Peers, Significant Others and Food Psychology
We are very influenced by our significant others: partners, girlfriends, boyfriends, ex-lovers, close friends, and family. But we often do not consciously think about how they affect our health promotion. Some psychologists think that female same-sex couples are emotionally closer than other-sex couples, and some referred to many same-sex couples as "merged" or "fused." Because of this, they may have more influence over each other's behavior than a couple that is not so emotionally close.

- Do you think women in same-sex relationships are closer than mixed-sex couples? If so, has this affected any of your relationships? In what ways?
- Has your partner or an ex-lover been supportive of your efforts to get healthier? How? If not, how do others sometimes sabotage your efforts to get healthier?

Sociologist Corrine Reszek (2012), studied how couples influence each other's health behaviors and found three patterns:
1. "bad" together: each person influenced the other to engage in health-damaging behaviors
2. "good" together: each person supports the other in health promoting behaviors
3. One is the bad influence; the other is the promoter of health (in straight couples, half the time the man was the bad influence and the woman the health promoter; in same-sex couples this pattern was found in one-third of couples).

Our close friendship networks also affect our health. We tend to adopt the health habits and "lifestyles" of our social network. In addition, we are more successful in changing our behavior if we have the support of our network. Many lesbian and bisexual women report that they would exercise more if they could find someone to go with them to the gym or for walks. Often they were afraid of going to gyms or recreational facilities alone because of fear of how they would be treated as older women, women of size, and lesbian/bisexual women.

- How do your close relationships affect your mood/stress levels, nutrition, and physical activity behaviors?
- How can you communicate with partners or close friends about your needs and prompt changes in your relational behaviors (e.g. going out to eat, meeting at bars, eating dinner on the sofa in front of the TV, etc.).

Take a break to move your body.

Intuitive Eating: The Voices Within

We are all exposed to many conflicting voices about our food choices and eating behaviors. So far we have talked about the external ones, from family and significant others. This section reviews some of the common ones that can reside in our own thoughts. According to Intuitive Eating experts Tribole and Resch, there are three negative and two positive voices that affect how we feel about food. Use the scale below to determine which voices are strongest for you, and to set up a plan to shift from negative to positive. Rate how often each voice appears in your life at this time.

Negative Voices:	Never/ Rarely	Sometimes	Frequently
The Food Police: an inner judge that sets rules, monitors your every move, and punishes you with guilt and shame about what you eat.			
The Nutrition Informant: an inner critic that claims to be about health, but nags you to count calories, weigh foods, check your weight, eat only fat-free, and so on. This underlies a diet mentality.			
The Diet Rebel: wants to be bad just to spite the other voices. Often there is shame and guilt later after the rebellious episode.			

Positive Voices:	Never/ Rarely	Sometimes	Frequently
The Food Anthropologist is a nonjudgmental observer of your own eating behavior and of foods. It helps you explore how foods make you feel.			
The Nurturer is your own internal healing voice that comes from your own gut and knows what you need to be healthy. This voice can help us love our own bodies as we age.			

What voice tends to be the loudest one for you?

If it's a negative voice, what are some strategies you can use to shift to more positive self-talk?

Physical Activity: What is the role of your social network and relationships on your physical activity? Do you prefer solitary activities or group activities? How can you use social networks to increase your activity and meet your physical activity goals?

Action Steps:

- Review one or more websites dedicated to healthy eating. For example, Michael Pollan (http://michaelpollan.com) , Marion Nestle (www.foodpolitics.com), Linda Bacon (www.lindabacon.org), or UCSF's Sugar Science site (www.sugarscience.org). These may give you ideas of foods that could take the place of inflammation producers. Select only the foods you already like, or have wanted to try.
- Think about whether your relationships are supportive of good health. And then practice talking with your significant other or close friends about what they could do to help you in your quest to be healthier. Have a discussion about how emotional eating might be present in your relationships if needed.
- Journal about the voices within (see the next page).
- Use your social network in some way to further your physical activity or stress-reduction goal.

Check out: Tell off one of the negative voices, whether its internal in your own head, or comes from someone in your social network or family.

Who's driving the bus?

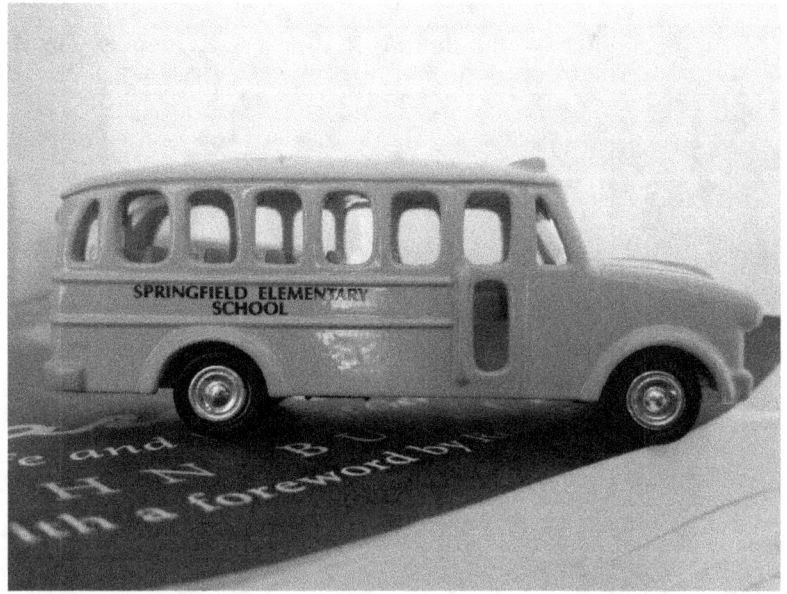

This activity came from DIFO facilitator Jan Thomas, and expands on the idea of voices that affect our behavior. Imagine you are in the bus, representing your life's journey. Are you fully in control? Are you the driver? Is anyone trying to be a backseat driver or affect where you go, how fast you go, etc?

Journaling about Who's Driving The Bus:
Where do you encounter negative voices in your life at this time? Do these voices come from the outside, or are they mainly an internal stories we tell ourselves?

What kind of messages do the voices tell you? List some here:

What other voices are talking to you about food and eating behavior? Which of these voices is the loudest one? How has that loudest voice affected you?

Develop a speech to respond to those negative voices. Maybe the speech comes from your Nurturer or the Food Anthropologist. Consider how you could remove the negative voices from your bus.

Tracking Goals

Goals	What I did this week:	Evidence: What I learned about this goal this week.
Physical activity goal:		
Nutrition goal:		
Stress reduction goal:		

Session 5: Dealing with Stress

Suggested Reading:
Chapter 3. Minority Stress section (31-33) and Chapter 16 (pp 132-136)
Chapter 19. Nutrition, Honor your hunger and making peace with food (pp 155-156)

Breathing to Arrive

Check In
- Share conversations with significant others or friends about supporting your health.
- Share any new insights from daily tracking of goals or the "who's driving the bus" activity.

What Stresses You?
Stress is part of the human condition, and we all have some stress all the time. In this program, we deal mostly with the stress that comes from stereotypes about our identities or communities. In the research literature, it is often called "minority stress." Stress can be insidious and invisible. We live with it for too long, and we don't even see it anymore. It becomes "normalized." This session focuses on making the stress visible so it can be dealt with.

Stress Worksheet
The goal of this activity is to make the stress visible, not to re-hash old stories or open old wounds. Just acknowledge where the big stressors have been in your life, in the past and now. These may come from stereotypes about your ethnicity, religion, age, sexuality, or many other factors. Just make a list of them without lots of detail, but pay attention to what feelings come up for you. The point is not to relive those experiences, just to note that they happened.

Stress from the outside world: What experiences have you had with discrimination, harassment, violence, or other differential treatment because of your sexuality, gender, race, disability, or other difference?

In the Past:

Currently:

Stress turned inward: To what degree do you, or have you in the past, felt shame, guilt, or that you were "less than" others? Or felt that you were to blame for the stress? Name the factors that have caused feelings of shame or guilt (parent's expectation, religion, peer pressure, media, etc.).

In the Past:

Currently:

Current Intensity of Stress:

How much stress are you currently experiencing as a result of these experiences? Put an X between no stress (0) and almost unbearable stress (100)

0 --100

From what sources:

What other stresses do you have in your life, not necessarily related to your identities or communities?

Take a break to move your body.

Coping With Stress

We all learned ways to cope with the stress, often during childhood. Some of those coping mechanisms have not worked so well for us now, or are even health-damaging. In this section, you will list some of the methods you have used to cope with stress in the past, and now. Rate the methods as health promoting (reduces the stress and nurtures the body, mind, spirit), neutral ways (reduces the stress with no harmful or positive effects on body, mind, spirit), or generally health-damaging (reduces stress but causes short or long-term harm to body, mind, spirit).

HEALTH PROMOTING METHODS

1.

2.

3.

4.

NEUTRAL METHODS

1.

2.

3.

4.

HEALTH-DAMAGING METHODS

1.

2.

3.

4.

What action steps can you take to shift the health-damaging methods to neutral or health promoting coping strategies? In your group, share the health promoting strategies with each other. Where and how do you get to a feeling of inner peace or calmness when you are stressed?

The Antidote to Minority Stress: Pride and Resilience

The concept of "pride" was developed to counteract those internalized messages. Instead of feeling bad for being different, we can reframe our thinking into pride for having survived homophobic families, churches, and schools; dealing with that racist teacher, and finding the courage to be who we really are. This applies to our physical appearance as well as our sexual and gender identities. We can take pride in embracing our bodies and challenge all the forces in our environment that try to shame us. When someone says, "You don't look your age," respond that you are proud to be whatever age you are. We need to challenge fat phobia, heterosexism, ableism, racism, and other shaming forces whenever we can (and forgive ourselves if we just don't have the energy or strength to do it every time because it would be a fulltime job to challenge all the crap that is thrown at us daily).

- Where do you feel a sense of pride in your current life? How can you extend that pride to other aspects of your life?

Nutrition: Honor Your Hunger

Some of us have been on automatic pilot when eating for so long that we don't even recognize the signs of being hungry versus full. If you have difficulty sorting out the physical sensations of hunger from emotional and other cues, try tracking hunger cues for a few days, using the chart below. Every time you reach for a snack or start thinking about a meal, pull out this chart.

Time	Hunger Rating Before	What I Ate	Hunger Rating After

Use a 0 to 10 scale for hunger. We suggest a scale you can use, where 5 is the middle point or neutral (not hungry or full). A 0 to 1 means "starving." A 2-3 means ravenous or really hungry, and a 4 is mild hunger pangs (stomach gurgles, growls). On the other side of the scale, a 6 means satisfied, a 7, full, but 8-9 means stuffed and 10 means feeling sick because of overeating. If these words do not resonate with you, create your own scale using words that fit your own personal experience better.

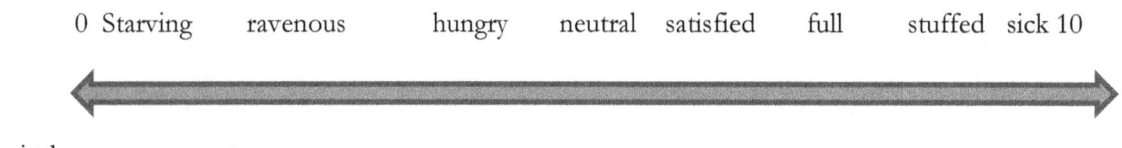

0 Starving   ravenous   hungry   neutral   satisfied   full   stuffed sick 10

Physical:

Emotional:

Put your own words along the line above. Closest to the line, put terms that relate to the physical sensations of hunger and fullness, and below them, any words that relate to emotional hunger. When you track hunger, try to focus on the physical cues. This will help you sort out when you are eating for emotional reasons rather than physical hunger.

Physical Activity

What kind of physical activities help you to reduce stress? For some, it is as simple as standing up and shaking off the stress or wiggling. For others, it may be taking a walk. This week, explore the types of movements that help you reduce stress and introduce more calmness to your life.

Action Steps:

- Track stress this week. Pay attention to how stress impacts your health. Note how much each major source of stress is related to minority stress.
- Complete the Mindful Responses to Stress worksheet.
- Use the hunger rating scale for at least three days in the next week and journal about your efforts to assess your physical hunger.

Check Out: What am I most proud of today? What have I survived that shows me where I am resilient and strong?

Hunger Rating Scale

Day: _____

Time	Hunger Rating Before	What I Ate	Hunger Rating After

Notes:

Day: _____

Time	Hunger Rating Before	What I Ate	Hunger Rating After

Notes:

Day: _____

Time	Hunger Rating Before	What I Ate	Hunger Rating After

Notes:

Tracking Goals

Goals	What I did this week:	Evidence: What I learned about this goal this week.
Physical activity goal:		
Nutrition goal:		
Stress reduction goal:		

Mindful Responses to Stress

This activity was developed by Carley Hauck, a wellness coach and consultant in the San Francisco Bay Area who teaches classes on mindful eating (www.intuitivelywell.com). The next page has a diagram that Carley drew from Jon Kabat-Zinn's work on mindfulness and stress reduction that helps you figure out how you usually respond to stress, and helps you to shift to a more mindful and stress-reducing reaction.

Think about the things that often cause stress for you in your life. What is the external event that happens? Maybe your partner wants to process some aspect of your relationship. Maybe your mother is laying a guilt trip on you about not visiting more often. Perhaps your boss is sending you conflicting messages. Write down 2-3 common sources of stress in your life below to use in this exercise.

Now, choose one of those stressful situations and go through the table on the next page. Identify the thoughts and feelings that come up for you, and then track whether you usually have an automatic reaction (most of us do until we make an effort to change). Consider whether you often engage in poor coping, the self-destructive patterns that may lead to health problems, or the more adaptive coping skills. Start taking small steps toward a mindful response to stress and shifting poor coping to adaptive coping.

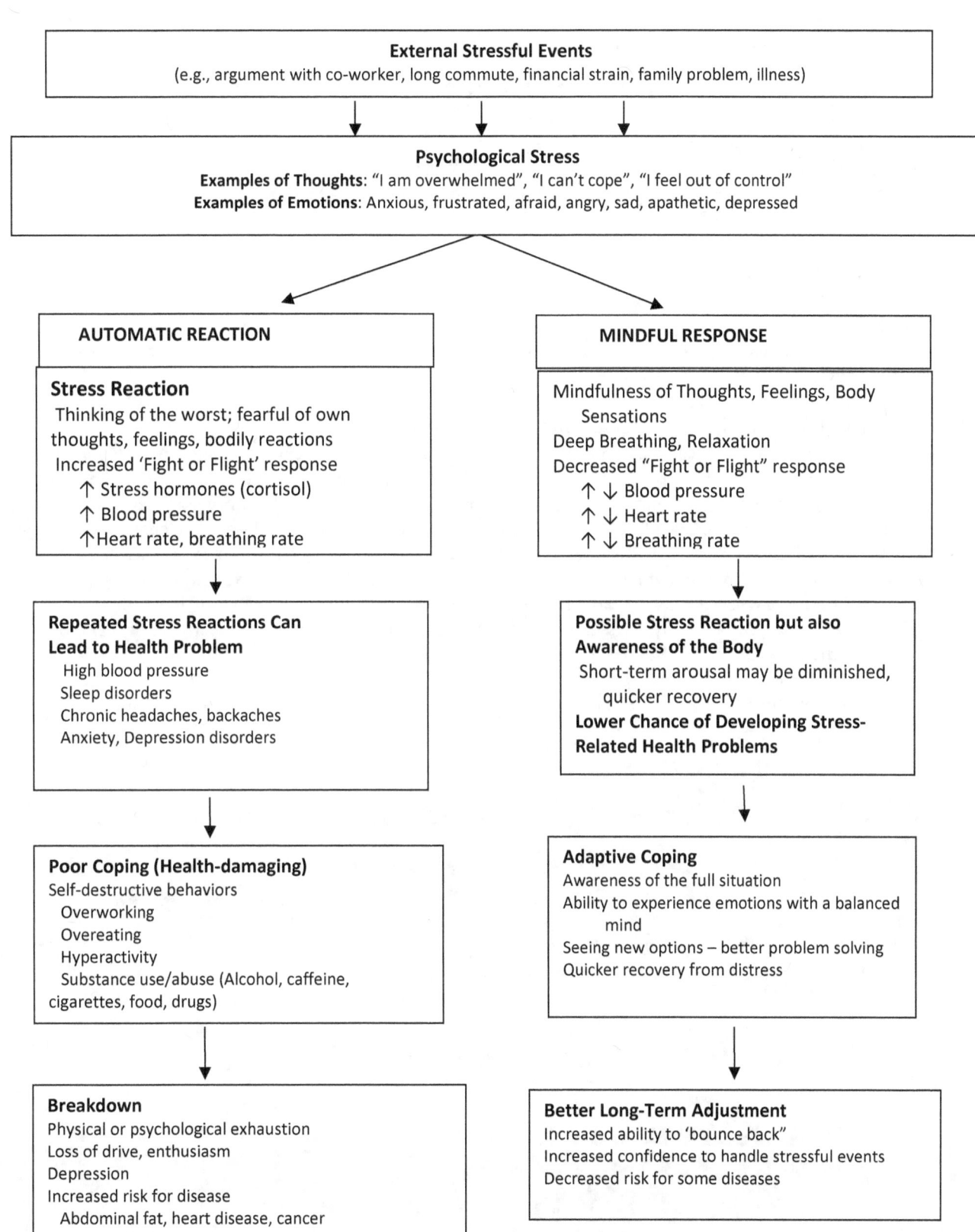

External Stressful Events
(e.g., argument with co-worker, long commute, financial strain, family problem, illness)

Psychological Stress
Examples of Thoughts: "I am overwhelmed", "I can't cope", "I feel out of control"
Examples of Emotions: Anxious, frustrated, afraid, angry, sad, apathetic, depressed

AUTOMATIC REACTION

Stress Reaction
Thinking of the worst; fearful of own thoughts, feelings, bodily reactions
Increased 'Fight or Flight' response
↑ Stress hormones (cortisol)
↑ Blood pressure
↑ Heart rate, breathing rate

Repeated Stress Reactions Can Lead to Health Problem
High blood pressure
Sleep disorders
Chronic headaches, backaches
Anxiety, Depression disorders

Poor Coping (Health-damaging)
Self-destructive behaviors
Overworking
Overeating
Hyperactivity
Substance use/abuse (Alcohol, caffeine, cigarettes, food, drugs)

Breakdown
Physical or psychological exhaustion
Loss of drive, enthusiasm
Depression
Increased risk for disease
Abdominal fat, heart disease, cancer

MINDFUL RESPONSE

Mindfulness of Thoughts, Feelings, Body Sensations
Deep Breathing, Relaxation
Decreased "Fight or Flight" response
↑ ↓ Blood pressure
↑ ↓ Heart rate
↑ ↓ Breathing rate

Possible Stress Reaction but also Awareness of the Body
Short-term arousal may be diminished, quicker recovery
Lower Chance of Developing Stress-Related Health Problems

Adaptive Coping
Awareness of the full situation
Ability to experience emotions with a balanced mind
Seeing new options – better problem solving
Quicker recovery from distress

Better Long-Term Adjustment
Increased ability to 'bounce back'
Increased confidence to handle stressful events
Decreased risk for some diseases

Diagram adapted from Kabat-Zinn, J. (1990). *Full Catastrophe Living*. Random House: New York.

Session 6: Health Risk and Protective Factors in Lesbian/Bisexual Women's Communities

Suggested Readings:
Chapter 4, 6 (skim)
Chapter 18 (skim)
Chapter 19, Feeling your fullness (page 157)

Breathing Meditation

Check In
How did the tracking of stress go in the previous week? Any insights on the effects of stress on eating, physical activity, or mood?

Research on the Health of Older Lesbian/Bisexual Women
If we developed the self-destructive coping strategies that many lesbian/bisexual use, such as smoking, drug use or drinking, we probably increased our risk for health problems. Luckily, it is never too late to change our coping strategies to behaviors that are easier on the body, mind, and spirit, and improve our health. In this session, we will focus on the so-called "lifestyle factors" that affect our risk for illness. The chart below comes from a study of California women (Boehmer et al, 2012) and shows that lesbian/bisexual women have higher rates of smoking and drinking, but tend to get more physical activity than heterosexual women. Bisexual women showed more health risk behaviors than lesbians. This has been found to be true in several other studies as well: there may be more stress associated with a bisexual identity than a lesbian identity. The main reasons for the increased stress are that biphobia sometimes comes from lesbian communities, and bisexual women are less likely to feel connected to lesbian communities that provide support for its members. Few studies report on these behaviors for transgender women, or for lesbian/bisexual women of color.

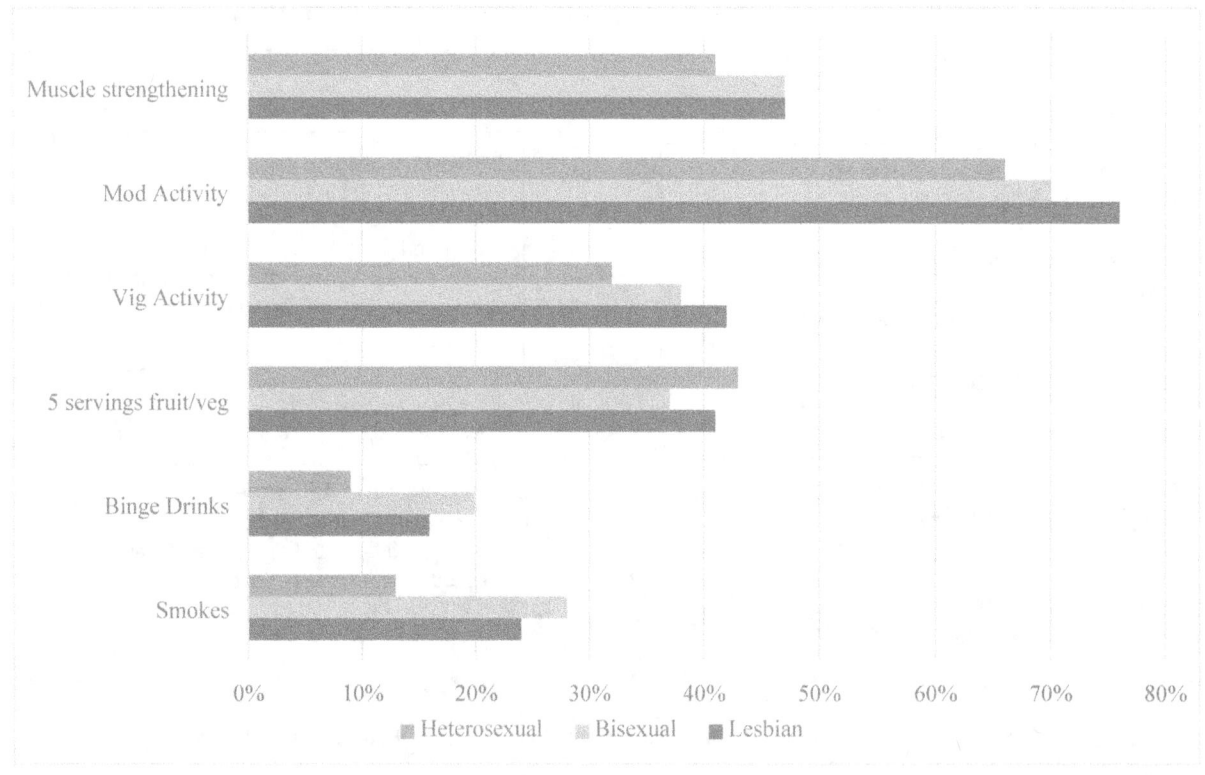

The top five factors are protective—things that promote health; the bottom two are examples of risk factors, or those things that can lead to damage to health. At the end of this section you will find a checklist for you to assess your own health risk and protective factors.

A Powerful Protective Factor: Physical Activity

One of the most potent protective factors for many physical and mental health problems is physical activity; that is, any kind of movement. Chapter 18 reviews the benefits of physical activity. Here we will focus on the barriers to engaging in physical movement. Complete the worksheet below and discuss in your group to get more ideas for ways to overcome the barriers.

True?	Barrier	Ways to Overcome
	My neighborhood is not safe.	
	There are no gyms/rec centers near me.	
	I don't have time to work out.	
	I feel self-conscious about the way I look.	
	I don't have the right clothes, shoes, or equipment.	
	I don't like to do this alone.	
	I feel self-conscious undressing in a locker room with straight women.	
	I feel uncomfortable in a gym with men	
	It is too expensive to join a gym, rec center, or get the equipment I need.	
	Physical activity causes pain.	

Others: list them here:	

Take a break to move your body.

Intuitive Eating: Feeling Your Fullness

Last time we talked about what it feels like to be hungry. This week it's time to start relearning when you are full. Be compassionate with yourself during this process. It took a long time to lose your intuitive eating voice, so it will take a while to get it back. Feeling your fullness relies on conscious, or mindful, eating. Tribole and Resch recommend two steps in developing this mindfulness. Try this during at least one meal this week.

Step 1: Pause in the middle of the meal to check in with your body. Ask yourself:
- How does it taste? If you are not enjoying this meal or snack, you can stop now. Are you eating it just because it is there?
- Am I still hungry? If so, keep eating, or choose something else to eat.

Step 2: Pause again near the end of the meal to assess your level of fullness. Remember that it is ok to leave food on your plate, or eat it all. Your cue is whether your stomach is full, not the food or the plate. You can use the following scale to track fullness for a while, until you can feel your own hunger and fullness naturally.

Time	What I just ate	Fullness rating

For now, rate yourself using the scale you developed or the one below. How hungry/full you are right now?

<--->

0 starving   5 neutral   10 sick

Notes about fullness:

242

Revisiting the Stages of Change

We are about half-way through the program, so it's a good time to think about your motivation for your three goals. Have you been consistent about tracking? Has your motivation shifted or are you still stuck? Are you feeling half-hearted about any of your goals? Rate where you are right now on the 3 goals you set.

Stage	What it means	Nutrition	Physical Activity	Stress
Pre-contemplation (not ready)	This is before you seriously started thinking about getting healthier. Now that you have considered being healthier, you can never go back to this stage.			
Contemplation (ready)	The process of thinking about getting healthier, but not yet doing anything. You started this program, so you are probably in contemplation on many health behaviors.			
Preparation	This is the step of making a plan to get healthier. You may have started looking into gyms, reading about healthier foods, looking for farmer's markets, or seeking a therapist.			
Action	In this stage, you try out your plan and see how it works. You may have to work out obstacles and challenges.			
Maintenance	Once you have a plan that works, you have to stay motivated to keep to the plan. Because there are temptations all around us, we need to monitor our behaviors. This means paying attention to your body, building in time to shop, cook, and getting physical activity every day.			
Slips	We will succumb to temptations now and then. Use a slip as a lesson—what do we learn about our triggers? What do we need to do differently? Or maybe just forgive ourselves and move back to the action phase and start again. A slip is not failure, it is merely being human. Community can help us get back on track.			

Action Steps:

- Complete the checklist on health and protective factors at the end of this section and reflect on your own health. What can you do to reduce the risk and increase the protections? Generate at least three ideas to try out.
- Rate your fullness for at least 2 meals in the next week and journal about your discoveries. What did you notice when you used the fullness ratings? Are you often aware of when you are full, or do you use external cues, like whether the plate is empty?
- Try one of the strategies you came up with to overcome a barrier to physical activity. Watch the video Moving For Our Health again and select a few of these to do daily this week.

Check Out: What is one action you can commit to taking this week to increase your physical activity?

Identifying Your Risk Factors/Enhancing your Protective Factors

The major chronic physical health problems that increase in frequency as we age: diabetes, heart disease, hypertension, stroke, and cancer, have some very similar risk factors, and we can take lifestyle measures that will help to reduce our risk for all of these conditions. But protective factors are equally important and you can get healthier by doing these as well as avoiding risk factors. Here is a risk/protective factors check list. You do not have to share any of this information with the group.

Yes	No	Risk factor
		Do you smoke?
		Do you drink 7 or more drinks of any kind of alcoholic beverage each week?
		Do you often drink 3 or more drinks at one sitting?
		Do you use any illegal substances or prescription drugs in a way that is not prescribed and that affect you in a negative way?
		Protective factor
		Do you have a supportive community? People you can count on?
		Do you live in a neighborhood where you feel safe walking and socializing?
		Are you in a stable, nurturing, and safe relationship with a significant other?
		Do you at least 15-20 min per day of moderate or vigorous activity?
		Do you have a mostly optimistic or easy-going way of responding to the world?
		Do you have access to healthy, whole foods within a mile of where you live?
		Do you have any practices or rituals that help you to achieve inner peace?

If you answered yes to smoking, drinking, or drug use questions, please refer to the readings in the first part of the book or look at the website for more information. Consider how you can reduce your risks and beef up your protective factors. List some strategies below:

Tracking Goals

Goals	What I did this week:	Evidence: What I learned about this goal this week.
Physical activity goal:		
Nutrition goal:		
Stress reduction goal:		

Session 7: Dealing with Pain, Fatigue, and Loss

Suggested Readings:
Chapter 6 (skim)
Chapter 18: think about reducing pain with physical activity and stress reduction activities
Chapter 17: Getting satisfaction from food (pp. 159-161)

Breathing Meditation

Check In
What did you discover about tracking your fullness last week? How is your motivation level for working on your goals?

Stress and Pain, Grief, Loss
Pain is the body's warning that we have reached some limit and need self-care. Some lesbian and bisexual women experience a great deal of pain because of minority stress and human stress. Pain can be related to physical health concerns like bad knees and cancer but it can also stem from mental health factors such as depression, and spiritual factors such as experiencing a loss of meaning in one's life. Grief is one specific type of emotional pain related to the loss of someone or something important to the person. When we retire, it might feel like a loss of meaning and purpose in life when we shift from a role as a worker to a new type of life. As we age, we are more likely to experience all of these factors that can put our bodies, minds, and spirits out of balance. They can negatively affect our nutrition, physical activity, and sleep quality.

Physical Pain. Pain can come from physical health ailments. Cochran and Mays (2007) studied California women's reports of some conditions that can result in pain and found differences by sexual orientation as shown in the chart below. Lesbian and bisexual women reported more disability, arthritis, chronic pain, chronic fatigue, and back pain than heterosexual women. Bisexual women had more headaches and asthma. What do you think accounts for these differences?

Disorder	Heterosexual	Lesbian	Bisexual
Migraines/headaches	19%	18%	26%
Asthma	9%	13%	19%
Arthritis	21%	34%	18%
Back problems	14%	23%	27%
Functional health limitations	21%	31%	38%
Chronic pain	12%	19%	19%
Chronic fatigue, fibromyalgia	5%	9%	12%

Grief (Emotional Pain). What types of grief might be different or more intense for lesbian/bisexual than for heterosexual women? Examples might include family and friend rejection at the time of coming out; loss of the heterosexual dream life; not being able to bring partners to family events; loss of children or close friends; loss of a beloved pet. Often, the emotional pain is intensified because others fail to recognize the pain associated with a breakup of a partner because they did not understand that it was a relationship like a heterosexual marriage, or because they did not recognize the depth of the connection with the pet.

Lesbian and bisexual women might experience more grief over the perceived loss of health or mobility, because of the higher rates of disability and feeling a greater need for independence than heterosexual women. If she does acknowledge the need and seek help, imagine how health care providers and service delivery systems may treat lesbian/bisexual older women with disabilities and or larger bodies or butch appearances--the number of stigmatizing identities can result in poor treatment.

Reframing Activity: Think of a person, pet, or a thing you have lost recently, like some aspect of your health or a job. Now think of all of the reasons why this thing or person was so important to you. Give gratitude for having that person/pet/thing in your life. What would your life have been like without this person, pet, or thing? How lucky you were to have experienced that joy!

It's easy to get caught up in the negatives. The news media is full of stories of anti-gay violence and discrimination, sexual assault, women's lower wages, weight-shaming, and ignoring or making fun of older people. But the flip side is that we have made great progress as a society in terms of acceptance of women, older adults, and sexual minorities. Lifespan has increased and older adults have greater possibility of active and quality lives. Focusing on the positives will help put our lives in perspective and make the negatives feel less devastating.

- What helps you to feel more positive about your life? [turning off the TV, reducing exposure to negative people, getting out into nature] Make a list of these activities.

- In times of turmoil, who or what do you turn to? What helps you out of times of trouble?

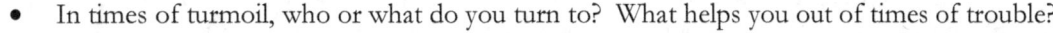

Research shows that mild physical activity is as effective as many prescription drugs for relieving pain, grief, and mild depression symptoms. Walking, particularly in nature, can be healing. Swimming or water aquatics are also gentle activities that may relieve pain. Physical pain often stems from muscle tension, so anything that relaxes or gently stretches the muscles may help to reduce pain.

- What has worked for you in the past in relieving pain?

- How can you use those practices more mindfully to keep pain from getting too uncomfortable?

Sleep Quality

A common complaint, particularly as we get older, is the inability to get a restful night's sleep. Stress, pain, grief, loss, and many health-damaging behaviors can have great impact on sleep. Most people need between 7 and 8 hours of sleep each night. If deprived, even slightly, we may have "micro-sleeps" or periods of falling asleep for 3-10 seconds during the day. These are a major cause of accidents and injuries. Sleep deprivation also affects other health outcomes:

- Vaccines don't work as well
- Blood sugar and other hormone regulation is impaired
- Cortisol levels increase (these are the stress hormones) and so does risk for hypertension
- Leptin decreases, disrupting hunger cues, so we eat more and crave foods more often. In one study of over 68,000 women over a 16 year period, those who slept less (5 hours per night) gained more weight than those who slept more, even though they did not consume more calories or get less exercise. The experts think the difference is that sleep deprivation changed their metabolic rate.

If sleep is an issue for you, check out the section on sleep hygiene in Chapter 16 and try some of the suggestions.

Intuitive Eating: Getting Satisfaction

The opposite of pain and loss is satisfaction and happiness. Eating should bring happiness, not guilt, remorse, or a sense of duty. Here are five steps to a satisfying culinary experience.

- **Step 1. What do you really want to eat**? Don't eat something just because it is there, or because you think you should eat it. Figure out what you really want and eat it in a mindful way. If you constantly say, "I don't know what I want to eat" you may need to repeat some of the earlier activities, like making lists of favorite foods and paying attention to your body.
- **Step 2. Focus on the sensual experiences of eating**. Mindful eating means being aware of the taste, aroma, texture, temperature, appearance, and volume of the food you are eating. Find out what really gives you pleasure and makes you feel satisfied (full), without painful after effects.
- **Step 3. Savor your food.** Make time for your meals; at least 15 minutes to sit down and do nothing but eat. Eat slowly so that you can fully engage your taste buds. Put down your fork every few minutes to feel your body and appreciate the taste. Track when you are getting full and stop before reaching "stuffed." Have a variety of foods on your plate to provide different nutrients and different sensory experiences.
- **Step 4. "If you don't love it, don't eat it, and if you love it, savor it."**
- **Step 5. Check in regularly to see if foods still taste good**. If you eat a lot of the same food, over time it may lose its appeal. Researchers call this "sensory-specific satiety." Once it stops giving you pleasure, maybe you only want to eat that first pleasurable bite and then stop. Or replace it with a new food experience.

Action Steps:

- Track pain in the next week. What are the major types and sources of pain that you experience: physical, emotional, or spiritual? What seems to trigger these pain experiences? You can use the pain tracking tool at the end of this section.
- Track what you were grateful for each day. If challenges arise, express gratitude for the chance to grow and problem-solve. Try a gratitude practice every day for the next week:

Check Out: What am I grateful for today and why?

Ideas for Gratitude Practices

Try completing each sentence at least once a day:

I am grateful that I am a woman today because _____.
I am grateful that I am lesbian/bisexual today because _____.
I am grateful that I am an older woman today because _____.

If you don't want to inject an identity into your gratitude exercise, try these:

I am grateful that I am me today because _____
I am grateful that I am alive today because _____

This activity will be more effective if you develop your own gratitude mantra about what factors in your life bring you joy. Write it below: If some person is involved, the power of the gratitude is doubled if you tell the person directly that you are grateful for his/her presence in your life.

Angeles Arrien's book on Living in Gratitude suggests that you give thanks for four types of gifts each day. Give gratitude for:
- What you learned today (learnings)
- The kindnesses extended to you by others or circumstances or that you extended to others
- The things that protected you from harm
- The things/people that brought you joy

Think about today: can you identify one source of gratitude for each of these four components of life?

Tracking Pain

For each day of the next week, track what triggered pain, how intense it was, and how you responded to it. Did your response lessen the pain? On retrospect, what are other strategies you could use for addressing these types of pain.

Day	Emotional Pain	Physical Pain	Spiritual Pain
Monday			
Tuesday			
Wednesday			
Thursday			
Friday			
Saturday			
Sunday			

Tracking Goals

Goals	What I did this week:	Evidence: What I learned about this goal this week.
Physical activity goal:		
Nutrition goal:		
Stress reduction goal:		

Session 8: Emotional Eating

Suggested Readings:
Chapter 16 (skim)

Breathing Meditation

Check In
What did you notice about pain when you tracked it for a week?
How did the gratitude practice go? Was it hard to reframe pain and loss into gratitudes?

Responding to Stress/Injustice without Food
Emotional eating begins very early in life, from the time we are offered the breast or bottle when we were crying, being offered a cookie when we fell and bumped our heads, or were given an ice cream cone to celebrate getting an A on a test. We were practicing emotional eating when we "cleaned our plates" to please a parent or partner. We learned to associate the comfort of a loving family with the food we eat, as well as the distress of a dysfunctional family with the traumas of family meals. Food is offered as evidence of love, a reward, or a means of comforting all sorts of ills (feed a cold!). For some, eating became a way of coping with unwanted or feared sexual feelings or emotional responses to being gender different. We had no one we felt safe to talk to about our attractions to girls or discomfort with our bodies, so we stuffed our fears and guilt with food. We stuffed our emotions with ice cream when our partners were not invited to work-related social events. When life feels unfair and we feel powerless, we eat to comfort ourselves. Emotions are so wrapped up with eating that we often no longer recognize when we are eating to sooth an emotion rather than a physical hunger.

So far, we have talked about emotions resulting in emotional eating, but sometimes eating can cause an emotional response as well. Can you fill in the blank in this statement:

"I felt guilty because I ate_____."

If so, you had an emotional response to eating. It's time to give up the guilt and show yourself some compassion. Emotional eating is on a continuum from pleasurable eating to punishing eating. See if you can ease yourself up toward the pleasure end of the continuum.

> Sensory gratification (eating for the pleasure and satisfaction of the food)
>
> Comfort eating (mild emotions)
>
> Distracted eating (eating to avoid feeling something like boredom, guilt, or anxiety)
>
> Sedation (eating yourself into a near coma)
>
> Punishing eating (a pattern of overeating followed by severe guilt). This extreme form of emotional eating may lead to an eating disorder.

Think about what situations may lead to experiencing different points on this continuum of emotional eating. List some of them below:

Take a break to move your body.

Emotional eating is usually not associated with binging on broccoli! Why do you think we tend to choose high fat and high sugar foods when we are stressed? How can we reduce the inflammation brought on by comfort foods? Let's start by tracking what emotions trigger emotional eating. Think about the past six months when you fill this out.

I often eat when	Never	Rarely	Sometimes	Often
I feel bored				
I want to procrastinate				
I need to bribe myself to do something				
I want to reward myself				
I feel excited				
I need to feel comfort/soothing				
I want to show or receive love				
I am frustrated				
I am angry				
I feel stressed				
I feel anxious				
I feel depressed or sad				
I want to feel connected				
I want to lose control				
I feel I was treated unfairly				
I feel someone did not value my sexuality, gender, or relationship				
I feel embarrassed or humiliated				
I feel guilty				
I feel "out of control"				
Other:				

Did you see a pattern? Are you in touch with what emotions trigger eating, or do you need to track this more closely? What was missing from this list for you?

Action Steps:
- Try filling out the emotional eating scale every day for a week to see what emotions come up for you, or use the daily tracking tool you developed. Extra copies of the emotional eating scale appear at the end of this section.
- Is there a pattern? Do certain emotions come up regularly? What can you do to begin to break the pattern?
- Try the "What's in the U-Haul" exercise to identify the emotional baggage you might be carrying around that affects your health.

Check Out. State one emotion that seems to be associated with overeating for you and one thing that you can try this week to change the pattern.

Emotional Eating Tracking

Today I ate when	Never	Rarely	Sometimes	Often
I feel bored				
I want to procrastinate				
I need to bribe myself to do something				
I want to reward myself				
I feel excited				
I need to feel comfort/soothing				
I want to show or receive love				
I am frustrated				
I am angry				
I feel stressed				
I feel anxious				
I feel depressed or sad				
I want to feel connected				
I want to lose control				
I feel I was treated unfairly				
I feel someone did not value my sexuality, gender, or relationship				
I feel embarrassed or humiliated				
I feel guilty				
I feel "out of control"				
Other:				

Today I ate when	Never	Rarely	Sometimes	Often
I feel bored				
I want to procrastinate				
I need to bribe myself to do something				
I want to reward myself				
I feel excited				
I need to feel comfort/soothing				
I want to show or receive love				
I am frustrated				
I am angry				
I feel stressed				
I feel anxious				
I feel depressed or sad				
I want to feel connected				
I want to lose control				
I feel I was treated unfairly				
I feel someone did not value my sexuality, gender, or relationship				
I feel embarrassed or humiliated				
I feel guilty				
I feel "out of control"				
Other:				

Today I ate when	Never	Rarely	Sometimes	Often
I feel bored				
I want to procrastinate				
I need to bribe myself to do something				
I want to reward myself				
I feel excited				
I need to feel comfort/soothing				
I want to show or receive love				
I am frustrated				
I am angry				
I feel stressed				
I feel anxious				
I feel depressed or sad				
I want to feel connected				
I want to lose control				
I feel I was treated unfairly				
I feel someone did not value my sexuality, gender, or relationship				
I feel embarrassed or humiliated				
I feel guilty				
I feel "out of control"				
Other:				

What's in the U-Haul?

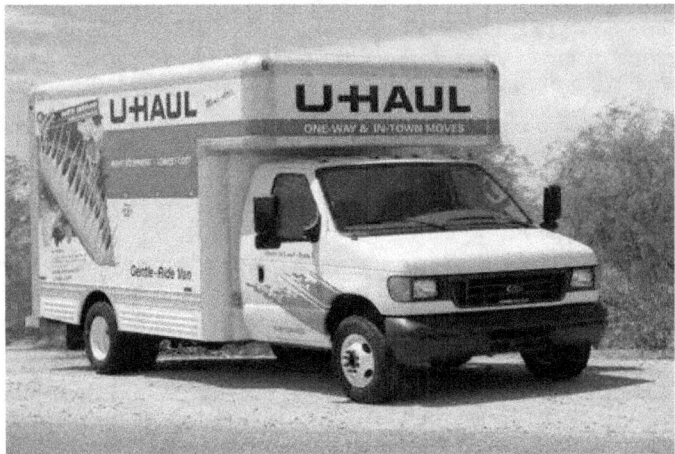

click to enlarge

A few sessions ago, we explored the concept of who's driving the bus. Now let's look at the other baggage we carry around with us. We all know the jokes about lesbians and the U-Haul. We develop emotional attachments quickly, pack them up and move them in with us. Sometimes when a relationship is over (whether with a person or a thing, like food, alcohol, tobacco, shopping, hoarding, etc), we do not get rid of this traumatic event. Instead, we continue to haul it around with us. So here is a chance to take inventory of the crap that's still packed in the U-Haul. You need to make room for new, healthier behaviors and relationships. What needs to go to the dump now? You can use this exercise broadly and think about all aspects of life that need some spring-cleaning, or focus on the baggage related to food, physical activity, and stress.

What I need to let go of: What it will take to part with this?

Goals	What I did this week:	Evidence: What I learned about this goal this week.
Physical activity goal:		
Nutrition goal:		
Stress reduction goal:		

Session 9: Emotional Eating Part II

Suggested Readings:
Review your own notes on emotional eating from last week

Breathing Meditation

Check In:
What did you discover about emotional eating this week? Spend a little extra time on the check in this week to be able to explore the issues that arose for you as you examined the role of emotions on eating behaviors.

Emotional Eating and Emotional Baggage
Discuss any insights you had when doing the U-Haul exercise this week. Are you carrying around emotional baggage that you were not consciously aware of? What impact does this have on your life? To turn the discussion to positive action, spend some time brainstorming with your group about other ways to deal with emotions besides eating. What can you try in the next few weeks when you feel the emotional responses that tend to trigger over-eating or eating things that are not healthy for your body. List as many of these alternative actions as you can below:

Movement/Breathing Break: Take a little longer movement break this week, and incorporate another stress-reduction breathing activity. You may need to stop frequently for stress-relieving breathing as you work through issues related to emotional eating.

Using Humor to Deal with Stress

One way that lesbian and bisexual women (and their GBT family members) have dealt with stress is through humor. If we can laugh, we can deal with our stress better. In this part of the group, share your favorite lesbian/bisexual women's stories, jokes, books, or comedy routines that make you laugh. As the group shares, make a reading/viewing list for yourself below:

Action Steps:

- This week, find a buddy to check in with you about your thoughts on these two sessions on emotional eating. This can be a challenging topic for many women, so make sure that you express what is going on for you and engage in extra self-compassion and self care.
- Try at least two things from the alternative actions list to deal with emotions this week.

Check Out: Name one thing that made you laugh this week.

Progress in Tracking Alternatives to Emotional Eating

Record your experiences in trying out alternatives to emotional eating. What activity did you try, and how did it make you feel?

Goals	What I did this week:	Evidence: What I learned about this goal this week.
Physical activity goal:		
Nutrition goal:		
Stress reduction goal:		

Session 10: Taking Charge of Our Health

Suggested Readings:
Chapter 16. Health literacy section (pages 140-141)

Breathing to Arrive:

Check In
Did you find any new patterns in emotional eating? What activities did you try out to substitute for emotional eating and how did they work?

Health Care Seeking of Lesbian/Bisexual Women
Today we will focus on health care access and quality of care issues. As we have discussed in other sections, lesbian and bisexual women have slightly higher risk for several mental health problems, alcohol, tobacco, and drug problems, and some physical illnesses, such as asthma. We are also more likely to be disabled. This means that particularly as we age, we may need to access healthcare services even more often than heterosexual women.

Some studies suggest that lesbian/bisexual women are more likely to delay seeking help after having symptoms of an illness. Many experts think this is because of past negative experiences in health care—lesbian and bisexual women are treated differently, more roughly, ignored, made fun of, or have had their partners dismissed or ignored. In a few rare cases, healthcare providers have not allowed same-sex partners to visit a loved one in the hospital and have not shared vital health information even when the partner had legal documents to protect their families. Some transgender people have been denied healthcare all together. Unfortunately, most healthcare professionals have not received any training about LGBT issues, and they may be uncomfortable, unaware, or even negative about caring for lesbian and bisexual women. This means that there is more pressure on you to tell your provider what you need. We will talk about two issues today: Coming out to health care providers and health literacy. If you do not already have a primary care provider, there is a checklist at the end of this section to help you screen providers for their knowledge and sensitivity to LGBT issues.

Disclosure
- Are you out to your primary care provider?
- If yes, how did you come out to that health care provider and what was the response?
- If you are not out, what is keeping you from coming out?

Communicating with a healthcare provider
At the end of this section, you will find a one page handout and on getting the most out of a healthcare visit. If you plan ahead, write out all of your questions, and bring printed copies to the visit, you are more likely to get your questions answered (see form at end of this section). Things to discuss with your healthcare provider include:
- What regular preventive screenings do I need?
- What legal documents, if any, do I need to protect myself and my family?
- How does the healthcare provider screen referrals…are they LGBT friendly?

Use of Alternative and Complementary Health Services
Because of suspicion or fear about the medical model that has pathologized us in the past, many lesbian/bisexual women choose to use alternative and complementary health practices to address their health concerns. These include herbal products, acupuncture and acupressure, chiropractic medicine, naturopaths, and meditation, among others. These practices can enhance our health, but it's difficult to find accurate

information about which practices are good for what kind of health problem. One good resource is the National Center for Complementary and Alternative Medicine (NCCAM). Many of these practices are body positive and are ways to reconnect our minds and bodies and track bodily experience.

- What alternative/complementary practices have you tried and how have they helped you?
- Do you have any books, websites, or other resources to share?
- Some people engage in spiritual practices to create more balance, inner peace, self-compassion, or other positive qualities. How do you foster that type of growth for yourself?

Action Steps:
- Compile your health history and develop a system (electronic or paper) for keeping all health information together. There is a sample of this form at the end of this section, but download it from the web if you want to make an electronic health record for yourself.
- Start creating a new story about your own health that includes plans for tracking health behaviors and symptoms, getting back on track if you experience setbacks, rewarding healthy behaviors and not punishing oneself for slips to unhealthy behaviors.
- Review the legal documents needed to protect yourself and your family, and develop a plan for getting the documents you need if you do not already have them.

Check Out. What is one thing you would like to say or do on your next health care visit?

LGBT Welcoming and Inclusive Services Checklist:
Screening a healthcare provider agency

Yes	No	Agency Policies and Procedures
		They have a nondiscrimination policy for clients or patients
		The mission statement is inclusive of LGBT people
		Client confidentiality policies include how to deal with LGBT people who do not want information about sexuality or gender on their records
		Written notice is given to clients about when and for what reason information about them may be disclosed to a 3rd party
		Staff Training/Conduct
		All staff had basic training on LGBT people and issues at least once
		Some staff get advanced training
		All staff treat LGBT clients with respect and honor confidentiality
		Staff members know how to intervene when other clients or patients act in discriminatory manner to LGBT clients/patients
		Inclusive Language: Forms/Assessments/Treatment
		Written forms have inclusive language and encourage disclosure
		Assessments are inclusive and encourage discussion of whether gender or sexuality issues need to be addressed in treatment
		Case management, treatment, and aftercare plans include issues related to sexual and gender if appropriate
		There is some recognition of LGBT people in the brochures, posters, written materials, newsletter, magazines, etc.

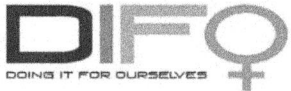

Guide for Efficient Healthcare Provider Visits

Bring at least 3 hard copies of your written questions when you go for a visit. Put one on top of the forms you fill out in reception, and bring the others with you into the exam room. If your primary healthcare provider does not have the copy you put with the intake forms, give him/her another copy right away to guide the conversation.

Rationale: people can read faster than they can listen, and when we tell stories, we tend to get off track. Writing this out ahead of time forces you to focus on the main issues, and list and prioritize the things that are not as critical to cover. Having the written form also increases the chances that the healthcare provider will record your issues accurately in your medical record without having to rely on memory.

What is the symptom(s) or issue that brought you here today? Specify when it started, where it is located, the intensity and frequency of the symptoms. If relevant, mark the spot on the body outline below—front and back views

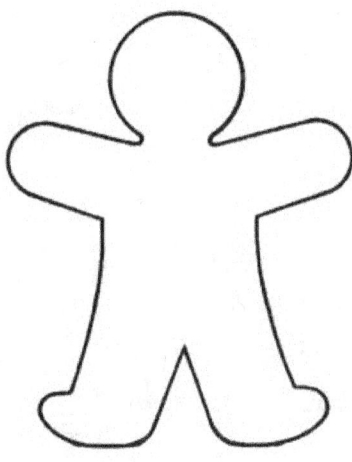

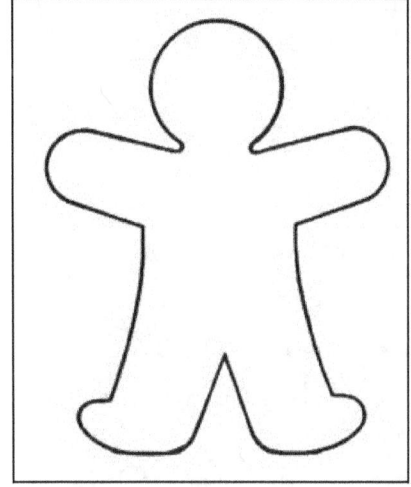

Front   **Back**

What other questions do you want to address this visit? Make a list of your questions in order of priority, with the most urgent on the top.

MEDICAL RECORD FORM

Today's Date _____

Legal Name _____ Birth date _____/_____/_____ Age _____

Preferred Name _____

Address _____Apt # _____ City _____State ____ Zip _____

Phone #1 _____ (mobile) Phone #2 _____(home)

Email _____

Occupation _____ Employer_____

Birthplace _____ Primary Language_____SS#_____

HAVE YOU EVER HAD OR ARE YOU HAVING PROBLEMS WITH ANY OF THE FOLLOWING? IF YES, PLEASE NOTE IF THE PROBLEM IS CURRENT OR PAST

_____ 1. Skin Problems

_____ 2. Eyes, Ears, Nose, Throat Conditions

_____ 3. Asthma

_____ 4. Tuberculosis

_____ 5. Lung Problems

_____ 6. Heart Disease

_____ 7. Rheumatic Fever

_____ 8. Chest Pain

_____ 9. High Blood Pressure

_____ 10. Blood Clots or Vein Problems

_____ 11. Breast Problems (lumps, soreness, discharge, cancer)

_____ 12. Gastrointestinal Pain or Problems

_____ 13. Bladder or Kidney Infections

_____ 14. Urinary Pain or Burning

_____ 15. Diabetes

_____ 16. Thyroid Problems

_____ 17. Anemia or other Blood Disorder

_____ 18. Hepatitis or Liver Disease

_____ 19. Cancer (specific organ)

_____ 20. Joint or Muscle Pain

_____ 21. Severe Headaches or Migraines

_____ 22. Fainting or Dizzy Spells

_____ 23. Immune System Disorders (HIV, Lupus, CMV, Multiple Sclerosis)

_____ 24. Other: _____

EXPLAIN (DATES OF PROBLEMS AND TREATMENT):

_____

_____

ALLERGIES: Do you have any allergies to any medications or substances (penicillin, sulfa, aspirin, iodine, gluten, doxycycline, latex, etc.)?

_____

CURRENT MEDICATIONS (INCLUDING HORMONES): Please list:

_____

CURRENT SUPPLEMENTS/VITAMINS/HERBS: Please list:

_____

HOSPITALIZATIONS/ SURGERIES: List dates, condition, treatment:

_____

_____

DISABILITIES: Please list

_____

Have you had a cholesterol test in the past 5 years? _____ If so, when? _____

Have you had any of the following vaccines? (Check if yes) _____ Hepatitis B _____ HPV

FAMILY HISTORY: Have any members of your family had (write in relationship and age of onset):
_____ Heart Disease _____
_____ Breast Cancer _____
_____ Stroke _____
_____ Other Cancer (what type?) _____
_____ High Blood Pressure _____
_____ High Cholesterol _____
_____ Diabetes _____
_____ Blood clots _____
_____ TB _____
_____ Other

_____
(_____ Family health history unknown _____ Father's history unknown ___ Mother's history unknown)

EMOTIONAL HEALTH:
Do you have any unusual stress in your life at this time?

_____
Do you have a history of emotional health problems?

_____

Have you recently been in a situation that feels unsafe or harmful to you?
_____
Have you in the past or are you currently experiencing emotional, sexual or physical abuse or violence?

_____

Are you interested in counseling or other well-being referrals? _____

HABITS: Smoke tobacco_____/ day   Alcohol _____   Other drug use _____
                     Coffee/tea/soda _____/ day   Sleep _____ hrs./night
Describe your eating habits. _____
Do you have or have you had an eating disorder? _____
Is food or eating a source of anxiety for you? _____
Exercise (type and amount): _____

GENDER:
How do you identify? (check one or more)
_____ Woman   _____ Trans   _____ Intersex   _____ Man

_____ Gender queer (or describe your gender) _____Preferred pronoun: _____

SEXUAL ACTIVITY:
Are you currently sexually active with a partner/partners? _____

If no, have you ever had sexual contact with a partner in the past? _____

If yes, is/are your current partner/partners: _____ Female _____ Male _____ Trans _____ Intersex

If having vaginal sex with males, do you use contraception? _____

Do you have any sexual concerns or problems? _____

Do you have any questions or concerns regarding sexual pleasure or orgasm?

_____

_____

Do you use any methods to protect yourself from sexually transmitted infections?

_____

Have you ever had a screening for sexually transmitted infections?

_____

WHAT (IF ANY) CONTRACEPTIVE   WHEN/HOW LONG? PROBLEMS? METHODS YOU
HAVE USED:

_____

_____

GYNECOLOGICAL:

Age menstrual periods began _____ Menopause at age _____

First day of last menstrual period _____ Are periods regular? _____

How many days from the first day of one period to the first day of the next period? _____

How many days do you bleed? _____ Do you ever bleed between periods? _____

During your period do you have excessive bleeding, pain, cramping, or vomiting? _____

Has there been any recent change in your menstrual period? _____

Do you have pre-menstrual symptoms or problems? Describe: _____

Number of pregnancies _____ Live births (dates) _____

Miscarriages/stillbirths (dates) _____ Abortions (dates) _____

Any complications related to pregnancy? _____

Date of last PAP smear _____ Result _____

Date of last Mammogram _____ Result _____

HAVE YOU EVER HAD ANY OF THE FOLLOWING? CHECK IF YES.

_____ Abnormal Pap Smear
_____ Colposcopy
_____ Cryosurgery
_____ Cone Biopsy, LEEP or Laser Surgery
_____ Uterine Fibroids
_____ Endometriosis
_____ Ovarian Cysts
_____ Vaginal Infections (Yeast/Bacterial)
_____ Sexually Transmitted Diseases or Infections (Chlamydia, Gonorrhea, Herpes, Genital Warts, Syphilis, Hepatitis, Trichomonas)
_____ Pelvic Inflammatory Disease

EXPLAIN (GIVE DATES OF PROBLEMS AND TREATMENT): _____

_____

WHO SHOULD BE INVOLVED IN DISCUSSIONS ABOUT YOUR HEALTH?

Names: _____ **Relationship:** _____

Does this person have power of attorney for healthcare for you? **YES   NO**

List any legal documents related to your health that your healthcare providers need to know about:

IS THERE ANYTHING ELSE YOU WANT TO SHARE? _____

Tracking Goals

Goals	What I did this week:	Evidence: What I learned about this goal this week.
Physical activity goal:		
Nutrition goal:		
Stress reduction goal:		

Session 11: Health and Community

Suggested Readings:
- Chapter 12 (skim)
- Choose a chapter in the book that you are most interested in but have not yet read

Breathing Meditation

Check In
Share any thoughts you had this week on coming out to health care providers, or on tracking any of your health goals. If you read a new chapter in the book, share the one or two things you learned.

The Power of Community
Some research has explored the role of community on our health, and the results are impressive. In one study, feeling a sense of belonging to one community had health benefits that were as dramatic as stopping smoking. People who feel connected to community live longer, are happier, and feel healthier. We will discuss two kinds of community today: the one where you live and the communities you choose. We will start with the physical neighborhoods where you live now. Discuss:

- Is your neighborhood safe for you as a woman, a lesbian or bisexual woman, a woman of color, and so on? In what situations do you feel unsafe, if any?

- Do you feel a sense of belonging to the place? Or spots within the neighborhood like a church, spiritual organization, club, and so on?

- Does your neighborhood promote health? Does it have places to walk, low cost gyms or swimming pools or rec centers, does it have affordable healthy food options?

- Is this the community you want to stay in as you age? Are there resources to support aging?

Break for movement.

Communities of Choice
These are the groups of people based on a shared interest or identity that we choose to affiliate with. Spend a few minutes making some notes, then discuss these questions in groups of 3 so you can go in more depth.

- Thinking across your lifetime, what communities have been the most powerful for you? Where have you felt the greatest sense of belonging and connection?

- How have those communities shifted or changed over time?

- How have those communities contributed to your health; in positive or negative ways?

- As you age, what role do you see community playing in your life? What do you need to be doing now to have the kind of ideal community that you want for the future?

Action Steps
- Think more about community and what you would like to do to strengthen or modify your community support in the near future

Check Out: Share one thing that you would like to remember from today's session.

Session 12: Celebrating with Pride!

Breathing Meditation

Planning for the Future: A Longer Check In

Congratulations on reaching the end of this phase of DIFO. The formal weekly meetings are over after today, but there are many ways you can stay connected and continue the work on your own or with others. Our first activity today will be to review where we are and reflect how DIFO helped us achieve our goals.

- o   What progress have we made as a group and as individuals?
- o   How has DIFO helped? What worked best for you?
- o   What could have been better?

Future Goal-Setting

Now go back to session 1, and review your own individual goals. Note whether you achieved this goal partly or completely, and indicate whether you will continue to work on this goal.

Goal	Achieved? Evidence?	Next steps

Make notes to yourself about how you would like to revise your goals now, and what you will work on in the next month or two. Also, prepare any statements you would like to make to close this experience with your other group members. Sharing your gratitude and positive experiences can be a powerful way to end a group.

Notes:

Gratitudes and Closure

The final activity is to share with the other group members any gratitude you might feel at this time, and to say whatever you need to say to achieve a level of closure with this phase of your health-improvement plan. This might include sharing your future goals or making commitments to continue working on the current goals.

Now Go Celebrate!

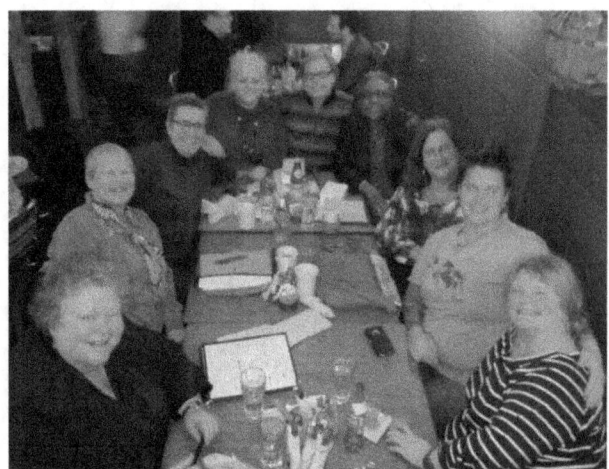

DIFO Group Celebration, Jan 2014

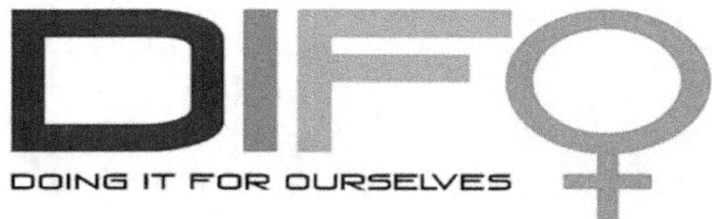

DOING IT FOR OURSELVES

Dear DIFO Group Member,

Thank you for participating in this project with a goal of creating lesbian/bisexual women's communities that are organized around health. You have contributed to this community building. I created this program out of my own perceived need for community where we can share our vulnerabilities and support each other as we age. Aging is hard enough without adding the stresses of being women and being lesbian/bisexual, poor, disabled, women of color, and all the other sources of stress and oppression that we have discussed in this program. It's impossible to go it alone.

I encourage to you to continue this work and keep on building communities of support with or without the DIFO label. Use these materials in any way that is helpful, share what you've learned, post to the website or contribute blogs, and do whatever you need to do to stay as healthy as you can. You are welcome to be in touch and let me know how this program or book can be improved. I will post the findings of our research on the website as they become available, so please check back frequently or contact me for updates.
Yours truly,

Mickey Eliason
meliason@sfsu.edu
http://difobayarea.org